MW01709531

Vertebral Tumors

Vertebral Tumors

Robert Gunzburg, MD, PhD
Senior Consultant
Department of Orthopedics
Edith Cavell Clinic
Brussels, Belgium

Marek Szpalski, MD
Chairman and Associate Professor
Department of Orthopedics
IRIS South Teaching Hospitals
Free University of Brussels
Brussels, Belgium

Max Aebi, MD, DHC, FRCSC
Chief of Staff
Department of Orthopaedic Surgery
Hirslanden-Salem Hospital

Professor and Co-Chair
MEM Research Center for Orthopaedic Surgery
University of Bern
Bern, Switzerland

Lippincott Williams & Wilkins
a Wolters Kluwer business
Philadelphia • Baltimore • New York • London
Buenos Aires • Hong Kong • Sydney • Tokyo

Acquisitions Editor: Robert Hurley
Managing Editor: David Murphy, Jr.
Marketing Director: Sharon Zinner
Production Manager: Bridgett Dougherty
Senior Manufacturing Manager: Benjamin Rivera
Design Coordinator: Teresa Mallon
Production Services: Nesbitt Graphics, Inc.

© 2008 by LIPPINCOTT WILLIAMS & WILKINS- a Wolters Kluwer business

530 Walnut Street
Philadelphia, PA 19106 USA
LWW.com

All rights reserved. This book is protected by copyright. No part of this book may be reproduced in any form or by any means, including photocopying, or utilized by any information storage and retrieval system without written permission from the copyright owner, except for brief quotations embodied in critical articles and reviews. Materials appearing in this book prepared by individuals as part of their official duties as U.S. government employees are not covered by the above-mentioned copyright.

Printed in the USA

Library of Congress Cataloging-in-Publication Data

Vertebral tumors / editors, Marek Szpalski, Robert Gunzburg.
p. ; cm.
Includes bibliographical references and index.
ISBN-13: 978-0-7817-8867-0
ISBN-10: 0-7817-8867-6
1. Spine–Tumors. I. Szpalski, Marek. II. Gunzburg, Robert.
[DNLM: 1. Spinal Neoplasms. WE 725 V5667 2007]
RC280.S72V47 2007
616.99'4711–dc22

2007033057

Care has been taken to confirm the accuracy of the information presented and to describe generally accepted practices. However, the authors, editors, and publisher are not responsible for errors or omissions or for any consequences from application of the information in this book and make no warranty, expressed or implied, with respect to the currency, completeness, or accuracy of the contents of the publication. Application of this information in a particular situation remains the professional responsibility of the practitioner.

The authors, editors, and publisher have exerted every effort to ensure that drug selection and dosage set forth in this text are in accordance with current recommendations and practice at the time of publication. However, in view of ongoing research, changes in government regulations, and the constant flow of information relating to drug therapy and drug reactions, the reader is urged to check the package insert for each drug for any change in indications and dosage and for added warnings and precautions. This is particularly important when the recommended agent is a new or infrequently employed drug.

Some drugs and medical devices presented in this publication have Food and Drug Administration (FDA) clearance for limited use in restricted research settings. It is the responsibility of the health care provider to ascertain the FDA status of each drug or device planned for use in their clinical practice.

To purchase additional copies of this book, call our customer service department at (800) 638 -3030 or fax orders to (301) 223-2320. International customers should call (301) 223-2300.

Visit Lippincott Williams & Wilkins on the Internet: at LWW.com. Lippincott Williams & Wilkins customer service representatives are available from 8:30 am to 6pm, EST.

10 9 8 7 6 5 4 3 2 1

Contents

Contributing Authors

M. Aebi, MD, DHC, FRCSC
Chief of Staff, Department of Orthopaedic Surgery
Hirslanden-Salem Hospital

Professor and Co-Chair
MEM Research Center for Orthopaedic Surgery
University of Bern
Bern, Switzerland

Stefano Bandiera, MD
Attending Surgeon
Department of Orthopaedics and Traumatology
Ospedale Maggiore
Bologna, Italy

Michel Benoist, MD
University of Paris VII
Paris, France

Mark H. Bilsky, MD
Department of Surgery, Memorial Sloan Kettering Cancer Center
New York, New York

Jean-Jacques Body, MD, PhD
Chief, Department of Medicine, CHU Brugmann

Professor of Medicine, Department of Medicine, CHU Brugmann
Université Libre de Bruxelles (U.L.B.)
Brussels, Belgium

Luca Boriani, MD
Resident, Rizzoli Institute
Post-Graduate School of Orthopaedics
University of Bologna Medical School
Bologna, Italy

Stefano Boriani, MD
Chief, Department of Orthopaedics;
Traumatology,
Spine Surgery
Ospedale Maggiore

Professore a Contratio
Post-graduate School of Orthopaedics
Universita di Bologna
Bologna, Italy

Michele Cappuccio, MD
Resident, Rizzoli Institute
Post-Graduate School of Orthopaedics
University of Bologna Medical School
Bologna, Italy

Brian J.C. Freeman, DM, FRCS (Tr & Orth)
Consultant Spinal Surgeon, The Centre for Spinal Studies and Surgery, Nottingham
University Hospitals NHS Trust
Queen's Medical Centre Campus

Professor of Spinal Surgery, Division of Orthopaedic and Accident Surgery, The University of Nottingham, Queen's Medical Centre
Nottingham, United Kingdom

Charles S. B. Galasko, MD
Emeritus Professor, Department of Orthopaedic Surgery, University of Manchester
United Kingdom

Alessandro Gasbarrini, MD
Attending Surgeon
Department of Orthopaedics and Traumatology
Ospedale Maggiore
Bologna, Italy

Pierre Guigui, MD
Professor of Orthopaedic Surgery
University of Paris VII
Beaujon Hospital
Clichy, France

Robert Gunzburg, MD, PhD
Senior Consultant, Department of Orthopaedics, Edith Cavell Clinic
Burssels, Belgium

Alexander G. Hadjipavlou, MD, MSc, FACS, FRCS(C)
Chief, Department of Orthopaedic Surgery, University Hospital of Heraklion
Heraklion, Crete,Greece

Professor, Department of Orthopaedic Surgery, University of Crete
Heraklion, Crete, Greece

Samuel W. Judd, MRCS
Clinical Research Fellow, The Centre for Spinal Studies and Surgery, Nottingham University Hospitals NHS Trust, Queen's Medical Centre Campus
Nottingham, United Kingdom

Andre J. Kaelin, MD
Chief, Department of Pediatric Orthopaedics, Children's Hospital
Professor, Departement de l'Enfant et de l'Adolescent, Medical School, University of Geneva
Geneva, Switzerland

K.N. Kakavelakis, MD
Department of Orthopaedic Surgery and Traumatology, University of Crete
Heraklion, Crete, Greece

P. Katonis, MD
Department of Orthopaedic Surgery and Traumatology, University of Crete
Heraklion, Crete, Greece

Tony S. Keller, MD, PhD*
Florida Orthopedic Institute
Research Foundation
Temple Terrace, Florida

Isador H. Lieberman, MD, MBA, FRCS(C)
Orthopedic and Spinal Surgeon, Center for Spine Health
Cleveland Clinic

Professor of Surgery
Cleveland Clinic Learner College of Medicine
Cleveland, Ohio

Michael A.K. Liebschner, MD, PhD
Professor, Department of Bioengineering
Rice University
Houston, Texas

Marc Lemort, MD
Chief of Radiology Department and MRI Unit
Institut Jules Bordet,
Université Libre de Bruxelles
Brussels, Belgium

Thibaud Lenoir, MD
Senior Resident of Orthopaedic Surgery, Hopital Beaujon
Paris, France

D. Michael Lovelock, PhD
Department of Medical Physics, Memorial Sloan Kettering Cancer Center
New York, New York

Stefania Paderni, MD
Attending Surgeon
Department of Orthopaedics and Traumatology
Ospedale Maggiore
Bologna, Italy

*Deceased

Roy A. Patchell, MD
Chief, Department of Neuro-Oncology,
University of Kentucky Medical Center
Lexington, Kentucky

Professor, Department of Neurology and
Neurosurgery, University of Kentucky
Medical Center
Lexington, Kentucky

E. Pateromichelakis
Department of Orthopaedic Surgery and
Traumatology, University of Crete
Heraklion, Crete, Greece

S. Rajasekaran, MD, PhD
Director and Head, Department of Orthopaedic
and Spine Surgery, Ganga Hospital
Coimbatore, India

Krzysztof B. Siemionow, MD
Resident, Department of Orthopedic Surgery,
Cleveland Clinic
Cleveland, Ohio

Marek Szpalski, MD
Chairman and Associate Professor, Department
of Orthopaedics, IRIS South Teaching
Hospitals, Free University of Brussels
Brussels, Belgium

Prof.dr.P.I.J.M. Wuisman, MD*
Department of Orthopaedic Surgery, Vrije
Universiteit Medical Center
Amsterdam, The Netherlands

Yoshiya Yamada, MD, FRCPC
Assistant Attending Radiation Oncologist
Department of Radiation Oncology
Memorial Sloan-Kettering Cancer Center
New York, New York

*Deceased

Preface

This book emerged from the well-established annual Brussels Spine Symposium of 2006 which presented an update on the current trends and state of the art in spinal tumor care. An overview of the occurrence, frequency, and clinical appearance of spinal tumors is given by M. Benoist (France), whereas Boriani (Italy) presents today's available classification systems for spinal tumors which serve as a base to standardize oncologic treatment modalities. Specific diagnostic issues in children and in imaging of spinal metastases are addressed by Kaelin (Switzerland) and Lemort (Belgium), respectively.

In a major chapter, several most actual and partially still debatable treatment modalities are discussed such as image-guided intensity modulated radiotherapy (Yamada), biphosphonates in spinal metastasis (Body, Belgium), as well as radiation and brachytherapy (Yamada). A special emphasis is put on the cement augmentation (kypho- and vertebroplasty), both from the biomechanical (Keller, USA) as well as the clinical point of view (Liebermann, USA). Patchell (USA) concentrates on decompressive surgery and a randomized trial in metastases surgery, a topic which is also addressed in a more comprehensive view by Galasko (UK) and Boriani by presenting a multinational prospective study.

The treatment of primary tumors, which are much rarer than metastases, is dealt with by experts who, in their clinical activity, focus on this pathology: Radical surgery for primary cervical and thoracolumbar spine tumors (Boriani, Italy); management of hypervascular tumors (Hadjipavlou, GR); and finally techniques of en bloc resection (Wuisman, NL). Liebermann (USA) and Freeman (UK) concentrate on two new techniques: Radiosurgery and intraoperative radionucleide localization of osteoid osteoma and osteoblastoma, respectively.

Rajasekaran (India) describes the intraoperative navigation with the ISO-C-arm to minimize collateral damages and increase precision of this complex surgery. Finally, Hadjipavlou presents a comprehensive overview of the outcome to be expected in spine tumors.

This book offers, in a condensed review, a spotlight on the present development and expectation of today's options in spinal tumor care.

Marek Szpalski
Robert Gunzburg
Max Aebi

Epidemiology of Spinal Tumors

Michel Benoist, Thibaud Lenoir, and Pierre Guigui

1

Spinal tumors may arise from primary local lesions or from distant malignancies, spreading to the spine. The majority of lesions are metastatic tumors, far more common than primary lesions. The management of malignant secondaries is different from that used in primary tumors, as these lesions, both benign and malignant, are frequently curable. This chapter focuses on the basic descriptive studies of the distribution and progression of spinal tumors in populations, with occasional references to studies of etiologic hypotheses. Local involvement of the spine may result from primary tumors of bone or from primary lesions arising in the spinal cord or in its coverings. The first part of this chapter considers the primary lesions. The metastatic tumors are discussed subsequently.

PRIMARY TUMORS

Primary tumors of the spine are very rare. They may develop in three locations: intramedullary, intradural-extramedullary, or extradurally.

Extradural Bone Tumors

Extradural tumors comprise principally primary bone tumors, nonosseous extradural primary tumors being exceptional. Their relative incidence reflects that of the skeleton in general. Certain tumors (chordoma, osteoblastoma) show a predilection for the spinal column, but they represent a small proportion of spinal tumors. The classification used in this chapter is similar to that advocated by Lichtenstein for bone tumors. This classification is based on histologic findings and differentiates hematopoietic tumors, chondrogenic tumors, osteogenic tumors, tumors of unknown origin, fibrogenic tumors, and notochordal tumors.

BENIGN PRIMARY BONE TUMORS

Chondrogenic Tumors

Osteochondroma

Spinal localization represents approximately 7% of this common benign tumor. It is usually observed in young patients younger than 20 years, affecting predominantly the lumbar spine, followed by thoracic sacrum and cervical spine. In the Mayo Clinic series, this tumor composes 22% of benign spinal tumors and 8% of all spine tumors (7).

Chondroma

Its typical localization is on the hands and feet. Composed of mature cartilage, the spinal localization is rare, representing approximately 4% of all chondromas and 5.7% of the benign spinal tumors disclosed in Dahlin's series (7).

Chondroblastoma and Chondromyxoid Fibroma

These tumors are rare. They are even more exceptional in the spine. They represent approximately 1% of the benign spinal tumors, usually occurring in the second decade of life (7).

Osteogenic Tumors

Osteoid Osteoma

Osteoid osteomas represent approximately 9% of all benign spinal tumors. They are usually located in the posterior arch of the vertebrae and encountered in the second decade of age, with a male predominance (7).

Benign Osteoblastoma

This tumor is observed predominantly in the spine, during the first 3 decades of life. Different from osteoid osteoma in its size and the absence of peripheral sclerotic bone, it represents 12% of all benign primary tumors of the Mayo Clinic series (7) and 22% of Weinstein's cases (39).

Tumors of Unknown Origin

Giant Cell Tumor

This tumor can produce metastasis, although it is cytologically benign. In the spine, sacrum location is predominant, occurring more frequently in women during the third and fourth decades of life. Giant cell tumors represent 16% of all benign spinal tumors in Weinstein's series (39) and 67% of the sacral benign tumors reported by Dahlin (7). Local postoperative recurrences may occur with this type of tumor.

Fibrous Histiocytoma

Fibrous histiocytoma is an exceptional benign spinal tumor. Seven cases have been reported in the literature.

Other Benign Tumors

Hemangioma

Hemangioma is a frequent asymptomatic tumor of the spine, representing 10% of benign lesions encountered in adults, with a female predominance (7).

Aneurysmal Bone Cyst

The cysts have a high propensity for the spine. Spinal localization represents approximately 30% of this type of tumor, occurring principally in adolescents and young adults. In Dahlin's series, its incidence was 2% of all spinal tumors (15).

MALIGNANT PRIMARY TUMORS

Hematopoietic Tumors

Hematopoietic tumors comprise lymphoma, solitary plasmacytoma, and myeloma. Lymphoma (23) may present as a systematic disease with skeletal manifestations, or as an isolated bone tumor. This neoplasm can occur at any age but is rare in children. Spine localization is not exceptional. Five cases of 51 malignant primary spinal tumors are disclosed in Weinstein's series (39). Dahlin (7) reported 46 cases in 542 patients. The thoracic spine is predominantly affected followed by the sacrum and the lumbar and cervical spine.

Solitary plasmocytoma (25) and myeloma (10) are the most frequent malignant primary tumors. Spinal localization represents 27% of all spine primary tumors and 34% of malignant primary tumors in the Mayo Clinic series (7). Solitary spinal plasmocytomas compose 29% of malignant primary tumors in Weinstein's report (39). The thoracic spine is the most common site, followed by the lumbar and cervical spine. They predominate in men and are rare before the fifth decade.

Chondrosarcoma

Chondrosarcomas can be primary or secondary to osteochondromas. They occur in adults, with a male predominance, representing approximately 10% of malignant spinal tumors. An adequate control of the disease is mandatory to prevent recurrences.

Osteosarcoma

The spinal localization affects primarily the sacrum, followed by lumbar, dorsal, and cervical spine. Principally observed in young male patients, it represents approximately 10% of malignant spinal tumors (7).

Ewing Tumor

Spinal localization is rare (5% of malignant bone tumors). It is principally encountered in the second decade of life, with a male predominance. The sacrum is the usual site, followed by the lumbar, thoracic, and cervical spine (30).

Malignant Giant Cell Tumor

Malignancy can be primary or after treatment of a benign giant cell tumor. Spinal location is rare (0.4% of malignant spine tumors), occurring during the third or fourth decade of life.

Chordoma

Chordomas develop from the remains of the primitive notochord. They have a high propensity for the distal end of the spinal column, affecting the sacrococcygeal area in one half of the patients, usually males younger than 30 years. They represent 30% of malignant spinal tumors (7).

Fibrosacroma

Fibrosarcomas are rare (3% of malignant spinal tumors) with no sex predominance, affecting mainly the sacrum. The age distribution is linear through the second to the sixth decade (7).

Intradural Tumors

Intradural spinal tumors are less common than brain tumors. Their annual incidence is estimated to be 2.5 per 100,000 (14). The epidemiologic description is divided into intramedullary tumors and extramedullary intradural tumors.

Intramedullary Spinal Gliomas

These gliomas represent approximately one third of intradural tumors. Astrocytomas and other less-differentiated but glial-derived tumors account for 50% of all lesions of this category. The most frequent location is the lumbar spine, followed by the thoracic and cervical regions. They have a poor prognosis, with risks of recurrences and progression. Ependymomas are the second most common intramedullary tumor, representing roughly 30% of these lesions. They usually are located in the lumbar region because of their relation with the filum terminale. They have a long-term free survival after removal, with a risk of postoperative central cord pain. The remaining 20% of these tumors concern hemangioblastomas, followed by lipomas and dermoids. These tumors have no predilection for a given gender or age (5).

Extramedullary Intradural Spinal Tumors

The most common types are meningiomas and neurofibromas, which occur with equal frequency. They represent 70% of all these tumors. Sarcomas are the third cause, representing 10% of the total. Other less-common types are dermoids, epidermoids, angiomas, and rarely lymphomas or metastases. Meningiomas, neurofibromas, and sarcomas occur in middle-aged or elderly patients. A strong female predominance is reported for meningiomas, found more frequently in the thoracic region. Neurofibromas are evenly distributed along the spinal column. One third of neurofibromas are extradural, and two thirds, intradural. Meningiomas are mostly located intradurally. Their excision is usually curative. However, a risk of recurrence exists if a complete removal is not achieved.

METASTATIC DISEASE OF THE SPINE

Location of Metastases and Sites of Primary Tumors

The development of a spinal metastasis is generally a catastrophic complication for the cancer patient. Pain, fractures, and neurologic complications lead to a major alteration of the quality of life, with additional medical and often surgical therapies. Most metastases develop extradurally on bony structures. Nonosseous epidural malignancies are exceptional. Intradural extramedullary and intramedullary secondaries are rarely encountered. Perrin (28,29) analyzed the location of spinal metastases in four studies, with a total of 200 cases (2,11,28,31). The location of the metastases was extradural in 94% to 98% of the cases. Spinal osseous metastases are the most frequent spinal tumors. It is estimated that they occur 20 times more often than primary tumors (28). In nearly half of the patients with solid carcinomas, bone metastases will develop, the spine being the most frequent skeletal location.

Autopsy studies have been performed to evaluate the rate of spinal metastases for various tumors. Drury et al. (9) studied the spread of carcinoma to the vertebral bodies by the long vertebral slice technique. They disclosed vertebral secondaries in nearly one third of all patients with carcinoma and in almost one half of those dying with distant metastases. The incidence of spinal metastases resulting from autopsy examination was subsequently reported by Wong et al. (40). Spines from 832 deceased patients with a terminal diagnosis of malignant neoplasm were studied grossly, microscopically, and radiographically for evidence of tumors. Overall metastases were disclosed in 36% of patients dying of neoplastic disease. Approximately 16% of total metastatic deposits were occult and not visible on plain radiographs, calling for the use of further imaging studies for cancer patients complaining of spine pain. As stated by Perrin et al. (28), "It is axiomatic that a cancer patient with new-onset back or neck pain harbors spinal metastases until proven otherwise." The incidence of spinal secondaries in cancer patients with metastatic disease, including nonspinal bone metastases, has been estimated at up to 40% in clinical studies (19), which is close to the findings of autopsy studies.

The prevalence of primary tumors varies according to published reports. For example, in a summary of 2,748 cases reported by Kostuik (20) considering only solid tumors, breast, lung, and prostate compose the majority of spinal metastases, followed by renal, gastrointestinal, and thyroid carcinomas. In the autopsy studies, breast and lung accounted for the most frequent primary sites, followed by lymphoreticular malignancies, carcinoma of the uterine cervix, the bladder, and the pancreas. The prevalence of the tumor type varies depending on whether autopsy studies or clinically nonoccult metastases are considered. For example, patients with liver, lung, or gastrointestinal primary tumors may die before spinal metastases become clinically significant.

Spinal metastases may occur with no known history of a primary site. The figures were high in the older literature; however, the tremendous progress in imaging and investigating techniques has considerably reduced the number of patients in this category, which is estimated by Klimo (19) at approximately 10% of metastatic spinal patients. In more than 50% of these cases, the most frequent primary tumors disclosed histologically are lung, followed by prostate and kidney (17).

Most studies indicate that the thoracic spine is the most frequent location of the metastases, followed by the lumbar and cervical spine (4,17). The vertebral body is usually the initial site in its posterior half (16,19). The posterior elements are involved later. Metastases may involve only one level. In this case, the isolated malignant focus must be differentiated from a primary lesion, especially if the primary tumor is not known. However, studies have shown that metastases occur at multilevel, noncontiguous levels in 10% to 38% of cases (13,34).

Spinal metastasis may develop at all ages, with the highest incidence between 40 and 70 years of age, reflecting the increased risk of cancer during that period. In the series reported by Constans (6) and by Gilbert (13), the risk of spinal metastases was higher in men than in women, probably reflecting the higher incidence of prostate cancer compared with breast cancer.

PATHOPHYSIOLOGY

Secondary spinal tumors may arise in several ways. Hematogenous spread is the most frequent pattern of metastasis. Tumor cells penetrate blood vessels most frequently through capillaries. Blood vessels can subsequently release tumor emboli into the arterial system. Tumor cells entrapment in the capillary beds of the bone marrow of the vertebral bodies is the first step of the secondary tumor growth. It has been speculated that a rich concentration of growth factors in the bone marrow stroma of the vertebrae is a predisposing factor, stimulating the local proliferation of tumor cells (1).

Hematogenous spread also may follow the venous system. Batson (32) demonstrated that the vertebral venous plexus drains the thoracic, abdominal, and pelvic viscera, when intra-abdominal pressure is increased, such as during straining and coughing (34). Direct extension through the intervertebral foramina via the venous channel may also occur, as observed in pediatric spinal metastases and lymphoma (18).

Intrinsic factors inherent to the tumor cells may play a role. Primary malignant tumors are not composed of uniform cells but contain subpopulations of cells with particular predispositions to survive and grow in medullary spaces. The development of spinal metastasis is a highly complex process involving interplay of the host response and tumor cell properties. Discussion of this process is clearly beyond the scope of this chapter.

Complications

The biologic behavior of the metastatic cells is not always similar to that of the primary tumor (20). A rapid development may cause destruction of the vertebral body, epidural invasion, and cord compression. It has been estimated that 5% of all patients with metastatic disease on whom an autopsy is performed have the tumor invading the extradural space (2). Approximately half of the cases of metastatic epidural compression arise from breast, lung, or prostate cancer. Variations of incidence of neurologic deficits exist according to the site of the primary disease. In the series reported by Gerszten et al. (12), the most frequent primary tumor causing cord compression was breast (22%) followed by lung (15%) and prostate (10%). The overall incidence of the site of the cord compression by primary tumor was 15% cervical, 68% thoracic, and 16% lumbosacral in the series reported by Gilbert et al. (12).

A population-based study of metastatic spinal cord compression (MSCC) described the incidence, the management, and the outcome of MSCC in the cancer population of the Canadian province of Ontario (22). Episodes of MSCC and the treatment used for each episode were identified by linking electronic hospital discharge records and cancer center records to Ontario's population-based cancer registry. The cumulative frequency of MSCC was described in 121,435 patients who died of cancer in the previous 5 years (1990–1995). Overall, the cumulative probability of developing at least one episode of MSCC was 2.5%, with great variation among different types of cancer ranging from 0.2% in cancer of the pancreas to 7.9% in myeloma.

Vertebral collapse as a result of an osteolytic metastatic lesion is the first step of epidural invasion, causing extreme pain and neurologic deficit. Collapse may be prevented by radiation or surgical prophylactic stabilization, depending on the mechanical properties of the metastatic spine. Tanechei et al. (36) studied risks factors and probability of vertebral collapse in metastases of the thoracic and lumbar spine in 100 patients with secondary malignancies. The criteria of impending collapse justifying prophylactic treatment were: 50% to 60% involvement of the vertebral body, with no destruction of other structures, or 25% to 30% involvement with costovertebral destruction in the thoracic spine. Probability of collapse for the lumbar and thoracolumbar spine was 35% to 40% involvement of the vertebral body or 20% to 25% involvement with destruction of the posterior elements. Early detection of risk factors of vertebral collapse to undertake treatment before neurologic injury occurs is an important factor of survival. In the already mentioned population-based study of MSCC, the overall median survival after the first episode of MSCC was 2.9 months (22).

In addition to the symptoms caused by the anatomic distortion and functional impairment of the spine, it should be mentioned that systemic metabolic emergencies may complicate metastatic disease of the spine. Hypercalcemia is the most frequently encountered of the acute medical problems. Patients with solid tumors and bone metastases compose the major group, including primarily breast, lung, kidney, and myeloma (26,27). Hypercalcemia is caused by an increased bone resorption. Its severity is not necessarily correlated to the extent of metastatic bone destruction, which can be limited to the spine (21). About 20% to 30% of patients with metastases develop hypercalcemia, constituting a metabolic emergency, and a threat to life without an appropriate treatment.

SURVIVAL AND OUTCOME

Prognosis in metastatic spinal disease is dependent on several interrelated factors. Takuhashi et al. (36) developed a scoring system for the preoperative evaluation of metastatic spine prognosis. Six parameters were used.

1. The general condition
2. The number of extraspinal bone metastases
3. The number of spinal metastases
4. The metastases to the major internal organs (lungs, liver, kidneys and brain)
5. Primary site of the cancer
6. Severity of spinal cord involvement.

Each parameter ranged from 0 to 2 points, with a total of 12 points. According to these authors, the prognosis could not be predicted from a single parameter; they recommend excisional operation in those cases scoring higher than 9 points, and a palliative operation for those scoring less than 5 points. As pointed out by Kostuik (20), probably the most important determinant is the tumor type. For example, breast carcinoma has a much better overall prognosis than pulmonary carcinomas, predominating in men with a survival that can be measured in weeks.

Severity of spinal cord compression is the other main determinant parameter. Sioutos et al. (33) studied factors affecting survival in 109 patients with thoracic spine metastases and cord compression. In more than two thirds of the patients, lung, prostate, and breast were the primary sites. The overall median survival was 10 months. Factors affecting survival included

1. Primary tumor site
2. Preoperative neurologic status: patients who were ambulatory before surgery survived longer than did nonambulatory patients

3. Number of vertebral bodies involved: patients with only one vertebra involved survived longer than did patients with multiple levels involved.

In a more recent study, Janson (17) stressed the difficulty of selecting appropriate MSCC patients for posterior decompression and stabilization and of verifying those who will die early.

REFERENCES

1. Argnello F, Baggs RB, Duerst RE, et al. Pathogenesis of vertebral metastasis and epidural cord compression. Cancer 1990:65:98–106.
2. Barron KD, Hirano A, Araki S, et al. Experiences with metastatic neoplasms involving the spinal cord. Neurology 1959;9: 91–106.
3. Batson OV. The function of the vertebral veins and their role in the spread of metastases. Ann Surg 1940;112:138–149.
4. Byrne TN. Spinal cord compression from epidural metastases. N Engl J Med 327:614–619.
5. Cassidy J, Ducker TB, Dienes EA. Intradural tumors. In: Frymoyer JW. The Adult Spine: Principles and Practice, 2nd ed. Philadelphia: Lippincott, Raven, 1997:1015–1029.
6. Constans JP, Divitiis E, Donzelli R et al. Spinal metastases with neurological manifestations: review of 600 cases. J Neurosurg 1983; 59: 111–118.
7. Dahlin DC. Bone Tumors: General Aspects and Data on 6221 Cases, 3rd ed. Springfield, Ill: Charles C Thomas, 1981.
8. Dodds PR, Caride VY, Lytton B. The role of vertebral veins in the dissemination of prostate cancer. J Urol 1981;126:753–755.
9. Drury RAB, Palmer PH, Highman WY. Carcinomatous metastases to the vertebral bodies. J Clin Pathol 1964;17:448–457.
10. Durr R, Wegener B, Krodel A, et al. Multiple myeloma of the spine. Spine 2002;27:320–325.
11. Edelson RN, Deck MD, Posner JB. Intramedullary spinal cord metas0tases: clinical and radiographic findings in nine cases. Neurology 1972;22:122–131.
12. Gerszten P, Welch W. Current surgical management of metastatic spinal disease. Oncology 2000; 14:1013–1024.
13. Gilbert RW, Kim JH, Posner JB. Epidural spinal cord compression from metastatic tumor: diagnosis and treatment. Ann Neurol 1978;3: 40–51.
14. Guidetti B, Mercuris, Vagnozzi. Long-term results of the surgical treatment of 129 intramedullary spinal gliomas. J Neurosurg 1981;54: 323–330.
15. Hay M. Aneurysmal bone cysts of the spine. J Bone Joint Surg (B) 1978;60:406–411.
16. Jaffe WL. Tumors and Tumorous Conditions of the Bones and Joints. Philadelphia: Lea & Febiger, 1958:589–618.
17. Janson KA, Bauer HCE. Survival, complications and outcome in 282 patients operated for neurological deficit due to thoracic or lumbar spinal metastases. Eur Spine J 2006;15:196–202.
18. Klein SL, Sanford RA, Muhlbauer MS. Pediatric spinal epidural metastases. J Neurosurg 1991;74: 70–75.
19. Klimo P. Kestle JRW, Schmidt MH. Clinical trials and evidence based medicine for metastatic spine disease. Neurosurg Clin North Am 2004; 15:549–564.
20. Kostuik JP. Differential diagnosis and surgical treatment of metastatic spine tumors. In: Frymoyer JW, ed. The Adult Spine: Principles and Practice, 2nd ed. Philadelphia: Lippincott-Raven, 1997:989–1016.
21. Lafferty FW. Pseudohyperparathyroidism. Medicine 1974;45:247–260.
22. Loblaw DA, Laperrierre NY, Mackillop WJ. A population based study of malignant spinal cord compression in Ontario. Clin Oncol 2003; 15:211–217.
23. Lyon S. Primary spinal epidural non-Hodgkin's lymphoma: report of eight patients and review of the literature. Neurosurgery 1992;30:675–680.
24. Marsch BW, Bonfiglio M, Brady LP, et al. Benign osteoblastoma: range of manifestation. J Bone Joint Surg (A) 1975;57–74.
25. McLain T, Weinstein JN. Solitary plasmocytomas of the spine: a review of 84 cases. J Spinal Disord 1989;2:69–74.

26. Muggia FM, Heinemann HO. Hypercalcemia associated with neoplastic disease. Arch Intern Med 1970;73:281–290.
27. Mundy GR. Calcium and cancer. Life Sci 1978; 23:1735–1744.
28. Perrin RG, Laxton A. Metastatic spine disease: epidemiology, pathophysiology and evaluation of patients. Neurosurg Clin North Am 2004;15: 365–373.
29. Perrin RG, Livingston KE, Aarabi R. Intradural extramedullary spinal metastases: a report of 10 cases. J Neurosurg 1982;56:835–837.
30. Rex M, Breh GJ. Ewing's sarcoma of the mobile spine. Spine 2005;30:769–773.
31. Rogers L, Heard G. Intrathecal spinal metatases (rare tumors) Br J Surg 1958;45:17–20.
32. Shives TC, Dahlin DC, Sim FH, et al. Osteosarcoma of the spine. J Bone Joint Surg (A) 1986; 71:1158–1165.
33. Sioutos PJ, Arbit E, Meshulam CF, et al. Spinal metastases from solid tumors: analysis of factors affecting survival. Cancer 1995;76:1453–1459.
34. Stark R, Henson R, Evans S. Spinal metastases: a retrospective survey from a general hospital. Brain 1982;105:189–213.
35. Sundaresan N, Rosen G, Huvus AG, et al. Combined treatment of osteosarcoma of the spine. Neurosurgery 1988;23:714–719.
36. Tanechei H, Kaneda K, Takeda N, et al. Risks factors and probability of vertebral body collapse in metastases of the thoracic and lumbar spine. Spine 1997;22:239–245.
37. Tokuhashi Y, Matsuzaki H, Toriyama S, et al. Scoring system for the preoperative evaluation of metastatic spine tumor prognosis. Spine 1990; 15:1110–1113.
38. Valderrama JAF, Bullough PG. Solitary myeloma of the spine. J Bone Joint Surg (B) 1968;50: 82–90.
39. Weinstein JN, McLain RF. Primary tumor of the spine. Spine 1987;12:843–851.
40. Wong DA, Fornasier V, MacNab I. Spinal metastases: the obvious, the occult and the impostors. Spine 1990;15:1–4.

Classifications of Bone Tumors of the Spine

2

Stefano Boriani, Stefania Paderni, Alessandro Gasbarrini, Michele Cappuccio, Luca Boriani, and Stefano Bandiera

ABSTRACT

Background

Any classification discards details and therefore modifies reality, but classifications are needed in medicine to create categories associated with similar behavior and evolution. This is mandatory for the decision-making process.

Methods

We describe currently accepted classifications of primary and secondary tumors of the spine.

Results

The basic classification of spine tumors is histologic, but for the decision-making process, a scale of aggressiveness is needed.

Conclusions

The Enneking staging system (10) proved to be a reliable method to understand the biologic behavior of primary bone tumors. Many scoring systems have been proposed for grading metastases, but no consensus has been reached. A flow-chart is proposed to articulate the patient's priorities with treatment options.

INTRODUCTION

Primary bone tumors of the spine are rare, often unsuspected, and misdiagnosis or late diagnosis is an unfortunate reality in many cases. Conversely, bone metastases in the spine are much more frequent: a 20% to 70% incidence of spine metastasis is reported in the evolution of the more common solid tumors. The magnitude of clinical problems due to spine metastases is revealed by the incidence of paraplegia in the population (8.5 per 100,000) versus traumatic spinal cord injuries (three to five per 100,000) (24). The main concern in the treatment of spine metastases is preserving mechanical and neurologic function (and deleting pain), whereas an oncologically appropriate treatment (based on early diagnosis and staging) can substantially improve the prognosis in primary bone tumors.

Classifications are needed in medicine to create categories associated with similar behavior and evolution, to set up proper decision-making processes. Any classification discards details and therefore modifies reality, but this generalization is mandatory to decide the treatment and evaluate the results.

PRIMARY TUMORS

According to the classification proposed by Schajowicz (20,21) and accepted by the World Health Organization, bone tumors are divided according to their histogenesis (Fig. 2.1).

BONE TUMORS

Differentiation or histogenesis	Benign	Low-grade (LG) malignancy	High-grade (HG) malignancy
Fibrous and histiocytic	Histiocytic fibroma Benign fibrous histiocytoma GCT Desmoid fibroma	Grades 1, 2 fibrosarcoma	Grades 3, 4 fibrosarcoma MFH
Cartilagineous	Exostosis Hemimelic epiphyseal dysplasia Chondroma Chondroblastoma Chondromyxoid fibroma	Grades 1, 2 central chondrosarcoma (CHS) Peripheral chondrosarcoma Periosteal chondrosarcoma Clear cell chondrosrcoma Fibrocartilagineous mesenchymoma	Grade 3 central chondrosarcoma Mesenchymal chondrosarcoma
Osseous	Osteoma Osteoid Osteoma Osteoblastoma Fibrous dysplasia Osteofibrous dysplasia	Parosteal osteosarcoma Periosteal osteosarcoma LG central osteosarcoma	Classical osteosarcoma Hemorragic OS Small cell OS
Emopoietic			Lymphoma Plasmacytoma
Vascular	Hemangioma Lymphangioma	Hemangioendothelioma	Hemangiosarcoma Hemangiopericytoma
Nervous	Neurinoma Neurofibroma		Ewing's sarcoma (?)
Adipose	Lipoma		Liposarcoma
Mixed		Adamantinoma	Malignant mesenchymoma
Notochordal		Chordoma	

FIGURE 2.1 Histogenetic classification (with some minor changes) of the World Health Organization by Schajowicz et al. (1972) for tumors of the skeleton.

The neoplastic conditions originating from osteoblasts are osteoid osteoma and osteoblastoma, if benign, and osteosarcoma, if malignant. Tumors originating from chondroid cells are chondromas and chondrosarcomas. Those deriving from angioblasts are angiomas and angiosarcomas. Chordoma, a typical tumor of the spine, arises from notochordal remnants. Further tumors originating from osteoclasts, vascular wall fibrous tissue, and mesenchymal neuroangiogenic components are also included.

More conditions, mostly dysplastic or hyperplastic, whose etiology may or may not be known, are the so-called "tumorlike" or "pseudotumoral" lesions (Fig. 2.2), known as such because they may resemble tumors and are often involved in a discussion of differential diagnosis. The most frequent tumorlike condition in the spine is the aneurysmal bone cyst, a hyperplastic reaction of the vascular structures, creating huge cavities filled with membranes and blood.

- Bone cyst
- Aneurysmal Bone Cyst
- Mucous Cyst
- Progressive Teleangiectatic Osteolysis
- Langerhans cell Granuloma (Histiocytosis X)
- Osteosis due to primary hyperparathyroidism
- Giant cell reparative granuloma
- Tumorlike periosteal ossification

FIGURE 2.2 So called "tumorlike" or "pseudotumoral" bone conditions.

The classification of soft tissue tumors according to their histogenesis was proposed by Fletcher (12) and approved by the World Health Organization. Soft tumors are not frequent in our series. Involvement of vertebrae by perivertebral soft-tissue tumors is mostly due to tumors originating in the nervous system (neurinoma and its malignant counterpart, schwannoma) and therefore mostly observed in neurosurgical departments. In our series, tumors of fibrous and smooth muscular histogenesis are included. Aggressive fibromatosis, a histologically benign condition generated by fibrous cells, has a tendency for local recurrence and therefore is best treated with en bloc resection. Its malignant counterpart is the fibrosarcoma. Retroperitoneal fibrous and smooth muscular tumors (fibrosarcoma and leiomyosarcoma, respectively) are likely to invade the spine by continuity and pose delicate problems for surgical treatment.

These classifications give little information to the surgeon, who needs elements to understand the biologic behavior. Further, the lack of logically organized paradigm makes it confusing to evaluate the results of treatment for primary spine tumors. Without a common terminology (11),difficulties exist in sharing information and comparing results. The result is that the same procedure (e.g., intralesional excision) is performed for different spine tumors without regard for histology and aggressiveness (19).

The Enneking staging system was set up (10) to grade the aggressiveness of the tumors and to decide on this basis which is the most appropriate surgical margin for any tumor and therefore the extent of surgical en bloc or intralesional excision. A surgical staging system has been proposed for planning the surgical procedure to achieve such margins (6).

The combination of Enneking staging (10) and WBB staging (6) aims to

- avoid high-morbidity surgery when not necessary (for example, in stage 2 benign or in metastatic tumors);
- achieve the appropriate margin by correctly performed en bloc resections in selected cases; and
- improve the knowledge of these tumors by comparing uniform reports on outcomes of homogeneously treated series,

Enneking Staging System

Enneking (10) proposed in 1980 a classification for bone and soft-tissue tumors that can be adopted for the spine. This classification is based on clinical and laboratory data, imaging, and histology. The combination of all these elements helps to assess the natural history of the disease. Several tumors can occur in different stages, confined inside the compartment of origin or spreading, and the treatment should be pertinent. For each stage, a specific surgery is indicated: intralesional (piecemeal excision or en bloc violating the tumor), marginal (en bloc along the pseudocapsule), wide (outside the pseudocapsule), radical (excision of the entire compartment, if the tumor is intracompartmental).

The terms "vertebrectomy" (removal of all the elements of the vertebra), "corpectomy," and "somectomy" (removal of the vertebral body) have no significance from an oncologic viewpoint if they are not specified according to the terminology previously mentioned.

All the surgical procedures generally done for a functional purpose (cord decompression, fracture stabilization), with or without partial (piecemeal) removal of the tumor, are called "palliative." In general, it is intended only to make a diagnosis, decrease pain, and possibly improve function.

The oncologic staging proposed by Enneking (9,10) divides benign tumors into three stages (S1, S2, and S3) and localized (nonmetastatic) malignant tumors into four stages (IA, IB, IIA, and IIB). Two further stages include metastatic high-grade intra- and extracompartmental malignant tumors (IIIA and IIIB, respectively). This classification is based on clinical features, radiographic pattern, CT scan/MRI data, and histologic findings. It was formerly described for long-bone tumors and applied to spinal tumors in some reports (2–4,16).

BENIGN TUMORS

The first stage of benign tumors (S1, latent, inactive; Fig. 2.3) includes asymptomatic lesions, bordered by a true capsule, which is usually seen as a sclerotic rim on plain radiograms. These tumors do not grow or grow only very slowly, like hemangiomas or fibrous dysplasia. No treatment is required, unless palliative surgery is needed for decompression or stabilization. Benign tumors, stage 2 (S2, active; Fig. 2.4), grow slowly, causing mild symptoms. Osteoid osteoma, osteoblastoma, and some early giant cell tumors can be observed at this stage. The tumor is bordered by a thin capsule and by a layer of reactive tissue, sometimes found on plain radiograms as an enlargement of the tumor outline. Bone scan is positive. An intralesional excision can be performed with a low rate of recurrence (2). The incidence of recurrences can be reduced further by local adjuvants (cryotherapy, embolization, radiation therapy). The third stage of benign tumors (S3, aggressive; Fig. 2.5) includes rapidly growing benign tumors: the capsule is very thin, discontinued, or absent. The tumor invades neighboring compartments, and a wide reactive hypervascularized tissue (pseudocapsule) is often found, sometimes permeated with neoplastic digitations. Bone scan is highly

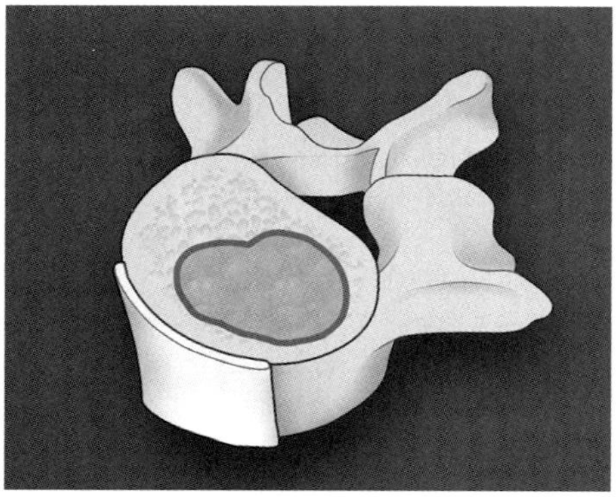

FIGURE 2.3 Stage 1 benign tumor (so-called "latent" or "inactive").

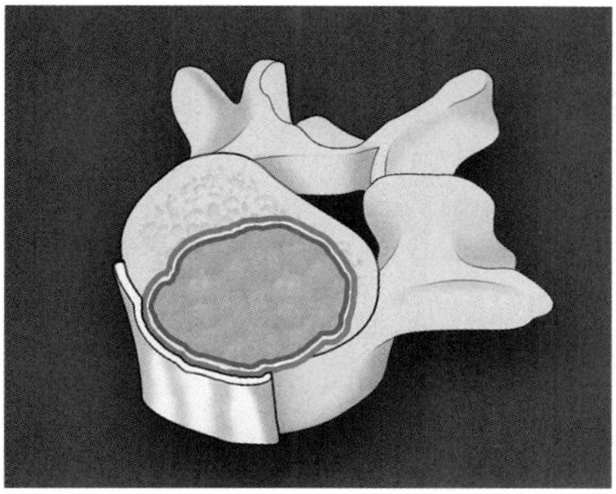

FIGURE 2.4 Stage 2 benign tumor. So-called "active" lesion.

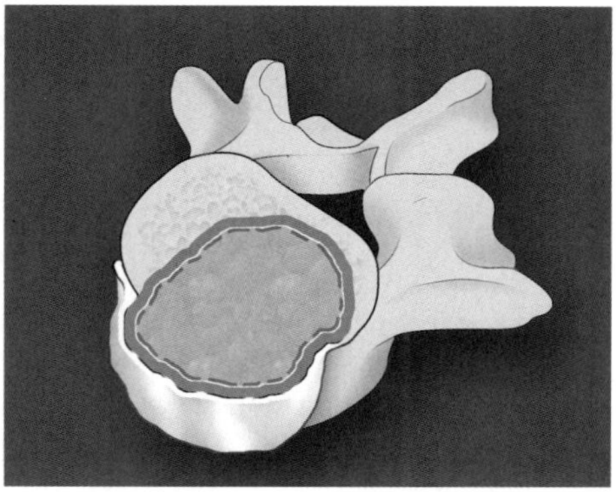

FIGURE 2.5 Stage 3 benign "aggressive" tumor. The extracompartmental growth is remarked.

positive; fuzzy limits are seen on plain radiographs, the CT scan shows extracompartmental extension, and the MRI clearly defines a pseudocapsule and its relation to the neurologic structures. Intralesional excision (curettage), even if augmented by radiation, can be associated with a significant rate of recurrence (7,17). En bloc excision is the treatment of choice. Most giant cell tumors, some osteoblastomas, and many hemangioendotheliomas are found at this stage.

MALIGNANT TUMORS

Low-grade malignant tumors are included in stage I (Fig. 2.6a), subdivided into IA (the tumor remains inside the vertebra) and IB (the tumor invades paravertebral compartments). No true capsule is associated with these lesions, but a thick pseudocapsule of reactive tissue permeated by small microscopic islands of tumor is seen. A resection performed along the pseudocapsule often leaves residual foci of active tumor; megavoltage radiation or proton-beam therapy can be added to reduce the risk of recurrence (23). The treatment of choice–if feasible–is a wide resection. High-grade malignancies are defined as IIA and IIB (see Fig. 2.6b). The neoplastic growth is so rapid that the host has no time to form a continuous reactive tissue. Continuous seeding occurs with neoplastic nodules (satellites). Moreover, these tumors can have neoplastic nodules at some distance from the main tumor mass (skip metastases). These malignancies are generally seen on plain radiographs as radiolucent and destructive and, in many cases, are associated with a pathologic fracture. Invasion of the epidural space is rapid in stage B, particularly in small cell tumors (Ewing sarcoma, lymphomas) characterized by semifluid tissue, able to occupy the epidural space after infiltrating the cortical border of the vertebra.

The margins of the resection must be wide (it is not possible to achieve a "radical" margin in the spine if the tumor invades the epidural space). To achieve a radical margin in a tumor confined to the compartment, the whole vertebra should be resected (including the cord), and courses of radiation and chemotherapy (according to the tumor type) must be considered for local control and to reduce the risk of distant spread. Sometimes the anatomic constraints prevent achieving an appropriate margin.

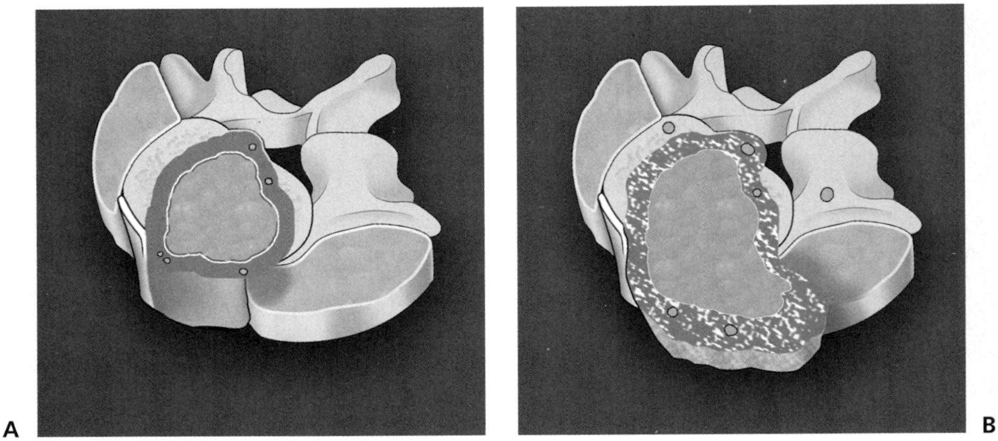

FIGURE 2.6 **A:** Stage IA low-grade, intracompartmental malignant lesion. A small tumoral island can be found within the pseudocapsule. **B:** Stage IIB high-grade, extracompartmental malignant lesion. The tumor growths outside the compartment and a small island of tumor can be found far from the main tumor mass (skip metastasis).

Stages IIIA and IIIB describe the same lesions as IA and IIB, but are associated with distant metastasis.

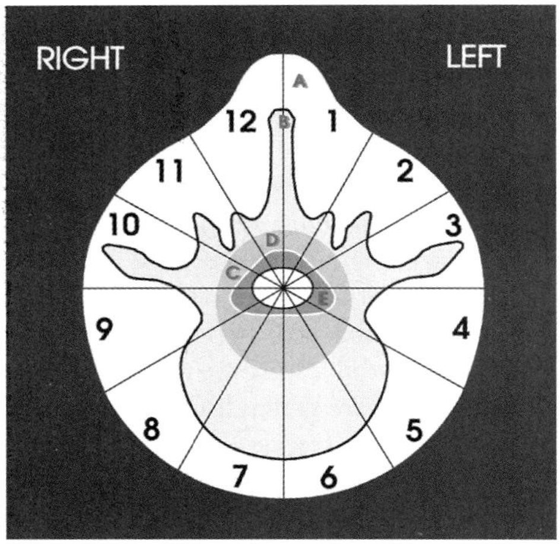

FIGURE 2.7 WBB (Weinstein–Boriani–Biagini) surgical staging system. The transverse extension of the vertebral tumor is described with reference to 12 radiating zones (numbered 1 to 12 in clockwise order) and to five concentric layers (A to E from the prevertebral to the dural involvement). The longitudinal extent of the tumor is recorded.

Surgical Staging

For correct application of the described grading, a complete preoperative workup must be performed. The first attempt at staging spine primary tumors for surgical purposes was done by Weinstein (28) in 1987 and was later modified in collaboration with the Rizzoli Institute. This staging system—now called the WBB system from the names of the authors (Weinstein, Boriani, Biagini) (1,5,6)—proposes to divide the vertebrae on the transverse plane into 12 radiating zones (numbered 1 to 12 in clockwise order) and into five layers (A to E from the prevertebral to the dural involvement). The longitudinal extent of the tumor is recorded by identifying the specific vertebrae involved. This system (Fig. 2.7) allows a more rational approach to surgical planning, provided that all efforts are made to perform surgery along the required margins. The basic concept is a clock face with radiating zones around the longitudinal axis of the involved vertebra (represented by the spinal cord/cauda equina), which allows the crucial planning necessary in performing en bloc resections. To separate the spinal cord or cauda equina or both from the tumor, the surgeon is compelled to resect each sector(s) of the vertebra along the proposed planes (e.g, it is impossible to perform an en bloc resection of a vertebral body without first removing the posterior arch: the margins are the pedicles). Conversely, if the tumor occupies an eccentric area, the surgeon is often compelled to remove the healthy contralateral parts of the vertebra, dislocate the dural sac, and perform radiating sections by use of an osteotome and other appropriate instruments.

This staging system has been subjected to several clinical evaluations (2–4,16).

METASTASES

Spine metastatic deposits in bone can be classified according to the organ of tumoral origin and the tumor histiotype. Region of occurrence (cervical, thoracic, lumbar, sacrum), radiologic pattern (lytic, osteosclerotic, permeative, geographic, and so on), and neurologic symptoms are further criteria to differentiate.

Several classifications of spine metastases have been published in the most recent literature. The large number of different proposals is justified by the frequency of the disease and by the increasing need for appropriate treatment to improve the quality of life. Most propose a score for each considered parameter and suggest a treatment based on mathematical addition. Several preoperative scoring systems have been proposed to classify patients affected by spine metastases and to decide the appropriate treatment (14,15,25–27).

Harrington (14,15) divides patients who have spinal metastases into five categories, depending on the extent of neurologic compromise or bone destruction:

Class I: No significant neurologic involvement,

Class II: involvement of bone without collapse or instability,

Class III: major neurologic impairment (sensory or motor) without significant involvement of bone,

Class IV: vertebral collapse with pain due to mechanical causes or instability but without significant neurologic compromise, and

Class V: vertebral collapse or instability combined with major neurologic impairment.

Indications for treatment according to this staging system are as follows. Patients who are in class I or II generally obtain relief from pain with chemotherapy or other medical treatment, or, if unsuccessful, from local radiation therapy. Those in class III usually respond to treatment with radiotherapy alone. If the neurologic compromise is of acute onset and relatively rapid, the radiotherapy should be augmented by systemic administration of steroids.

When metastatic tumor has destroyed enough bone to result in vertebral collapse and progressive pain in the spine due to mechanical causes (class IV), or when that collapse has caused fragments of bone, ligament, or disk to compress the cord directly (class V), it is illogical to assume that any improvement can result from irradiation alone, no matter how radiosensitive the malignant disease itself may be.

Tokuhashi and colleagues proposed in 1990 (26) a system that is supposed to assess the prognosis of metastatic spine tumors. Six parameters were used:

1. the general condition,
2. the number of extraspinal bone metastases,

3. the number of metastases in the vertebral body,
4. metastases to the major internal organs (lungs, liver, kidneys, and brain),
5. the primary site of the cancer, and
6. the severity of spinal cord palsy.

Each parameter ranged from 0 to 2 points. The total score obtained for each patient can be correlated with the prognosis and is valuable in predicting it. The AA recommends an excisional operation on those cases who scored more than 9 points, whereas a palliative operation is indicated for those who scored less than 5 points.

In 2005 Tokuhashi (25) revised his system, giving more importance to the primary site of cancer (0 to 5 instead of 0 to 2). This allowed improvment of the prediction of the prognosis from 63.3% to 81.2%. In patients with a total score of 12 or more (predicted survival period, 1 year or more), excisional procedures are proposed. In patients with a total score of 9 to 11, excisional procedures are indicated in a single lesion without metastases to the major internal organs; palliative procedures are suggested in all other cases. Surgery is not indicated in patients with a predicted survival period of 6 months or less (score, 0 to 8).

Tomita (27) proposed in 2001 a scoring system for spinal metastases based on three prognostic factors:

1. grade of malignancy (slow growth, 1 point; moderate growth, 2 points; rapid growth, 4 points),
2. visceral metastases (no metastasis, 0 points; treatable, 2 points: untreatable, 4 points),
3. bone metastases (solitary or isolated, 1 point; multiple, 2 points).

These three factors were added to give a prognostic score between 2 and 10. A prognostic score of 2 to 3 points suggested a wide or marginal excision for long-term local control; 4 to 5 points indicated marginal or intralesional excision for middle-term local control; 6 to 7 points justified palliative surgery for short-term palliation; and 8 to 10 points indicated nonoperative supportive care.

The Karnofsky score (18) is a subjective measure of how well the patient is doing. It is useful to track it over time, to see ups and downs in the disease process. The Karnofsky score also sometimes is used as a criterion for entrance into a clinical trial.

- 100: Normal, no complaints or evidence of disease
- 90: Able to perform normal activity; minor signs and symptoms of disease
- 80: Able to perform normal activity with effort; some signs and symptoms of disease
- 70: Cares for self; unable to perform normal activity or to do active work
- 60: Requires occasional assistance but is able to care for most of own needs
- 50: Requires considerable assistance and frequent medical care
- 40: Requires special care and assistance; disabled
- 30: Hospitalization indicated, although death not imminent; severely disabled
- 20: Hospitalization necessary; active supportive treatment required; very sick
- 10: Fatal processes progressing rapidly; moribund
- 0: Dead

The systems proposed to dictate a prognosis and a treatment strategy are based on an arbitrary score attributed to selected parameters: the sum of these scores suggests the appropriate treatment. The score attribution is validated retrospectively on the outcome studies. Equal importance can therefore be attached to the various parameters considered in individual cases. For example, the histiotype of the primary tumor and the general conditions of the patient can have the same influence on the final score and therefore on selecting the treatment.

The validity of these systems and their ability to predict the patients' outcome is not discussed. However, the decision-making process for these patients is basically different in daily practice. Each patient follows his or her "personal" sequential process, which does not necessarily consider all the parameters every time, as some may be irrelevant in the decision-making process. For example, a patient in poor general conditions with a high "ASA" score (8) is usually not a candidate for surgery, irrespective of the histiotype of the primary tumor or the number of secondary localizations. For this patient, the most important parameter will therefore be the sensitivity of the tumor histiotype to adjuvant treatment. In the same way, a patient with acute and worsening spinal cord damage will undergo emergency palliative decompression and stabilization surgery without considering a more-demanding operation.

We should consider the patient and not just the disease, avoiding reducing the choice of treatment to an overly simplistic mathematical score. As an alternative to scoring systems, whose validity stands for series review and outcome evaluation, we propose a different methodologic approach: a decision-making process based on an algorithm (Fig. 2.8) that analyzes the case holistically, first considering the individual and his or her general conditions and only subsequently, the parameters of the metastases. Prospective studies are necessary to assess the validity, the reliability, and the reproducibility of this algorithm.

Algorithm for Decision-making Process

Once a spine metastasis is diagnosed, the decision-making process should start from the anesthesiologist assessment [ASA score (8)]: any treatment theoretically decided on a scoring system is not applicable if the ASA score is 4 or 5 for any reason, possibly independent of the disease we are dealing with.

If the patient cannot be operated on because of a high ASA score, nonsurgical options must be considered. Next, the sensitivity of the tumor histiotype to adjuvant therapies (chemotherapy, radiation, hormonal, immunologic) is considered. If the tumor does not respond to any form of treatment, the only option for the patient is pain relief.

If the patient can be operated on, the first element to be considered is the neurologic status. The surgical treatment of metastases is functional, finalized to improve the quality of life; the local control can be obtained with combinations of adjuvant treatments.

If neurologic compromise is present [for example, quantified by means of the Frankel score (13)], the possibility of recovery is evaluated on the basis of time elapsed from the onset of paraplegia.

If no neurologic recovery of the patient is possible, sensitivity to adjuvant treatments is reevaluated.

If the paralysis is incomplete and worsening, emergency decompressive surgery is suggested.

If no neurologic deficit is present, the decision-making process begins again from considering the sensitivity to adjuvant treatments.

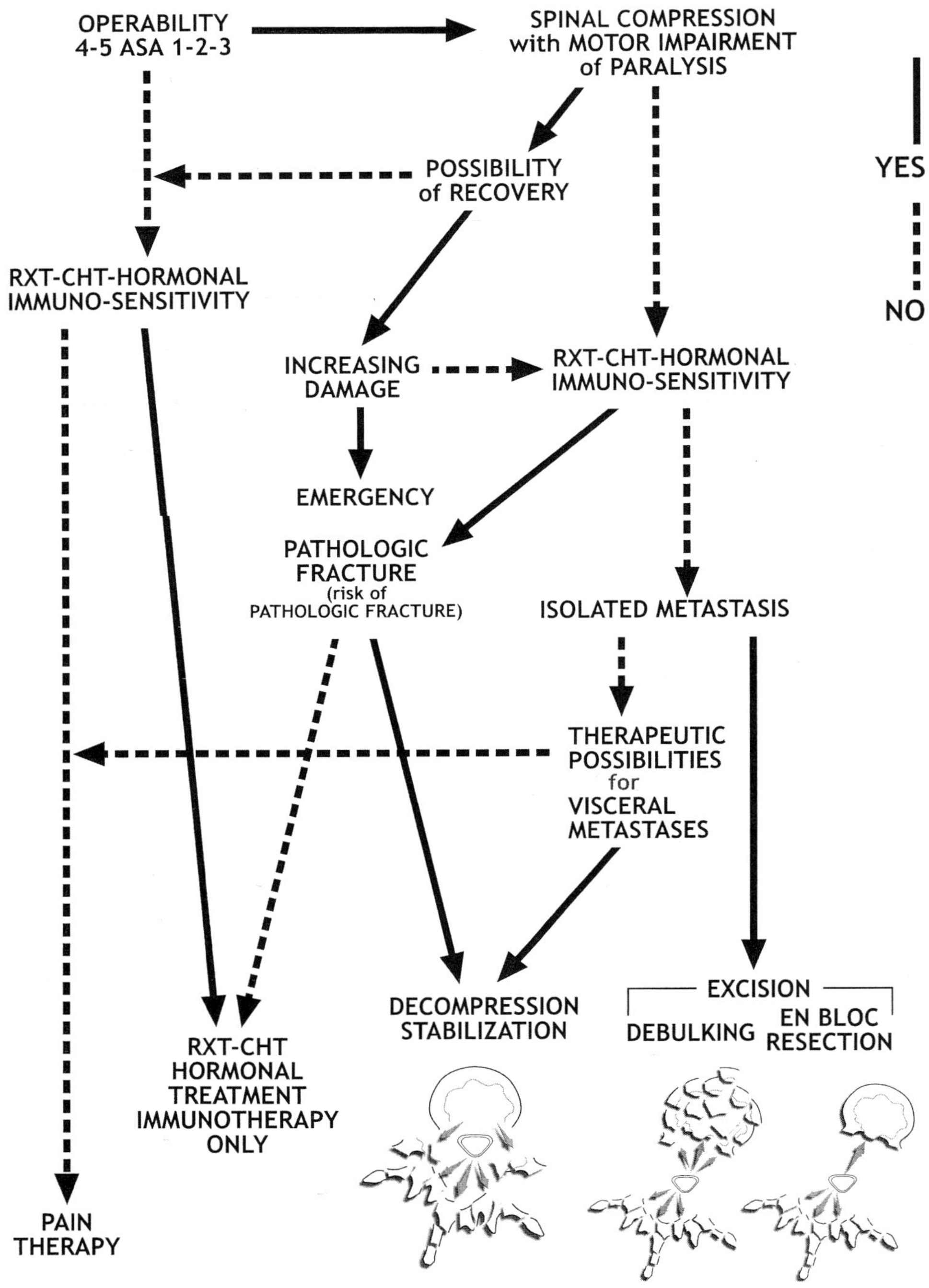

FIGURE 2.8 Algorithm for decision-making process of spine metastatic diseases. Continuous lines, yes; dotted lines, no.

If the tumor histiotype is not sensitive and the metastasis is solitary, resection of the lesion is chosen. But if the metastases are multiple, surgical planning including fixation (to prevent collapses) and decompression (to prevent spinal cord damage) is suggested. In case of disseminated disease, technically impossible to stabilize, the indication is for pain relief.

When no neurologic symptoms are present and the tumor is sensitive to some form of adjuvant treatment, impending or assessed pathologic fracture is evaluated. This parameter is decisive in making the choice between surgical treatment with decompression and stabilization or adjuvant treatment only.

Resection of the tumor may be performed by curettage (intralesional excision) or en bloc resection. En bloc tumor removal is the treatment of choice of primary low-grade malignant tumor and must be considered exceptional for metastases. In our experience, it should be reserved for hypervascularized tumors, like metastases from kidney carcinoma, and for metastatic sarcoma. The criteria of feasibility of such treatment (1) must be carefully considered as well.

The application of this algorithm to any single patient could represent a guideline for the decision-making process and help in making a wise decision in the treatment of spine metastases.

SUMMARY

Surgeons require a classification able to give information about the biologic behavior of the tumor, to standardize the decision-making process, and to assess prognosis related to the treatment performed.

In the United States, approximately 2,000 malignant tumors of bone are diagnosed each year (22). Of these, between 4% and 20% are primary spinal tumors. Therefore it would be very unusual and/or impossible for any one institution to acquire the necessary understanding or natural history of these tumors and their response to various forms of treatment. Therefore the authors would prefer that an international registry be organized through which centers with special interest in these cases work together. To this purpose, adopting the same terminology and a commonly accepted classification is mandatory. Only through a collaborative effort will enough information be obtained to make rational surgical and nonsurgical decisions for our patients.

REFERENCES

1. Boriani S, Weinstein JN, Biagini R. Primary bone tumors of the spine: terminology and surgical staging. Spine 1997;22:1036–1044.
2. Boriani S, Capanna R, Donati D, et al. Osteoblastoma of the spine. Clin Orthop 1992;278:37–45.
3. Boriani S, Chevalley F, Weinstein JN, et al. Chordoma of the spine above sacrum: treatment and outcome in 21 cases. Spine 1996;21:1569–1577.
4. Boriani S, De Iure F, Bandiera S, et al. Chondrosarcoma of the mobile spine: report on 22 cases. Spine 2000;25:804–812
5. Boriani S, Weinstein JN. Differential diagnosis and surgical treatment of primary benign and malignant neoplasms. In: Frymoyer JW, ed. The Adult Spine: Principles and Practice, 2nd ed. Philadelphia: Lippincott-Raven, 1997: 951–987.
6. Boriani S, Weinstein JN, Biagini R. Spine update: a surgical staging system for therapeutic planning of primary bone tumors of the spine: a contribution to a common terminology. Spine 1997;22: 1036–1044.

7. Campanacci M, Boriani S, Giunti A: Giant cell tumors of the spine. In: Sundaresan SN, Schmidek HH, Schiller AL, Rosenthal DI. Tumors of the Spine: Diagnosis and Clinical Management. Philadelphia: WB Saunders, 1990: 163–172.
8. Dripps RD, Lamont A, Eckenhoff JE. The role of anesthesia in surgical mortality. JAMA 1961; 178:261.
9. Enneking WF. Musculoskeletal Tumor Surgery. New York: Churchill Livingstone, 1983.
10. Enneking WF, Spanier SS, Goodmann M. A system for surgical staging of musculoskeletal sarcoma. Clin Orthop 1980;153:106–120.
11. Fidler MW. Radical resection of vertebral body tumours: a surgical technique used in ten cases. J Bone Joint Surg 1994;76 B:765–772.
12. Fletcher CD. The evolving classification of soft tissue tumours: an update based on the new WHO classification. Histopathology 2006;48: 3–12.
13. Frankel HL. Ascending cord lesion in the early stages following spinal injury. Paraplegia 1969;7: 111–118.
14. Harrington KD. Metastatic disease of the spine. In: Harrington KD, ed. Orthopaedic Management of Metastatic Bone Disease. St. Louis: CV Mosby, 1988:309–383.
15. Harrington KD. Metastatic disease of the spine. J Bone Joint Surg. (Am) 1986;68:1110–1115.
16. Hart RA, Boriani S, Biagini R, et al. A system for surgical staging and management of spine tumors: a clinical outcome study of giant cell tumors of the spine. Spine 1997;22:1773–1782.
17. Healy JH, Ghelman B. Osteoid osteoma and osteoblastoma: current concepts and recent advances. Clin Orthop 1986;204:76–85.
18. Karnofsky DA. Clinical evaluation of anticancer drugs: cancer chemotherapy. GANN Monogr 1967;2:223–231.
19. Magerl F, Coscia MF. Total posterior vertebrectomy of the thoracic and lumbar spine. Clin Orthop 1988;232:62–69.
20. Schajowicz F, Ackerman LV, Sisson HA. Histological Typing of Bone Tumors. Geneva: World Health Organization, 1972.
21. Schajowicz F, Sissons HA, Sobin LH. The World Health Organization's histologic classification of bone tumors: a commentary on the second edition. Cancer 1995;75:1208–14.
22. Silverberg B, Lubera J. Cancer statistics. CA Cancer 1987;37:12.
23. Suit HD, Goiten M, Munzenreider J, et al. Definitive radiation therapy for chordoma and chondrosarcoma of base of skull and cervical spine. J Neurosurg 1982 56:377–385.
24. Sundaresan N, Krol G, DiGiacinto GV, et al. Metastatic tumors of the spine. In: Sundaresan N, Schmidek HH, Schiller AL, et al., eds. Tumors of the Spine: Diagnosis and Clinical Management. Philadelphia: WB Saunders, 1990:279–304.
25. Tokuhashi Y, Matsuzaki H, Oda H, et al. Revised scoring system for preoperative evaluation of metastatic spine tumor prognosis. Spine 2005;30: 2186–2191.
26. Tokuhashi Y, Matsuzaki Y, Toriyama S, et al. Scoring system for the preoperative evaluation of metastatic spine tumor prognosis. Spine 1990;15: 1110–1113.
27. Tomita K, Kawahara N, Kobayashi T, et al. Surgical strategy for spinal metastases. Spine 2001;26: 298–306.
28. Weinstein JN, McLain RF. Primary tumors of the spine. Spine 1987;12:843–851.

Specific Aspects of Spinal Tumors and Traumatisms in Children

Andre J. Kaelin

3

INTRODUCTION

Spinal tumors and traumatisms are specific in infancy, childhood, and adolescence. The main factor during this period of life is the remaining growth, but etiologies, mechanisms of lesions, types of lesions, and outcomes are very different. In adulthood, most of the spinal tumors are secondary locations or metastases; in young patients, those lesions represent a very large differential diagnosis of primary benign and malign tumors. Spinal cord plasticity allows important tumor development before triggering neurologic deficit; pain, back stiffness, and hamstring tightness are often the initial complaints.

If the mechanism of trauma involves high energy, complete imaging is usually performed, and obvious bone fractures are detected. In childhood, spinal lesions can occur after very low energy trauma, because of bone pathologic or constitutional fragility, delaying diagnosis; pain, back stiffness, and hamstring tightness are again the only symptoms. In case of nonresolving back pain in children, tumor and trauma lesion must be ruled out. We describe only the specific aspects of the care process in tumor and spine trauma in the immature spine. The indications for treatments are described, but techniques of treatments that are mostly the same as those in adults are not addressed.

SPINAL GROWTH

At birth, the mean sitting height measures 35 cm; at the end of growth, this parameter measures 88 cm for girls and 92 cm for boys. The length of the thoracic and lumbar spine is 20 cm at birth and 45 cm at maturity. These 25 cm of growth are shared by 34 apophyseal zones located cranial and caudal to each vertebral body for the anterior spine. In the posterior, a very complex system of apophyseal growth cartilage is situated on the spinous processes, the transverses processes, and the joints.

The neurocentral cartilage increases the size of the medullary canal. It stops its action around the age of 6 years old, and it is the first growth cartilage to ossify.

Balanced growth between the anterior and posterior and the right and left parts of the spine are necessary for keeping a normal morphology. The earlier a growth imbalance occurs, the greater are the risks of deformities. During the first year of life, we see the larger increase, 12.4 cm, and then the growth slows progressively in 3 years to 2.3 cm. At puberty (14 to 15 years for boys, and 12 to 13 years for the girls), the speed increases again at 4 cm per year for 2 years.

The remaining growth for boys at 5 years old is 9.3 cm in the thoracic area and 5.6 cm in the lumbar area; at 10 years old, 6 cm in the thoracic area and 3.6 cm in the lumbar area. For girls at 5 years old, the growth is 7.8 cm in the thoracic area and 4.7 cm in the lumbar area; at 10 years old, 4.2 cm in the thoracic area and 2.5 cm in the lumbar area.

At birth, the spine is very flexible because of the ligamentous laxity, but ligaments are still stronger than bone. In addition, because of the muscular hypotonia; poor active and passive spinal cord protection exists. Progressively, stability increases, and tone increases to the adult standard at the end of puberty.

At birth more than 50% of vertebral bodies are cartilaginous and very soft; ossification reaches the body limit when the child is prone to stand, giving mechanical support.

The morphology of the vertebral plateau is unique; it acts as articular surface and apophyseal growth plate (no epiphyseal nucleus is present). In the limbus area during puberty, a ring apophysis appears with an ossifying nucleus that represents a weak point in the vertebral stability.

The mineral content in children is as low as that in elderly people. Mineralization builds up to a peak in young adulthood, which is why low-energy trauma causes fractures so easily in children.

Posture and the repartition of body weight changes during growth. For the first months, the baby is unable to support its trunk; the head is not actively controlled. Sitting is possible once head control is acquired, but the spine is in global kyphosis. After the acquisition of erect position, the definitive spinal morphology with lumbar lordosis, thoracic kyphosis, and cervical lordosis is obtained after walking.

At birth, the head weight is 25% of the total body weight. This proportion decreases to 5.6% for an adult; heavy heads and weak cervical muscles explain the high risk to the cervical spine in infancy and childhood.

SPINE TRAUMA IN CHILDREN

Patients to the age of 18 years represent 20% of the population, but only 3% of spinal fractures occur in children, which is very low. In a survey in our hospital, the mean age is 11 years old, with two peaks at 9 and 12 years old. Of our patients, 44% have one-level fractures; 20%, two levels; 19%, three levels; and 17%, four levels and more. Most of the time, levels are contiguous. One-level fractures occur mainly in the cervical or lumbar area, and the multilevel fractures in the thoracic area. In 87 cases, the most common level is T6 (30 cases); 84% are wedges and stable fractures, and 16% are burst or combined fracture/dislocation. One patient is definitively paraplegic; one has a regressive nerve root deficit, and two died of polytrauma. Of our patients, 62% were treated functionally (rest, analgesic medication, physical therapy), 26% received also a brace for up to a year; and 12% were treated surgically (cervical, three; thoracic, two; lumbar, three), mainly with a posterior approach.

The etiologies of fractures during the growth period are very different from those in the young adult; each age period has a specific mechanism.

For neonates and young infants, spinal fracture and dislocation are very often associated with head injury; for all unconscious patients, not only cervical but also thoracic and lumbar fractures must be ruled out.

Newborn: Spinal Fractures

Prenatal fracture secondary to osteogenesis imperfecta in association with limbs, ribs, and skull fractures.

Birth trauma (fetomaternal dystocia or emergency delivery due to fetal distress) associated with shoulder or brachial plexus injury or both (Fig. 3.1)

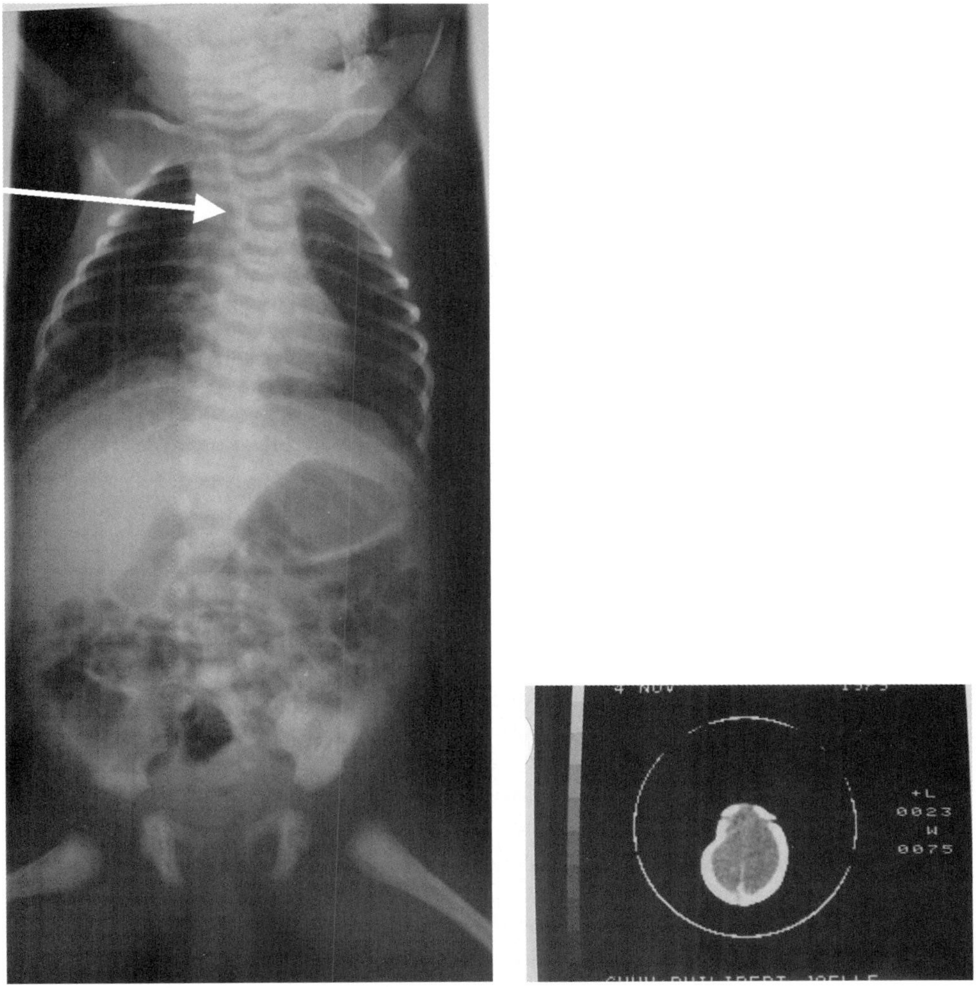

A B

FIGURE 3.1 Traumatic delivery, breech presentation. Spinal trauma, fracture at D4 level, paraplegia, brachial plexus injury, and skull fracture.

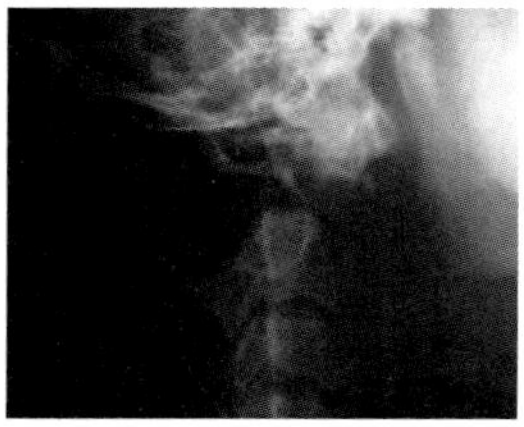

FIGURE 3.2 A 2-year-old child, strapped in a car seat, involved in a car accident at 100 km/h with quick deceleration. C1–C2 axial dislocation caused death.

Infant: Spinal Fractures

Fall from low height

Deceleration traction trauma in cervical and high-thoracic area (Fig. 3.2) (baby installed in a baby seat with four-point fixation), in low thoracic and lumbar area (baby installed in a baby seat with abdominal seat belt)

High-energy polytrauma (car accident)

Battered-baby syndrome (association with head, limbs, skin lesion)

Children: Spinal Fractures

Street trauma

Playground accident

Sports accident

High-height fall

Adolescents: Spinal Fractures

Sports accident

Motor vehicle accident

The type of trauma and the morphology of children's spines lead to specific lesions.

1. SCIWORA (Spinal Cord Injury Without Radiographic Abnormalities) is rare for children younger than 8 years. Very important flexion/extension movement or axial traction on the hyperlaxe cervical spine causes a direct spinal cord lesion or ischemic lesion. Complete or partial paraplegia appears immediately or could be delayed by some hours. Radiographs and computed tomography (CT) scan are normal. If no magnetic resonance imaging (MRI) modification is found, the outcome is very good; if the MRI shows edema or a hemorrhage, the risk of permanent lesion is high. Rest and immobilization of the cervical spine give a better chance of neurologic recovery.
2. High cervical fracture and dislocation (C1 to C3) occur in small children, mainly shacked babies and patients with pathologic hyperlaxity and Down syndrome. Morphologic anomalies of the dens are very frequent and should not be interpreted as fractures. Flexion–extension stability is assessed with functional lateral radiographs; a distance of more than 4 mm between the dens and the arch of C1 is considered pathologic. Rotatory C1–C2 dislocation is often the cause of traumatic torticollis; a CT scan must be performed with an aligned head to avoid misinterpretation of the physiologic C1–C2 subluxation that appears with head rotation.
3. A Chance fracture occurs mainly in car accidents when children wear abdominal seat belts. A high-energy flexion mechanism on a fulcrum causes posterior element distraction with osseous or ligamentous disruption. Capsular, ligamentous, and disc lesion without bony lesion are very usual; misalignment of the spine can be missed on radiographs and/or CT scans performed in a supine position. For this type of trauma mechanism, MRI or functional radiographs (if the patient is conscious) must be performed. Intraabdominal lesions like duodenal and small intestine perforation or necrosis are very often associated with this type of Chance fracture (Fig. 3.3).

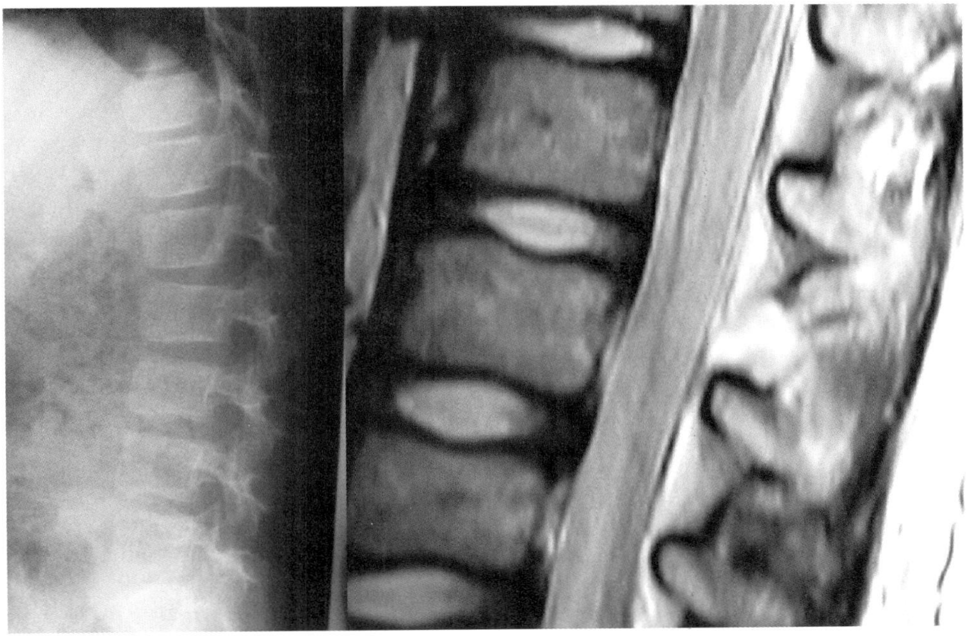

A

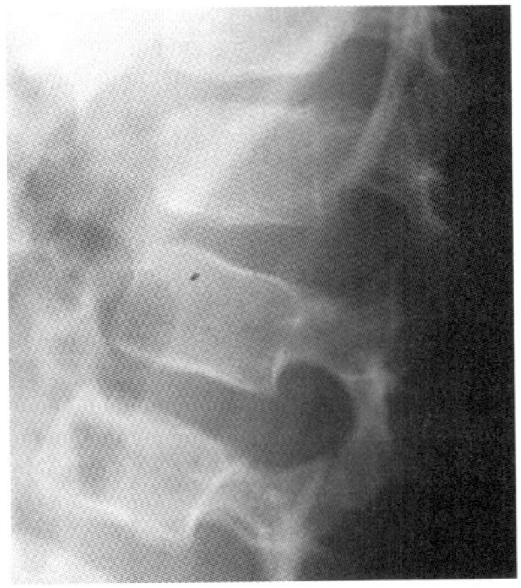

B

FIGURE 3.3 **A:** 10-year-old girl in a car accident with an abdominal seat belt. Duodenal perforation. Radiograph: slight opening of posterior part of the L2–L3 disc. MRI: no disc lesion, interspinous ligament edema. **B:** Dynamic flexion radiograph demonstrating L1–L2–L3 instability and soft tissue Chance lesion.

4. Between the ages of 6 to 12 years, multiple thoracic vertebral bodies fractures are very frequent after falls or sport injuries. D4 to D10 compression fractures are usual, involving three to five vertebrae. Growth monitoring is important to avoid progressive kyphosis due to epiphyseal cartilage damage (Fig. 3.4).
5. Compression fracture after low-energy trauma must trigger metabolic and morphologic workup to rule out juvenile osteoporosis or osteogenesis imperfecta.
6. Adolescents close to the end of growth can have a unique lesion: the ring apophysis fracture. Posterior ring apophysis dislocation can lead to cord compression and paraplegia. In an acute neurologic lesion, decompression in emergencies is indicated.

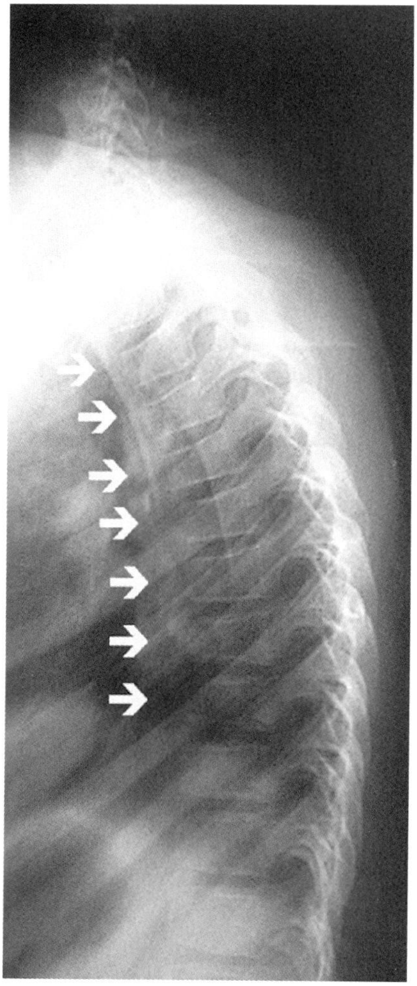

FIGURE 3.4 Typical multilevel thoracic fractures in adolescent with low- to mid-energy trauma.

Trauma history and accurate clinical examination including neurologic status are mandatory to define the ideal imaging techniques. Joint injuries are very frequent in cervical trauma and Chance fractures. CT scans must be performed in an emergency for this situation and for all children in a coma. MRI is the second choice.

Bone lesions usually heal quickly, and conservative treatment is the rule. Unstable articular capsule lesions need surgical stabilization.

Secondary growth disturbances appear when the epiphyseal plate is injured in preadolescent children. In children with traumatic paraplegia, severe scoliosis will develop.

BACK PAIN AND SPINAL TUMOR IN CHILDREN

Many epidemiologic enquiries address the occurrence of back pain in childhood. In meta-analysis studies, the cumulative prevalence is found in 30% to 50% of children and adolescents. In industrial countries, fewer than 10% of these patients have an established diagnosis (acute trauma excluded), which in decreasing order are as follows.

Kyphosis and Scheuermann	28%
Spondylolysis, spondylolisthesis	25%
Disc protrusion, hernia	12%
Tumor (benign, malignant)	10%
Infection	8%
Deformities (congenital, acquired)	6%
Other	11%

In persisting back pain, some questions are mandatory:

Is the pain present at night?

Has the intensity of the pain increased over time?

Do any medications relieve the pain?

Are any other alleviating or aggravating factors present?

Do you have any shooting pains or any weakness down your arms or legs?

Do you have any trouble with your bowel or bladder function?

Has your child had any recent fevers, a gait abnormality, or lost weight?

"Yes" answers must raise the suspicion of tumor around the spine. Clinical examination includes assessment of posture, balance, antalgic position and contracture, stiffness and rigid spine deformity, palpation of the full spine and pelvis, pain localization, skin examination looking for flakes, angiomas, and hair, gait analysis including tip-toe and heel walk, and full neurologic examination. Examination includes also abdominal and kidney areas.

Imaging is the major part of the diagnosis process:

- Plain radiographs detect spine deformities, sclerosis, and osteolysis.
- Bone scintigram is used aspecifically to locate the lesion.
- CT scan is the best imaging technique for the morphology of osseous lesions.
- MRI is the best imaging technique for the spinal cord, soft tissues and cartilage lesions, and bone edema. Venous and arterial patterns are best visualized with gadolinium injection.
- Ultrasound examinations are useful for intra- and retroabdominal masses.
- PET scan and CT-PET fused images are new imaging techniques, for which indications are not yet specifically defined.

Imaging leads to a strong suspicion of tumor. Definitive diagnosis is supported by open or needle biopsy unless a very typical image like osteo-osteoid and eosinophiliac granuloma.

Differential Diagnosis by Localization

Extraspinal	Teratoma, Wilms tumor, hepatoblastoma
Paraspinal	Soft tissue sarcoma, neuroblastoma, Hodgkin lymphoma
Dumbbell tumors	Neuroblastoma, neurofibromatosis
Bony vertebral tumors	Ewing (PNET), osteosarcoma, aneurysmal bone cyst (Fig 3.5), osteo-osteoid (Fig 3.6), osteoblastoma, osteochondroma, angioma, Langerhans cell histiocytoma (Fig. 3.7), metastasis, giant cell tumor
Anterior elements	Giant cell tumor
Intraspinal	Astrocytoma, ependymoma, meningioma (Fig. 3.8), medulloblastoma, malignant glioma, neurofibromatosis

Differential Diagnosis by Age

Younger than 5 years	Langerhans cell histiocytoma, Ewing (PNET), leukemia, neuroblastoma, Wilms
Younger than 10 years	Astrocytoma, ependymoma, meningioma, medulloblastoma, malignant glioma, neuroblastoma, teratoma, Wilms, Ewing (PNET), Langerhans cell histiocytoma
Older than 10 years	Soft tissues sarcoma, Hodgkin, lymphoma, neurofibromatosis, Ewing (PNET), osteosarcoma, aneurismal bone cyst, osteo-osteoid, giant cell tumor, osteoblastoma, osteochondroma, angioma, eosinophiliac granuloma, metastasis

Benign tumors are treated depending on symptoms, neurologic compromise, mechanical stability, and evolution.

Malignant tumor treatments are very challenging; chemotherapy is used to control risk of secondary localizations. En bloc resection is recommended but not always possible. Radiation therapy is applied for residual or unresectable tumors.

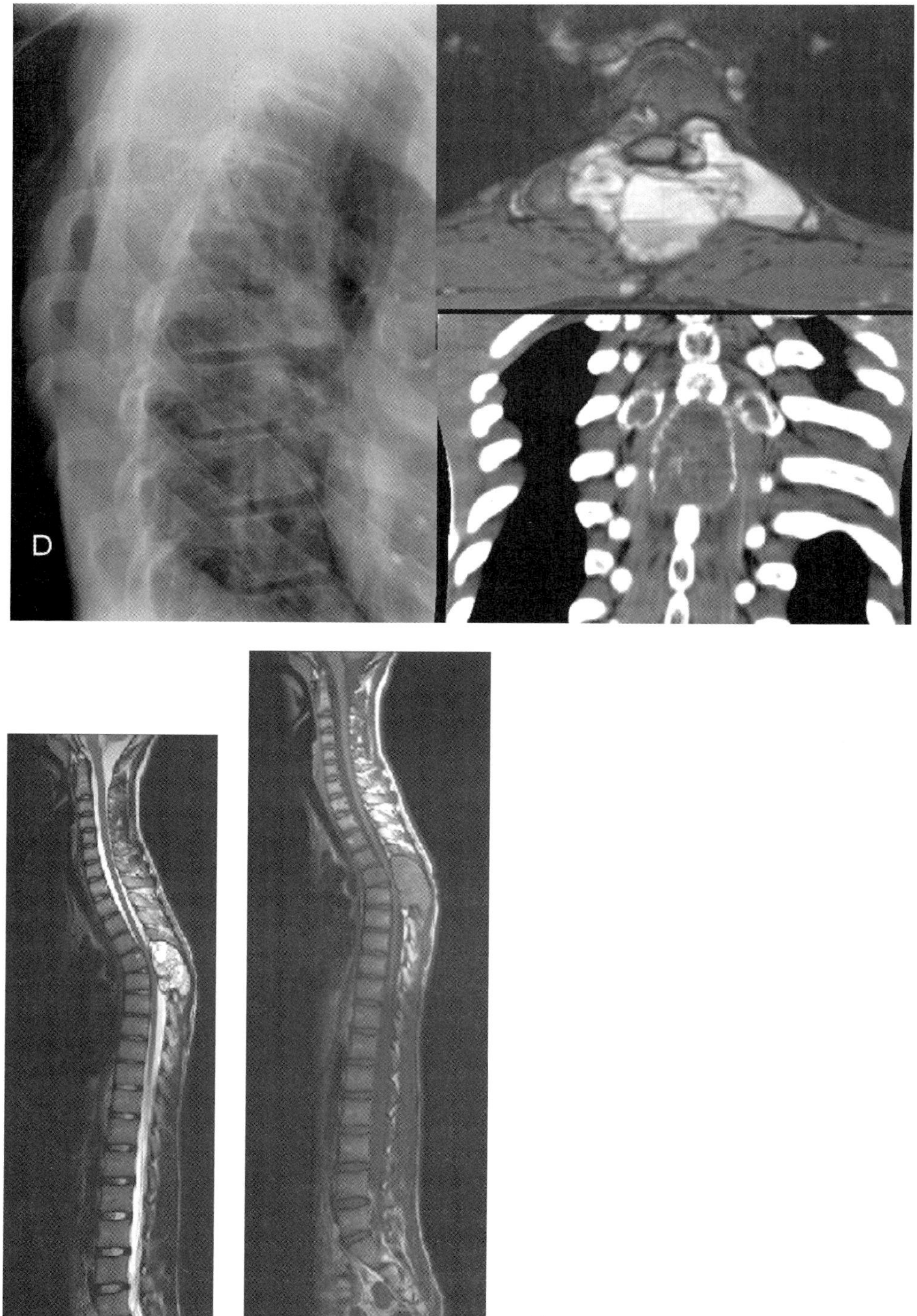

A B C

FIGURE 3.5 A 12-year-old patient, with a 6-month history of back pain, and 1 week history of ankle clonus and weakness; D5–D6 tumor lesion.

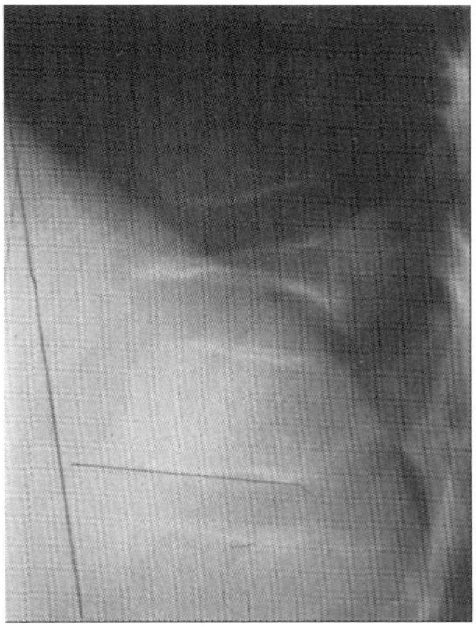

FIGURE 3.6 A 9-year-old boy with back pain for 3 weeks; vertebral body collapse and preserved disc height. The diagnosis is eosinophiliac granuloma (vertebra plana).

Spinal cord tumors need excision and adjuvant therapy if they have a high grade of malignancy. All the resection procedures must include a stable spine reconstruction, taking into account the residual growth.

Tumors of the spine are rare but must be included in the differential diagnosis of children with lasting back pain, spine stiffness, or neurologic symptoms. Imaging is the basis of lesion localization, and biopsy gives the final diagnosis.

Surgical treatment aims at local excision and stable reconstruction of the spine.

A 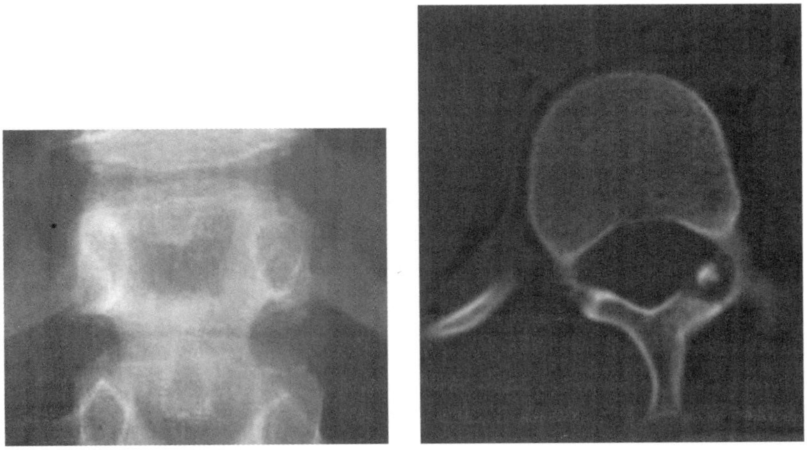 B

FIGURE 3.7 **A:** Typical radiograph of an osteoid osteoma with sclerotic (white) asymmetric pedicle. **B:** On the CT scan, the nidus is located in the deep cortex at the junction of the pedicle and the lamina.

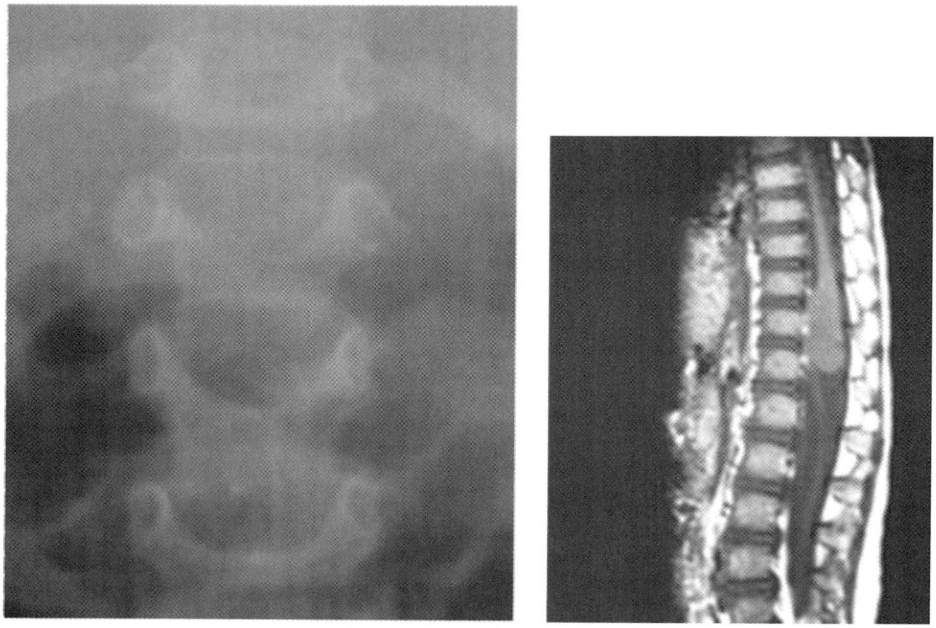

FIGURE 3.8 **A:** A 3-year-old boy with a history of 3 weeks of limping, slight hyperreflexia. Radiograph shows segmental increased interpedicular distance. **B:** MRI: very large conus tumor. Biopsy diagnosis: meningioma.

REFERENCES

Spinal Growth

Dimeglio A. Le Rachis en Croissance. Paris: Springer-Verlag, 1990.

Children's Spinal Trauma

Reynolds R. Pediatric spinal injury. Curr Opin Pediatr 2000;12:67–71.

Parisini P, Di Silvestre M, Greggi T. Treatment of spinal fractures in children and adolescents: long-term results in 44 patients. Spine 2002;27: 1989–94.

Santiago R, Guenther E, Carroll K, et al. The clinical presentation of pediatric thoracolumbar fractures. J Trauma 2006;60:187–192.

Pouliquen JC, Kassis B, Glorion C, et al. Vertebral growth after thoracic or lumbar fracture of the spine in children. J Pediatr Orthop 1997;17: 115–120.

Akbarnia BA. Pediatric spine fractures. Orthop Clin North Am 1999;30:521–536.

Lowry DW, Pollack IF, Clyde B, et al. Upper cervical spine fusion in the pediatric population. J Neurosurg 1997;87:671–676.

Goradia D, Blackmore CC, Talner LB, et al. Predicting radiology resident errors in diagnosis of cervical spine fractures. Acad Radiol 2005;12: 888–893.

Kaps HP, Badke A. Development of the spine after traumatic spinal cord injury in children and adolescents. Orthopade 2005;34:128–130, 132–136.

Wang MY, Hoh DJ, Leary SP, et al. High rates of neurological improvement following severe traumatic pediatric spinal cord injury. Spine 2004;29: 1493–1497.

Carreon LY, Glassman SD, Campbell MJ. Pediatric spine fractures: a review of 137 hospital admissions. J Spinal Disord Tech 2004;17:477–482.

Reddy SP, Junewick JJ, Backstrom JW. Distribution of spinal fractures in children: does age, mechanism of injury, or gender play a significant role? Pediatr Radiol 2003;33:776–781.

Launay F, Leet AI, Sponseller PD. Pediatric spinal cord injury without radiographic abnormality: a meta-analysis. Clin Orthop Relat Res 2005;433: 166–170.

Takata K, Inoue S, Takahashi K, et al. Fracture of the posterior margin of a lumbar vertebral body. J Bone Joint Surg Am 1988;70:589–594.

Spinal Tumor

Garg S, Dormans JP. Tumors and tumor-like conditions of the spine in children. J Am Acad Orthop Surg 2005;13:372–381.

Mirovsky Y, Jakim I, Halperin N, et al. Non-specific back pain in children and adolescents: a prospective study until maturity. J Pediatr Orthop B 2002;11:275–278.

Weinstein J, Boriani,S, Campanacci L. Spine neoplasms. In: Winstein S, ed. The pediatric spine: principles and practice, 2nd ed. Philadelphia: Lippincott, Williams & Wilkins, 2001:685–707.

Garg S, Mehta S, Dormans JP. Modern surgical treatment of primary aneurysmal bone cyst of the spine in children and adolescents. J Pediatr Orthop 2005;25:387–392.

Yeom JS, Lee CK, Shin HY, et al. Langerhans' cell histiocytosis of the spine: analysis of twenty-three cases. Spine 1999;24:1740–1749.

Ghanem I, Tolo VT, D'Ambra P, et al. Langerhans cell histiocytosis of bone in children and adolescents. J Pediatr Orthop 2003;23:124–130.

Weinstein J, Boriani S, Campanacci L. Spinal tumor. In: Weinstein S, ed. The Pediatric Spine: Principles and Practice, 2nd ed. Philadelphia: Lippincott, Williams & Wilkins, 2001:685–707.

Delamarter RB, Sachs BL, Thompson GH, et al. Primary neoplasms of the thoracic and lumbar spine: an analysis of 29 consecutive cases. Clin Orthop Relat Res 1990;256:87–100.

Boriani S, Capanna R, Donati D, et al. Osteoblastoma of the spine. Clin Orthop Relat Res 1992; 278:37–45.

Saifuddin A, White J, Sherazi Z, et al. Osteoid osteoma and osteoblastoma of the spine: factors associated with the presence of scoliosis. Spine 1998;23:47–53.

Floman Y, Bar-On E, Mosheiff R, et al. Eosinophilic granuloma of the spine.J Pediatr Orthop B 1997; 6:260–265.

Ozaki T, Flege S, Liljenqvist U, et al. Osteosarcoma of the spine: experience of the Cooperative Osteosarcoma Study Group. Cancer 2002;94: 1069–1077.

Bone Metastasis: Update on Imaging Workup

Marc Lemort

4

INTRODUCTION

Bone metastases of solid tumors and secondary involvement of bone by hematologic malignancies are among the most frequent causes of tumoral involvement of bone.

Techniques Available

Imaging of bone metastases may rely on nuclear medicine [bone scintigraphy or single-photon emission computed tomography (SPECT), positron emission tomography (PET), PET-CT, or SPECT-CT], on radiograph-based technologies (radiographs and CT), and on MRI. Even though we have this large choice of tools, early detection of these lesions and differential diagnosis with other pathologic conditions of bone are not so easy. To follow up the evolution of these lesions when using one of several of the many ways to treat these patients requires a rigorous approach and pertinent choice of the dedicated methods. The role of clinical evaluation and physical examination must be emphasized (disease context, biology, clinical signs). No imaging algorithm may be proposed without keeping that in mind.

NUCLEAR MEDICINE

Bone scintigraphy is a screening technique with a relatively poor specificity, because it studies the bone-forming reaction to the presence of the tumor but does not demonstrate the presence of tumor tissue itself. In addition, its sensitivity has been overestimated: bone scintigraphy is a relatively low-resolution technique and may miss small lesions or lesions that are purely lytic. An important point to improve the performance (particularly the specificity) of this technique is to ensure that reading is done by very experienced nuclear medicine specialists. Tomographic scanning by using SPECT and the combination with CT (SPECT-CT) may improve performance. Bone scintigraphy conversely has the advantage of being a whole-body screening method, with relatively low cost and low irradiation of the patient. It remains an important screening method, but needs control with a confirmatory examination when a suggestive abnormality is described. Most often, these confirmatory methods will be plain radiographs for the appendicular skeleton and x-ray CT for the axial skeleton, particularly the spine.

[^{18}F]fluoride positron emission tomography (PET) has been advocated as a more sensitive method. Spatial resolution and contrast-to-noise ratio are far better than with ^{99}Tc bone scintigraphy, but the method has a higher cost and requires use of a PET system that could be better used for true metabolic studies.

FDG-PET has the major advantage of imaging the tumor tissue, and not the sclerotic reaction of bone. It is based on the glucose avidity of the tumor due to increased metabolism. It is a whole-body method that detects not only bone lesions but also soft-tissue metastases. However, not all tumors in the bone are hypermetabolic. Prostate cancer is known to be poorly glucose avid, as are kidney cancer and some breast cancers before the tumor becomes more aggressive. PET-CT adds the localization power of x-ray CT and the time benefit of doing the attenuation correction by using CT data. PET is the best tool to detect bone lesions of lymphoma and lung cancer at staging or restaging. It is, however, under active evaluation for other tumors, notably advanced breast cancer, and may also be interesting in detecting early response to therapy.

RADIOLOGY

Plain radiographs remained for many years the basic method of confirmation and follow-up method for bone metastases. As a screening method, it was used under the form of a "skeletal survey" including the bones that were statistically most often involved: the axial skeleton and proximal appendicular bones. X-ray tomography was used in case of unclear findings. These methods have no place today.

The sensitivity of plain x-ray is poor (1). The detection is late when the lesion either disrupts the bone cortex, destroys more than 30% of trabecular bone (in a vertebral body), or is accompanied by a significant sclerotic bone reaction.

During the follow-up, plain radiographs do not report with detail the evolution of bone lesions: they may mimic disease worsening in case of sclerotic response to therapy or dissimulate a new lytic evolution in a densified bone.

Plain radiographs disappeared from most of the diagnostic algorithms for secondary bone lesions. They retain, however, some utility as a quick method to confirm complications such as a vertebral collapse in a patient with known bone metastases.

Computed tomography (CT) is a high-resolution, x-ray tomographic technique that permits a detailed analysis of the trabecular structure of bone and evaluation of the cortical integrity. The densitometric sensitivity is by far superior to that of the plain radiograph, and replacement of fat by tumor in the bone marrow may be directly seen, as well as the extension of the tumor in the soft tissues. New multidetector CT devices made it possible to investigate larger body parts in a short time, to freeze physiologic motion, and to reduce irradiation.

Magnetic resonance imaging (MRI) relies on magnetic properties of the hydrogen nucleus (proton) to produce images whose contrast is governed by multiple parameters (the most important being the relaxation times, T_1 and T_2). Images may be influenced by the different parameters, depending on the choice of the user. In most instances, several sequences with different weighting will be obtained in the same examination (see

Fig. 4.3). This leads to a tremendous increase in contrast between tissues in comparison with methods such as CT. The drawback is that the method is more difficult to achieve and interpret, is more operator dependant, and may lack specificity. Its sensitivity is high, and it is able to detect lesions at the stage of early invasion of the bone marrow, even before any destructive effect on the bone matrix.

Progress in MRI (multiple array coils, speed, and spatial resolution) allows consideration of covering larger body areas, or even the whole skeleton, with sequences that are sensitive to metastatic disease of bone. Diffusion contrast imaging (3) and dynamic contrast-enhanced MRI (DCE-MRI) (4) hold a promise for better specificity, particularly for differential diagnosis between tumoral and nontumoral vertebral compression fractures.

SIGNS OF BONE METASTASES AND DIAGNOSTIC PROBLEMS

Conventional Radiographs

Classically, bone metastases appear as lytic, sclerotic, or mixed lesions (the latter being the most frequent). A statistical association exists between lesion morphology and the primary site of the tumor. However, a large variation is found in the radiologic expression of bone metastases. Purely lytic lesions may be seen in cases of prostate cancer, for instance. The lytic or sclerotic character seems to be more in relation with tumor aggressiveness, mass effect, and local production of osteolysis-stimulating factors, as with response to therapy. It is the expression of the ability of bone to produce bone around the lesion. The presence of this bone-forming reaction is also the condition for positivity of bone scintigraphy, which is an indirect way to detect tumor. It is not so infrequent to find on CT large lytic lesions that are not visible on bone scintiscans.

Conventionnal radiographs detect sclerotic lesions more easily. The disappearance of these lesions with treatment could be misleading: it could be to the result of vanishing of the sclerotic changes due to lytic progression of the underlying lesion. Conversely, new sclerotic lesions appearing during treatment may be a sign of good response, with a sclerotic healing reaction around the lesion (5). In most cases, CT will give the right answer.

Conventional radiographs may remain an option in the follow-up of multiple bone lesions that are radiologically visible, complementary to a CT follow-up of targeted lesions (6).

Computed Tomography

CT allows us to detect both lytic and blastic lesions, even when small and limited to the spongious bone, without cortical disruption (Fig. 4.1 and 4.2). It also allows follow-up of targeted lesions over time and observation of early lytic evolution or appearance of sclerotic healing under treatment (Figs. 4.3 and 4.4). In our opinion, CT is the first-line examination for diagnostic confirmation and follow-up of most bone metastases (1,6).

Sclerotic changes, usually considered a sign of favorable response, may also be observed in patients receiving supportive treatment with bisphosphonates, a now common treatment in the management of metastatic disease of bone, and seem to be amplified in

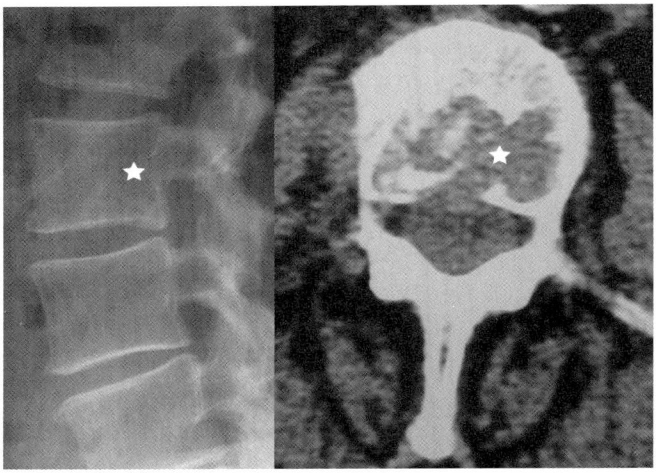

FIGURE 4.1

this case (Fig. 4.5). The sclerotic changes may induce an apparent worsening of the scintigraphic image that may be misinterpreted as a disease progression (so-called "flare" phenomenon). Sclerotic changes may also hide foci of lytic evolution of the disease. This can be demonstrated with CT (see Fig. 4.4).

Magnetic Resonance Imaging

MRI presently becomes the second-line examination for diagnostic confirmation when the clinical suspicion is high and other examinations are negative, or when it is necessary to search for a second metastatic localization in the spine, as for detection of

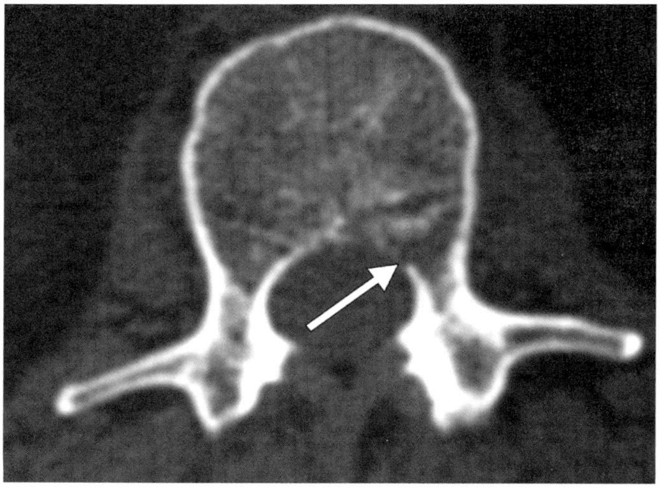

FIGURE 4.2

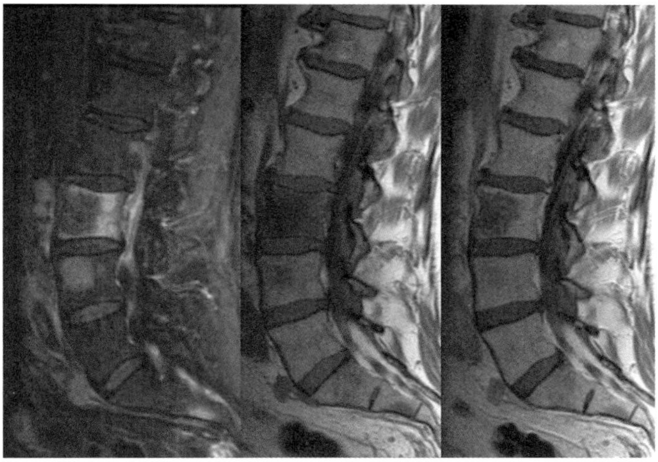

FIGURE 4.3

epidural extension (Fig. 4.6). This diagnosis of epidural extension is fundamental and must be considered a radiologic emergency event if no definite sign of radicular or medullar compression is present (7). These occur later, after a delay during which pain is the unique symptom, and a delayed diagnosis could have dramatic consequences on the quality of survival.

For bone, MRI may show very early infiltration when only subtle changes in the fat component of spongious bone are visible.

The fact that nearly 80% of the yellow bone marrow is constituted of fat offers a true natural contrast for detection of metastatic foci that are detectable by a reduced signal on T_1W images. Contrast enhancement will be better detected when using a fat-suppressed sequence. This also makes more detectable the high signal intensity of

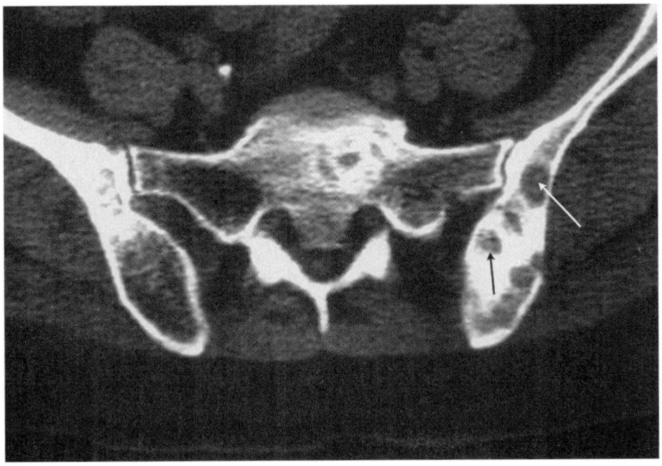

FIGURE 4.4

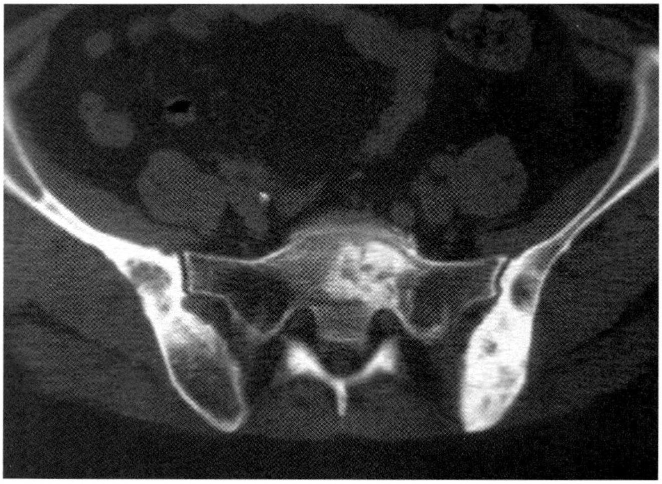

FIGURE 4.5

lesions on T_2W images [also with a short-inversion-time inversion recovery (STIR) sequence; see Fig. 4.3). Sclerotic lesions appear as low-signal areas on every sequence. Their appearance may vary depending on the remaining cellularity and water contents. Small blastic lesions may be hard to detect with MRI. The follow-up of lesions, particularly the lysis-to-sclerosis ratio, is easier with CT. MRI may be used even when metallic surgical hardware is present in the vicinity, which is rarely possible with CT (Fig. 4.7).

Finally, MRI allows us to find new arguments to differentiate metastases from other causes in the case of isolated vertebral collapse. Findings that favor the diagnosis of metastases are convexity of the vertebral shape, signal changes in the pedicles or posterior arch, epidural mass or infiltration, paravertebral soft-tissue mass, or bone metastases in noncollapsed vertebrae (8). In the case of an acute collapse, these arguments will not always be conclusive, and a follow-up will be needed. Apparent diffusion coefficient (ADC) measurements may be interesting for differential diagnosis (3).

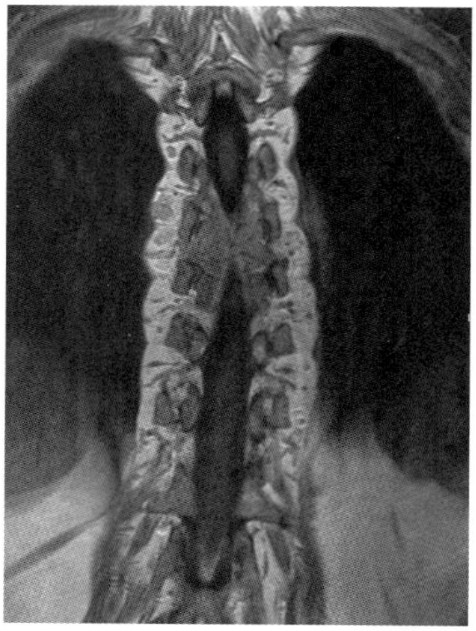

FIGURE 4.6

A PROPOSAL FOR A DIAGNOSTIC ALGORITHM

Figure 4.8 is a proposal for a diagnostic algorithm in the setting of primary diagnosis or follow-up of bone metastases. This algorithm is dependent on the presence or absence of suggestive clinical signs and does not include conventionnal radiographs, which could be skipped in most cases.

Such an algorithm is only a general template and must be modulated, taking into account the complete clinical data and the local or regional availability of techniques or expertise.

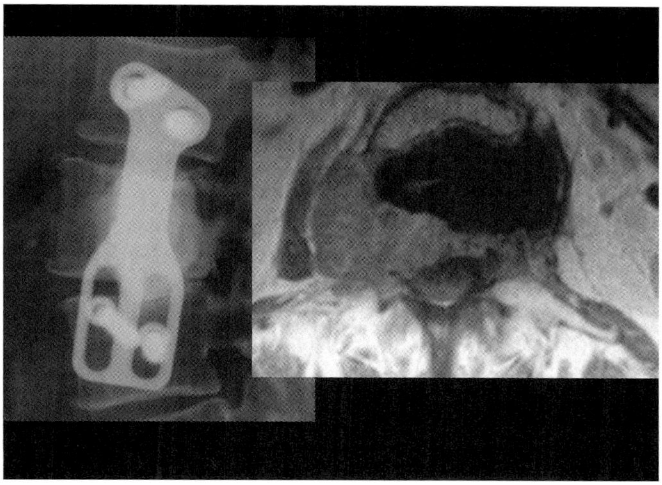

FIGURE 4.7

In addition to lung cancer, breast cancer with rising marker levels and lymphoma with suspected bone lesions also are indications for PET-CT scanning (depending on availability). Usefulness of a systematic search for bone lesions in an asymptomatic patient remains controversial. For breast cancer, it was recently shown that a systematical follow-up of patients with tumor markers and bone scintiscans does not add any survival benefit (9); in contrast, for non–small cell lung cancer, one may argue for systematic bone scintigraphy with confirmation technique (PET, MRI) as needed to avoid unnecessary aggressive therapy (estimated 14% to 22% of cases) (10).

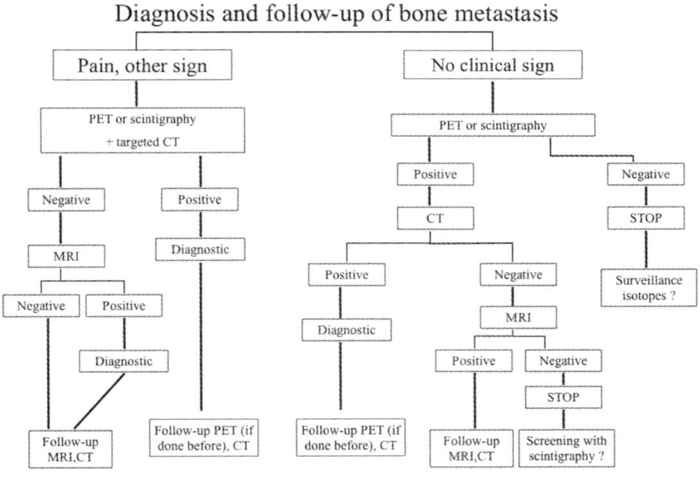

FIGURE 4.8

REFERENCES

1. Bellamy EA, Nicholas D, Ward M, et al. Comparison of computed tomography and conventional radiology in the assessment of treatment response of lytic bony metastases in patients with carcinoma of the breast. Clin Radiol 1987;38: 351–355.
2. Ghanem N, Altehoefer C, Hogerle S, et al. Comparative diagnostic value and therapeutic relevance of magnetic resonance imaging and bone marrow scintigraphy in patients with metastatic solid tumors of the axial skeleton. Eur J Radiol 2002;43:256–261.
3. Baur A, Dietrich O, Reiser M. Diffusion-weighted imaging of the spinal column. Neuroimaging Clin North Am 2002;12:147–160.
4. Chen WT, Shih TT, Chen RC, et al. Blood perfusion of vertebral lesions evaluated with gadolinium-enhanced dynamic MRI: in comparison with compression fracture and metastasis. J Magn Reson Imaging 2002;15:308–314.
5. Ciray I, Astrom G, Andreasson I, et al. Evaluation of new sclerotic bone metastases in breast cancer patients during treatment. Acta Radiol 2000;41:178–182.
6. Scutellari PN, Antinolfi G, Galeotti R, et al. Metastatic bone disease: strategies for imaging. Minerva Med 2003;94:77–90.
7. Levack P, Graham J, Collie D, et al. Don't wait for a sensory level: listen to the symptoms: a prospective audit of the delays in diagnosis of malignant cord compression. Clin Oncol (J R Coll Radiol) 2002;14:472–480.
8. Jung HS, Jee WH, McCauley TR, et al. Discrimination of metastatic from acute osteoporotic compression spinal fractures with MR imaging. Radiographics 2003;23:179–187
9. Sato N, Hino M, Sano M. Detection of bone metastases in routine follow-up after treatment for primary breast cancer. Breast Cancer 2003;10: 335–340.
10. Schirrmeister H, Arslandemir C, Glatting G, et al. Omission of bone scanning according to staging guidelines leads to futile therapy in non-small cell lung cancer. Eur J Nucl Med Mol Imaging 2004;28. (Epub ahead of print).
11. Peterson JJ, Kransdorf MJ, O'Connor MI. Diagnosis of occult bone metastases: positron emission tomography. Clin Orthop 2003;(415 suppl): S120–S128.
12. Rossleigh MA, Lovegrove FT, Reynolds PM, et al. The assessment of response to therapy of bone metastases in breast cancer. Aust N Z J Med 1984;14:19–22.
13. Lemieux J, Guimond J, Laberge F, et al. The bone scan flare phenomenon in non-small-cell lung cancer. Clin Nucl Med 2002;27:486–489.
14. Pollen JJ, Witztum KF, Ashburn WL The flare phenomenon on radionuclide bone scan in metastatic prostate cancer. AJR Am J Roentgenol 1984;142:773–776.
15. Pfluger T, Schmied C, Porn U, et al. Integrated imaging using MRI and ^{123}I metaiodobenzylguanidine scintigraphy to improve sensitivity and specificity in the diagnosis of pediatric neuroblastoma. AJR Am J Roentgenol 2003;181:1115–1124.
16. Bury T, Barreto A, Daenen F, et al. Fluorine-18 deoxyglucose positron emission tomography for the detection of bone metastases in patients with non-small cell lung cancer. Eur J Nucl Med 1998; 25:1244–1247.
17. Moog F, Kotzerke J, Reske SN FDG PET can replace bone scintigraphy in primary staging of malignant lymphoma J Nucl Med 1999;40:1407–1413.
18. Lonneux M, Borbath II, Berliere M, et al. The place of whole-body PET FDG for the diagnosis of distant recurrence of breast cancer. Clin Positron Imaging 2000;3:45–9.
19. Salminen E, Hogg A, Binns D, et al. Investigations with FDG-PET scanning in prostate cancer show limited value for clinical practice. Acta Oncol 2002;41:425–429.
20. Bellamy EA, Nicholas D, Ward M, et al. Comparison of computed tomography and conventional radiology in the assessment of treatment response of lytic bony metastases in patients with carcinoma of the breast. Clin Radiol 1987;38: 351–355.
21. Ghanem N, Altehoefer C, Hogerle S, et al. Comparative diagnostic value and therapeutic relevance of magnetic resonance imaging and bone marrow scintigraphy in patients with metastatic solid tumors of the axial skeleton. Eur J Radiol 2002;43:256–261.
22. Baur A, Dietrich O, Reiser M. Diffusion-weighted imaging of the spinal column Neuroimaging Clin North Am 2002;12:147–160.

23. Chen WT, Shih TT, Chen RC, et al. Blood perfusion of vertebral lesions evaluated with gadolinium-enhanced dynamic MRI: in comparison with compression fracture and metastasis. J Magn Reson Imaging 2002;15:308–314.
24. Ciray I, Astrom G, Andreasson I, et al. Evaluation of new sclerotic bone metastases in breast cancer patients during treatment. Acta Radiol 2000;41:178–182.
25. Body JJ, Mancini I. Bisphosphonates for cancer patients: why, how, and when? Support Care Cancer 2002;10:399–407.
26. Hilner BE, Ingle JN, Chelbowski RT, et al. American Society of Clinical Oncology 2003 update on the role of bisphosphonates and bone health issues in women with breast cancer. J Clin Oncol 2003;21:4042–4057.
27. Scutellari PN, Antinolfi G, Galeotti R, et al. Metastatic bone disease: strategies for imaging. Minerva Med 2003;94:77–90.
28. Roudier MP, Vesselle H, True LD, et al, Bone histology at autopsy and matched bone scintigraphy findings in patients with hormone refractory prostate cancer: the effect of bisphosphonate therapy on bone scintigraphy results. Clin Exp Metastasis 2003;20:171–180.
29. Levack P, Graham J, Collie D, et al. Don't wait for a sensory level: listen to the symptoms: a prospective audit of the delays in diagnosis of malignant cord compression. Clin Oncol (J R Coll Radiol) 2002;14:472–480.
30. Jung HS, Jee WH, McCauley TR, et al. Discrimination of metastatic from acute osteoporotic compression spinal fractures with MR imaging. Radiographics 2003;23:179–187.
31. Sato N, Hino M, Sano M. Detection of bone metastases in routine follow-up after treatment for primary breast cancer. Breast Cancer 2003;10: 335–340.
32. Schirrmeister H, Arslandemir C, Glatting G, et al. Omission of bone scanning according to staging guidelines leads to futile therapy in non-small cell lung cancer Eur J Nucl Med Mol Imaging 2004. (Epub ahead of print).

Overview of the Management of Metastastic Spine Tumors

Yoshiya Yamada and Mark H. Bilsky

5

ABSTRACT

The optimal management of tumors metastatic to the spine is controversial. At Memorial Sloan Kettering Cancer (MSKCC), a multidisciplinary team of surgeons, radiation oncologists, physiatrists, and neuroradiologists that make up the spine service assess patients according to neurologic and oncologic symptoms, mechanical stability, and extent of systemic disease (NOMS).

Neurologic considerations are based on the patient's degree of neurologic compromise. Oncologic factors include tumor histology and radiosensitivity and degree of epidural disease. Mechanical issues concern spinal stability. Systemic evaluation of the overall extent of disease and patient condition must always be factored into the decision-making process.

The NOMS paradigm is a systematic assessment of the clinical situation and is an easily understood system of categorizing patients, regardless of the specialty. A common lexicon for recommending treatment options has proven invaluable to provide patients with the most appropriate options for treatment.

INTRODUCTION

Cancer metastatic to the spine is commonly encountered in clinical practice. Recent advancements in the areas of surgery and radiation therapy have made a significant impact on the management of such patients.

More than 18,000 new cases of spinal metastases are diagnosed in North America each year, affecting more than 100,000 patients each year (1,2). The vast majority of secondary malignancy to the spine is extradural. More than 90% of patients initially have significant pain (3). Motor weakness, paresthesia, and myelopathy are also important problems that often affect patient quality of life. Despite the enormity of the problem, no real consensus exists on the optimal management of spinal metastases.

At MSKCC, patients are evaluated in a multidisciplinary manner, including experts from orthopedics and neurosurgery, radiation oncology, neuroradiology, and physiatry. Consequently, a multidisciplinary paradigm has been developed to evaluate each patient to guide management and decision making. This paradigm provides a systematic multidisciplinary structure to evaluate each patient in terms of neurologic, oncologic, mechanical, and systemic (NOMS) aspects (4). The pros and cons of each treatment modality are weighed in view of the specific clinical scenario to provide the most effective and appropriate palliation for each patient.

NEUROLOGIC STATUS

Neurologic status of the patient is of paramount importance. Surgical management is given first consideration for patients who first seen with rapid and recent onset of symptoms, particularly those associated with myelopathy or loss of function (5). Level one evidence, reported by Patchell et al. (6), confirmed the superiority of surgery over radiation therapy alone for patients with high-grade epidural cord compression. In this study, a significant benefit was found in favor of surgery in terms of ambulation, as well as other quality-of-life measures, and the study was stopped before accrual was completed. Radiation therapy may contribute to spinal cord edema in the setting of high-grade epidural cord compression, and should be used cautiously in such settings, keeping in mind the potential for exacerbation of symptoms in such situations. Corticosteroids are routinely used to minimize cord edema.

In situations without rapid escalation of neurologic symptoms or significant epidural disease, or when surgery is contraindicated for medical reasons, radiation therapy may offer good palliation. Both conventional radiation therapy and high-dose image-guided radiation are appropriate considerations. Radiation therapy, much less invasive than surgery, is often an appropriate modality to maintain optimal quality of life in patients with metastases.

ONCOLOGIC CONSIDERATIONS

Oncologic issues to consider include the histology (radiosensitive or radioresistant) and the extent of the tumor, both the paradural and paraspinal components. Lymphomas, myelomas, and leukemias are likely to respond rapidly to systemic therapy or conventional radiation therapy. Surgery may be indicated if a histologic diagnosis has not been made or if mechanical back pain requiring surgical stabilization is present. In the previously mentioned phase 3 study reported by Patchell et al. (6), the majority of patients had high-grade epidural tumors with relatively radioresistant histologies (non–small cell lung cancer and colorectal carcinoma). These patients will not respond in a timely fashion to radiotherapy, and surgery should be considered. As reported in the study, these patients have significantly worse outcomes when conventional radiotherapy is used, reinforcing the need for surgical decompression in cases of high-grade epidural spinal cord compression.

At MSKCC, epidural disease is classified as 0 (no epidural disease), 1 (mild to minimal epidural disease), 2 (moderate) cerebrospinal fluid (CSF) still seen on T_2 axial MRI images, or 3 (loss of CSF around the spinal cord) (see Fig. 5.1). Surgical decompression is given first consideration for patients with grade 3 compression. Patients with grade 0 to 2 compression may do well with radiotherapy and can be considered. Radioresistant tumors may require higher doses of radiation than conventional radiotherapy can safely provide to give high levels of tumor control. Often, the spinal cord will limit the ultimate dose that can be safely given with conventional radiation techniques. Katagiri et al. (7)

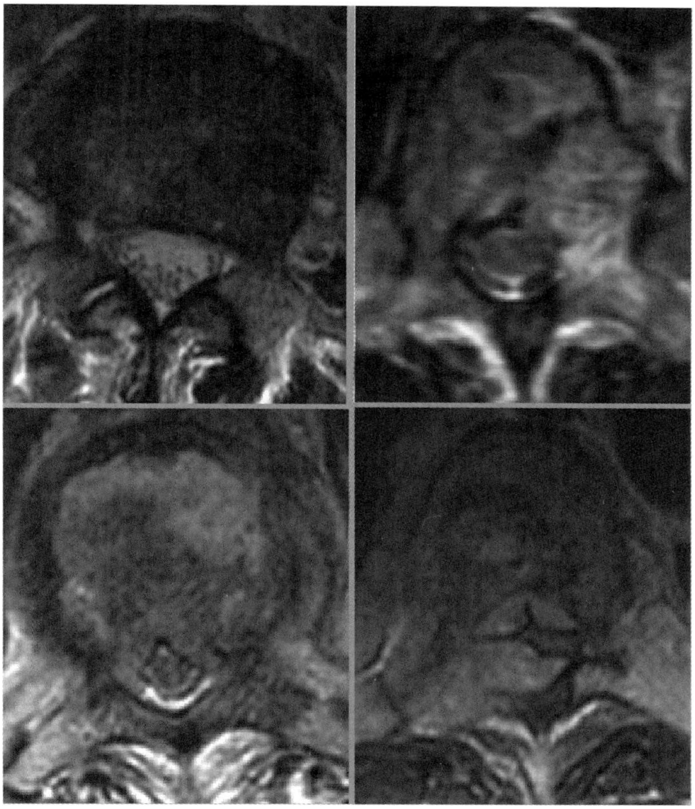

FIGURE 5.1 MSKCC epidural compression grading.

reported long-term data on the use of conventional radiotherapy for spinal metastases. Overall, approximately two thirds of patients responded favorably with radiotherapy alone. However, for unfavorable histologies, only 31% were thought to be treated successfully, whereas 72% of the favorable histologies were scored as having had successful treatment. Thus high-dose radiotherapy is likely to offer a greater benefit.

Image-guided intensity-modulated radiotherapy (IG-IMRT) is able to deliver very high dose radiation within 1- to 2-mm precision (8). With image-guided treatment, high-dose radiation can be given around the spinal cord with extreme accuracy. Intensity-modulated radiation techniques are able to spare nearby spinal cord of excessive dose, allowing the treatment of paraspinal tumors beyond what has traditionally been considered the tolerance of the spinal cord to radiation therapy. Gerszten et al. (9) recently reported the outcomes of 60 patients with renal cell carcinoma metastases, a relatively radioresistant histology, by using high-dose single-fraction radiotherapy with image-guided techniques. With a median follow-up of 37 months, 89% of patients have reported durable palliation. At MSKCC, our outcomes with high-dose single-fraction radiotherapy (median dose, 24 Gy) for radioresistant histologies such as melanoma and renal cell carcinoma are similarly high (100% local control), with a median follow-up of 14 months. Thus radioresistant histologies are considered for image-guided single-fraction radiation if they have not been previously irradiated and if significant epidural disease is not present. When a relatively radiosensitive histology, such as lymphoma or breast cancer, is presented, conventional radiotherapy (i.e., 3,000 cGy in 10 fractions) is considered. In cases of recurrence after prior radiotherapy in which surgery is not indicated or possible, image-guided hypofractionated radiotherapy is considered. In a recent report from our institution, approximately 60% of patients have been successfully salvaged with image-guided IMRT (10). Currently, the target dose is 3,000 cGy in five fractions. Outcomes in this patient cohort are suboptimal, and dose escalation is being considered to improve local control.

MECHANICAL INSTABILITY

Mechanical pain is best palliated with surgical fixation or vertebral body augmentation (kyphoplasty or vertebroplasty). Radiation therapy is effective in palliating tumor-related pain, but cannot help patients with mechanical spinal instability. These patients often need stabilization to have a reasonable expectation of palliation. Mechanical instability is ultimately defined clinically. Patients often complain of pain that is related to activity or is positional in nature, often worsening through the day. Often mechanical pain is relieved with lying down, relieving the mechanical stress on the spine. In contrast, tumor-related pain is typically worse at night and is not relieved by lying down. Although both tumor and mechanical instability can cause radiculopathy, a history of worsening radiculopathy with axial loads would point to mechanical instability. Corticosteroids may help both mechanical instability and tumor-related pain. A good response to corticosteroids is suggestive of a significant tumor component to the pain. Radiologic findings suggesting the vertebral body collapse, or destruction of the pedicle and articulating joint, or both, are also highly suggestive of mechanical instability. In cases of retropulsion of bony fragments into the spinal canal, surgery is preferred over radiation therapy. Although radiculopathy is not likely to improve with kyphoplasty, in cases with an intact posterior vertebral body wall, augmentation of the damaged vertebral body with methyl methacrylate can result in dramatic improvement in pain. In the setting of metastatic disease, the use of image-guided single-fraction radiotherapy with kyphoplasty has been reported with excellent results (11). Although clinical experience with this approach is still maturing, because it is minimally invasive and the pain relief often is rapid, it is an attractive option for patients with metastatic disease, mechanical instability, and potentially limited life expectancy.

Radical resections, such as en bloc resection of spine metastases, have been advocated in patients with oligometastatic disease (12). However, the excellent outcomes, both in terms of local control of disease and minimal toxicity with high-dose single-fraction IG-IMRT, call into question the need for very aggressive surgery such an en bloc resections and associated postoperative recovery in the setting of metastatic disease and limited expected survival (13).

SYSTEMIC DISEASE

The extent of systemic disease is also an important consideration when assessing the patient with metastases. Several systems have been suggested to try to prognosticate patient outcome (14–17). It is extremely difficult to predict the survival of any given patient. Physicians are notoriously inaccurate in assessing the probability of survival of patients with metastases. Nonetheless, in terms of quality of life, patients who are thought to have less than a 3- to 6-month expected survival may not live long enough to benefit from aggressive back surgery, when recovery from surgery is taken into consideration. Many patients with metastatic disease have multiple medical problems that make surgery risky and are not considered for surgery. However, consideration of surgery is given to patients with limited survival when a good likelihood exists that function can be restored, such as the ability to ambulate.

SUMMARY

Patients with spine metastases are often complicated and, in any case, require urgent management. The NOMS (Neurologic/Onocologic/Mechanical/Systemic) paradigm to assess patients in a multidisciplinary manner has been integrated successfully into the spine service at MSKCC. It provides a systematic framework to evaluate each patient in four critical domains. It is easy to apply across disciplines and provides a common frame of reference when considering optimal palliative therapy for patients with metastases.

REFERENCES

1. Black PMcL. Spinal metastases: current status and recommended guidelines for management. Neurosurgery 1979;5:726–46.
2. Gokaslan ZL, York JE, Walsh GE, et al. Transthoracic vertebrectomy for metastatic spinal tumors. J Neurosurg 1998;89:599–609.
3. Sorensen S, Hilweg-Lassen S, Mouridsen H, et al. Effect of high-dose dexamethasone in carcinomatous metastatic spinal cord compression treated with radiotherapy: a randomized trial. Eur J Cancer 1994;30A:22–27.
4. Bilsky MH, Lis E, Raizer J, et al. The diagnosis and treatment of metastatic spinal tumor. Oncologist 1999;4: 459–469.
5. Wang JC, Boland P, Mitra N, et al. Single-stage posterolateral transpedicular approach for resection of epidural metastatic spine tumors involving the vertebral body with circumferential reconstruction: results in 140 patients: invited submission from the Joint Section Meeting on Disorders of the Spine and Peripheral Nerves, March 2004. J Neurosurg Spine 2004;1:287–298.
6. Patchell RA, Tibbs PA, Regine WF, et al. Direct decompressive surgical resection in the treatment of spinal cord compression caused by metastatic cancer: a randomized trial. Lancet 2005;366: 643–648.
7. Katagiri H, Takahashi M, Inagaki J, et al. Clinical results of nonsurgical treatment for spinal metastases. Int J Radiat Oncol Biol Phys 1998:42:1127–1132.
8. Lovelock DM, Hua C, Wang P, et al. Accurate setup of paraspinal patients using a noninvasive patient immobilization cradle and portal imaging. Med Phys 2005; 32:2606–2614.
9. Gerszten PC, Burton SA, Ozhasoghi C, et al. Stereotactic radiosurgery for spinal metastases from renal cell carcinoma. J Neurosurg Spine 2005;3:288–295.
10. Wright JL, Lovelock DM, Bilsky MH, et al. Clinical outcomes after repeat irradiation of paraspinal tumors. Int J Radiat Biol 2005;63:S266.
11. Gerszten PC, Germanwala A, Burton SA, et al. Combination kyphoplasty and spinal radiosurgery: a new treatment paradigm for pathological fractures. Neurosurg Focus 2005;18:e8.
12. Tomita K, Kawahara N, Baba H, et al. Total en bloc spondylectomy for solitary spinal metastases. Int Orthop, 1994; 18:291–298.
13. Gerszten PC, Burton SA, Welch W, et al. Single-fraction radiosurgery for the treatment of spinal breast metastases. Cancer 2005;104:2244–2254.
14. Tomita K, Kawahara N, Kobayashi T, et al. Surgical strategy for spinal metastases. Spine 2001;26: 298–306.
15. Tokuhashi Y, Matsuzaki H, Oda H, et al. A revised scoring system for preoperative evaluation of metastatic spine tumor prognosis. Spine 2005;30:2186–2191.
16. Chow EK, Harris LE, Fung K. Successful validation of a survival prediction model in patients with metastases in the spinal column. Int J Radiat Oncol Biol Phys 2006;65:1522–1527.
17. van der Linden YM, Dijkstra SP, York EJ, et al. Prediction of survival in patients with metastases in the spinal column: results based on a randomized trial of radiotherapy. Cancer 2005;103: 320–328.

Image-Guided Intensity-Modulated Radiotherapy for Spinal Tumors: A Review

6

Yoshiya Yamada, D. Michael Lovelock, and Mark H. Bilsky

INTRODUCTION

Recent technologic innovations have the potential to make significant improvements in patient outcomes for those treated with radiation therapy. These new technologies include miniature linear accelerators mounted on a robotic arm (Cyberknife, Accuray, Sunnyvale, CA) or mounted in a ring gantry (TomoTherapy, Inc., Madison, WI), as well as improvements and modifications of more traditional gantry-based linear accelerators using gantry-based kilovoltage imaging systems such as the Novalis (Brainlab, Westchester, IL) or cone beam–capable machines such as Synergy (Elekta, Stockholm, Sweden) or Trilogy (Varian Medical Systems, Palo Alto, CA). These technologies all allow the accurate delivery of highly conformal high-dose radiation, by providing a reliable platform to give very high radiation near sensitive structures such as the spinal cord. The improved outcomes that are demonstrated with these technologies are starting to change the traditional treatment paradigm of spinal tumors.

A multidisciplinary approach to spine tumors is important to provide the optimal treatment approach. Systemic therapy, radiation therapy, and surgical interventions, on their own, often result in less than satisfactory outcomes for spine tumors. Surgical resections are often limited by adjacent normal structures, such as the dura. Also, patients with metastatic disease may not be able to tolerate aggressive surgery of the spine. A recently reported randomized trial found significant benefit with the use of surgical resection with conventional radiation therapy compared with conventional radiation alone for high-grade epidural spinal cord compression (1). However, for patients who do not have high-grade epidural cord compression, or who do not have other indications for surgery, management remains controversial. Although many important recent advances in systemic therapy have been demonstrated, systemic therapy for bony metastases is often is less effective than that in soft tissues.

Conventional radiotherapy has been used for many years in the management of spine metastases, with less than ideal results (30% to 50% durable control) (2). One important limitation is the dose, which must be limited to respect spinal cord tolerances. It is delivered by using a shaped photon beam produced by a linear accelerator mounted on a gantry, with a limited number of radiation beams (typically two beams that oppose each other from the anterior and posterior directions). The gantry rotates about the patient in a transverse plane, allowing the gantry angles to be chosen such that the beam passes through the target volume while avoiding critical structures. A structure such as the spinal cord is very difficult to avoid with radiation beams, because of its proximity to spinal tumors and its central location. Multiple beams from different directions may be used in an effort to miss the spinal cord; however, all beams must strike the target. It is difficult to miss the spinal cord without also underdosing part of a nearby tumor (3).

Although each beam deposits dose within the patient from its entry to its exit on the opposite side of the patient, the doses combine only within the volume of the target where the beams overlap. In regions of the body away from the target, the dose is much lower. Thus it is possible to deliver tumoricidal doses to the target while keeping doses to other structures no greater than one seventh of the target dose in an equally weighted seven-beam non-coplanar plan, for example.

INTENSITY-MODULATED RADIATION THERAPY

An important development in radiation therapy was the introduction of the multileaf collimator (MLC). It consists of pairs of opposing tungsten fingers, or leaves, and resides in the head of the treatment machine. The position of each leaf can be set such that the gap between the opposing leaves can be adjusted, both in width and position, anywhere within the radiation field of the machine. An MLC is equipped with up to 60 opposing leaf pairs. The width of each leaf, depending on the manufacturer, varies from 1 to 3 mm. The use of an MLC allows each field to be set up automatically with greater speed and better geometric accuracy than the custom collimators or blocks.

The most important consequence of multileaf collimation, however, is that it has enabled intensity-modulated radiation therapy (IMRT). This is one of the most significant advances in the field of radiation oncology in the past 20 years. By sliding in and out of an active radiation beam, a portion of the radiation field can be modified or modulated in intensity. Thus the MLC can be used to vary the integrated intensity of the photon beam as a function of position within the aperture. The result of multiple intensity-modulated beams is a cloud of radiation that conforms tightly to the three-dimensional (3D) characteristics of the target volume (Fig. 6.1)

The goal of highly conformal radiation therapy is to deliver a tumoricidal dose to the target while minimizing the dose to normal tissues. IMRT, when used in conjunction with a software tool known as inverse treatment planning, provides an approach through which this goal can best be achieved. With this approach, the 3D volumes of the target and critical structures are first defined by manually delineating them in a computed tomography (CT) scan. Further information on target extent may come from positron emission tomography (PET) or magnetic resonance imaging (MRI) scans, which can be fused with the CT scan.

Another important component of IMRT is the use of inverse treatment planning. Inverse treatment planning differs from the above by starting with the final dose distribution and working backward toward the intensities for each beam. Specific dose constraints are assigned to organs and volumes of interest. Such constraints may include specifying a minimal dose to the target and a minimal dose uniformity within the target. Doses to normal structures are constrained by limiting the maximal dose within these structures to acceptable levels. The inverse-planning algorithm is then run to find the intensity distributions for each beam, such that the sum of the distributions from each modulated beam best satisfies the specified constraints. For the treatment of paraspinal

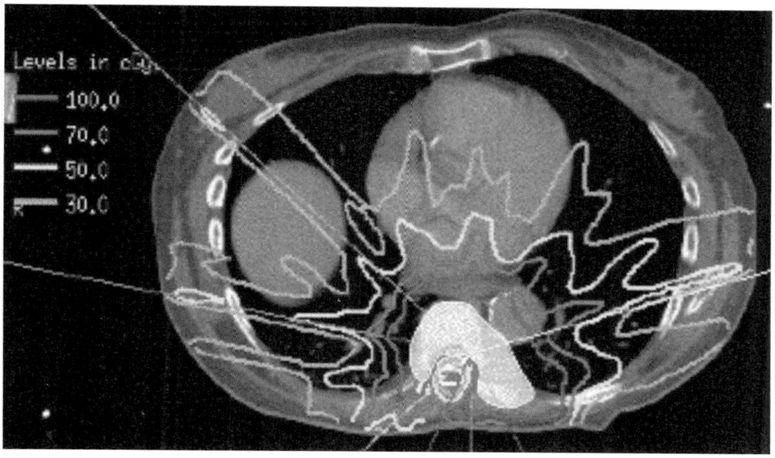

FIGURE 6.1 Highly conformal IMRT plan with sparing of the spinal cord. A myelogram was performed to identify the spinal cord.

disease, such optimized distributions may partially or completely wrap the spinal cord, while featuring steep dose gradients to allow maximal coverage of target near to the spinal cord, while keeping the cord dose below a safe limit.

Typically, with the use of IMRT, a sharp dose gradient of approximately 10% per millimeter can be achieved near the spinal cord (4). Thus if the spinal cord were even 2 to 3 mm from the edge of the target volume, 7,000 cGy could be delivered, whereas the maximum dose to the cord surface would be less than 5,000 cGy.

A technique called "dose painting" can be used in IMRT plans to provide higher doses of radiation to volumes with the highest population of tumor cells, while simultaneously giving areas less likely to harbor tumor cells a lower dose, matching radiation doses with biologic characteristics of the target volume. For example, a higher dose of radiation can be given to the target volume with gross disease (gross tumor volume or GTV), while a lower dose can be prescribed to the volume that may include microscopic disease (clinical target volume or CTV). Dose painting can be a useful technique to spare excessive dose to nearby critical structures.

IMMOBILIZATION

The tumor (and the patient) must remain stationary in the correct position throughout dose delivery. The techniques used can be grouped into two approaches. In the first, the patient is immobilized in a stereotactic body frame or immobilization cradle. In a study of patients treated with IG-IMRT, patient-positioning errors were measured after positioning patients into a customized noninvasive cradle. Up to 7 mm of positioning error was detected in 30 patients repositioned at least 10 different times. However, once image-guided corrections were performed with immobilized patients, an analysis of 650 images, the standard deviations, as determined by the imaging procedure, were 1.3 mm, 1.6 mm, and 2.1 mm in the anterior/posterior (ant/post), right/left, and superior/inferior directions. Immobilization was assessed by measuring patient shifts between localization images taken before and after treatment. From 67 ant/post image pairs and 49 lateral image pairs, the standard deviations were found to be less than 1 mm in all directions (5). It appears that once the necessary corrections in positioning are made, the spine can be reliably immobilized in the correct position for the duration of treatment to within ±1 mm of error. Stereoscopic infrared cameras are also used to track reflective markers attached to the patient to provide continuous monitoring while the beam is on. Less than 2 mm of variation is the norm.

A second approach is used when localization images can be taken frequently during the treatment without greatly lengthening the procedure. It is especially suited to procedures in which dual in-room kV units are available. The patient can be set up conventionally on the treatment-machine couch without additional immobilization. The positions of the bony structures are checked many times during treatment; thus any shifts in position can be detected and quickly corrected.

IMAGE-GUIDED PATIENT SETUP

Precise positioning of spinal targets can be accomplished by using an image-guided patient setup. Pretreatment localization images of the target are acquired just before treatment. These are registered with corresponding reference images to determine any setup error. These errors are then corrected, usually by making small translations to the treatment-machine couch. The traditional image-guided technique has been to use the megavoltage treatment beam to take an image of the bony anatomy. Potential problems of this approach include poor definition of the bony structures in the MV localization images, especially in larger patients. Gold fiducial markers that can be seen clearly in the localization images are often implanted into the spine to improve the registration accuracy. The reference image itself may also have relatively poor spatial resolution in the cranial–caudal direction. This can arise because it is constructed from the planning CT, which may have poor longitudinal resolution because of slice spacing.

Recent innovations in image guidance have greatly improved the bone and even soft tissues visualization of the patient in the treatment position. Most of the new techniques involve the use of kilovoltage imaging. One approach uses two or more kV sources mounted in the room. Radiographs with superior contrast resolution can be acquired and registered to correct rapidly any patient-setup errors. In another method, the kV source is mounted to the gantry of the treatment machine. Orthogonal localization radiographs of the patient are acquired by rotating the gantry to the appropriate angles. An important development is the ability to acquire volumetric pretreatment images. A volumetric or 3D image contains much more information than simple orthogonal 2D projection images. This allows any rotational errors of the patient setup to be readily detected, and it also makes robust automatic-registration procedures possible. Specialized treatment machines such as the Tomotherapy machine, and machines in which a CT scanner has been integrated into the treatment machine, have ben developed to acquire such images (Trilogy or Synergy). Cone-beam CT (CBCT) imaging is a new volumetric imaging technique that uses a gantry-mounted kV source and detector; thus it can readily be added to existing treatment machines. By making a full gantry rotation, the kV system acquires several hundred projection images. These are converted to CT-like axial slices in a process similar to the reconstruction used by conventional CT scanners. CB scans provide very high spatial resolution of bony structures. This will make possible the setup of paraspinal sites with submillimeter targeting errors.

IMAGE-GUIDED IMRT

In conventional radiation therapy, to account for potential treatment-related errors, a margin of extra tissue around the target must also be irradiated to therapeutic levels to ensure that the full dose of radiation is received by the target volume. This volume is referred to as the planning target volume (PTV) (6). These margins have typically been 1 to 2 cm or greater. A major disadvantage of large margins is that a much larger volume of normal tissue will be irradiated, and it is more likely that nearby normal tissues will receive a higher dose of radiation. This may lead to a higher level of toxicity and may ultimately limit the amount of radiation that can be safely delivered. This has significant implications for spinal tumors. Although the spine is relatively stable with respirations when proper immobilization is used, because relatively sensitive structures such as the spinal cord, esophagus, kidneys, and bowel are often in the immediate vicinity, reducing geometric errors is critical. A difference of 2 mm could make the difference in an acceptable maximal cord dose because a 20% dose differential could be realized. The advent of modern image-guided technology has allowed extremely accurate treatment by eliminating or greatly reducing setup errors to within 2 mm (5), allowing smaller margins around the target volume without sacrificing the probability of tumor control.

Real-time verification is critical when delivering high doses of radiation near the spinal cord. This is performed on patients already positioned and set up for actual treatment on the treatment couch. Images of each treatment field can be taken in the "beam's eye view" (the appearance of a particular radiation field through the isocenter taken from a particular beam's angle and compared with computer-generated images) and compared with actual images taken of the patient at the appropriate beam angle. The images can be evaluated manually or with automated algorithms to determine whether any corrections in the positioning will be necessary. The goal is to have the patient positioned for treatment in exactly the same position as the simulation body position and may involve X, Y, or Z shifts to match the expected position. This is because the simulation position was the one used for treatment planning and is the basis of the treatment plan. If the positioning does not exactly match the planning position, it is probable that radiation will be given to some structures in higher doses than intended or that critical volumes will be irradiated to lesser doses than intended. Real-time image-guided verification significantly reduces uncertainties associated with radiation therapy, allowing greater confidence that radiation is being administered to the patient in the exact manner as it was virtually planned inside a computer. With this improved precision, treatment margins can be reduced to within 2 mm without worry that the target may be missed (5). It will also reduce the volume of normal tissues exposed to high doses of radiation. High doses of radiation (either in absolute dose or in biologic effect with hypofractionation) can be administered with a high level of confidence that it is actually being delivered to the patient as intended. Based on the dose-relation paradigm, this should result in less toxicity and higher rates of tumor control.

SPINAL CORD TOLERANCE

The risk of radiation-induced myelopathy is thought to be a dose-dependent phenomenon. In the past, physicians have hesitated to give high-dose radiation to lesions near the spinal cord. The exact nature of spinal cord tolerance to radiotherapy has not been well elucidated. Nonetheless, it is generally accepted that a dose of less than 45 to 50 Gy in standard fractionation (180 to 200 cGy per fraction) is well within the radiation tolerance, given less than a 5% probability of myelopathy within 5 years (TD5/5). Some have suggested that the TD5/5 of the spinal cord is actually in the range of 60 Gy. Mixed photon and proton-beam radiation given at the Northeast Proton Center has reported acceptable toxicity giving up to 60 Gy to the surface of the cord and 56 Gy to the center of the cord (7).

The tolerance of the spinal cord to single-fraction radiation is unknown. Hemibody radiation for widely metastatic patients has been given up to 8 Gy in a single fraction to a very large field that included spinal cord and has been given to large numbers of patients without reported myelopathy (8). However, these patients typically had aggressive systemic disease, and survival was not expected to be high. Therefore follow-up may not be sufficiently long to appreciate myelopathy fully, which has traditionally been conceptualized has a late-occurring toxicity of radiotherapy. The MSKCC group has accepted 12 to 14 Gy to a point dose as a maximum dose to the spinal cord, as defined on myelogram. Gerszten et al. (9) have prescribed up to 20 Gy as a maximum dose to the spinal cord. Neither group has reported radiation myelitis. Because of the potential devastating effects of radiation myelitis, caution is always recommended when giving large doses of radiation near the spinal cord. The ALARA principle (as low as reasonably allowable) (10) has been the general approach to spinal cord dose. Therefore outcomes of spinal tumors have been suboptimal, except for radiosensitive histologies, such as lymphoma or myeloma, in which case, doses lower than cord tolerance typically result in relatively rapid and satisfactory outcomes.

INDICATIONS FOR IG-IMRT

The decision framework used at MSKCC to assess all patients with spine tumors includes neurologic (N), oncologic (O), mechanical stability (M), and systemic disease and comorbidities (S), referred to by the acronym NOMS. IMRT has not altered our surgical indications but has significantly improved local tumor control (O) for metastatic and primary tumors, both for operated-on and unoperated-on patients. The two primary indications for operation are high-grade epidural spinal cord compression (ESCC) with or without myelopathy (N) from radioresistant tumors (O) and mechanical instability (M) (11). In a patient population with metastases, patients with high-grade ESCC from radioresistant tumors often show progressive myelopathy after treatment with conventional external-beam radiation therapy. This was recently confirmed by Patchell et al. (1) in a prospective randomized trial comparing surgery and conventional radiation therapy with conventional radiation alone. The surgical arm showed significantly improved rates of maintenance and recovery of ambulation and survival compared with the RT group. Unfortunately, IG-IMRT is not an effective solution to radioresistant tumors causing high-grade spinal cord compression, because the marginal dose at the spinal cord would have to be reduced to avoid toxicity. This would potentially underdose the tumor at the spinal cord margin, where one theoretically requires the greatest tumor control. Additionally, tumors responsive to IG-IMRT do not acutely show a significant reduction in tumor volume creating ongoing spinal cord compression. For these reasons, patients with high-grade ESCC with radioresistant tumors undergo surgery before IG-IMRT.

The second strong surgical indication is mechanical spine instability (M). No amount of radiation will stabilize an unstable spine. Instability is broadly defined as movement-related pain. Instability pain is defined by the spinal level with radiographic correlates. For example, thoracic instability pain is typically pain on extension of the spine, such as lying flat in bed, which straightens the thoracic kyphosis. Radiographically, these patients often have a pathologic burst or compression fracture, with extension into a unilateral joint. Unstable spines require surgery for decompression and stabilization.

Instability pain must be distinguished from biologic pain. Biologic pain is night or morning pain that is seemingly related to the diurnal variation in endogenous steroids and is often sensitive to exogenous steroid administration. Instability pain is defined by the spinal level with radiographic correlates.

Although patients with high-grade ESCC (N) from radioresistant tumors (O) and mechanical instability (M) require surgery, local tumor control is dependent on effective adjuvant therapy. High-dose IMRT made possible with image-guided technology gives an improved measure of tumor control compared with standard external-beam radiation therapy for radioresistant tumors, such as renal cell carcinoma, melanoma, chordoma, and chondrosarcoma. IG-IMRT is effective for patients as initial therapy or postoperatively in patients with surgical indications. Because of the ability to give high-dose radiation and spare the spinal cord, this technology can also be applied to recurrent tumors after failed prior external-beam radiation to the spinal cord.

IG-IMRT AT MSKCC

At MSKCC, the use of IG-IMRT has been applied to three treatment paradigms to assess safety and efficacy. Single-fraction therapy, 18 to 24 Gy, has been used principally for radioresistant metastatic tumors in patients with oligometastatic disease who have not been previously irradiated. Hypofractionated radiation (20 Gy in four to five fractions) has been used to retreat recurrent metastatic tumors after failed conventional external-beam radiation treatment. Standard fraction therapy (66 Gy in 37 fractions) has been used to treat primary spinal tumors, such as chordoma and chondrosarcoma, in accordance with proton-beam doses delivered for similar histologies (12). Regardless of the fractionation scheme, IG-IMRT provides the ability to deliver potentially tumoricidal doses to the tumor while sparing spinal cord tolerance.

Based on this paradigm, hypofractionated and single-fraction IMRT was first performed at MSKCC by using a noninvasive step-in immobilization cradle with stereotactic localization. Lesions were registered to stereotactic coordinates based on localization rods imbedded into the frame (13). It became apparent that despite the use of stereotactic localization, a final portal image-guided check was essential, as setup errors greater than 2 mm were commonly encountered. Errors of this magnitude are unacceptable because of the extremely close proximity of the spinal cord in most spinal and paraspinal lesions. An error greater than even 2 mm could very well result in overdosing the cord by more than 20% or underdosing the tumor or both. Therefore a completely imaged-guided system was incorporated, which no longer used localization rods. Initially, image-guided techniques were based on megavoltage portal imaging. Improvements in technology, such as digital portal imaging, and more recently kV imaging, infrared tracking, and 3D cone-beam CT have greatly facilitated this process. kV imaging offers a much more detailed image, particularly in the bone. 3D cone-beam CT is performed with the kV imager rotated 360 degrees around the patient by using the kV unit mounted on the gantry of the linear accelerator. This allows real-time verification of the isocenter by using a 3D dataset, which can be automatically registered with the treatment-planning CT image set, which represents the gold-standard imaging in terms of setup and positioning. The advantage of cone-beam CT is that it is able to provide positioning data of lesions without the use of marker seeds, especially in the soft tissues, where 2D fluoroscopic imaging is unable to identify lesions unless markers are placed. Therefore 3D imaging is less critical for paraspinal lesions. However, without 3D datasets, rotational errors may be very difficult to appreciate with 2D images.

Single-fraction IG-IMRT provides significant patient and oncologic benefits in terms of convenience and potentially returning patients to systemic therapy more quickly, compared with standard conventional external beam delivered in 10 to 15 fractions. More important, IG-IMRT appears to provide significantly better local tumor control compared with conventional-dose radiation, particularly for radioresistant tumors, such as melanoma, renal cell, lung, and colon carcinomas. In a recently reported case series from MSKCC, 45 nonsurgical patients were treated with IG-IMRT for radioresistant tumors (14). The median tumoral dose to the planning target volume was 21 Gy, with a range of 18 to 24 Gy. The maximum spinal cord dose was 12 Gy, and cord average was 4 Gy. Three (8.7%) patients had local tumor failure with recurrence of symptoms, 11 (27%) patients died of disease, and 31 (67%) patients were alive with no evidence of disease. At a median 7-month follow-up, no patient experienced myelopathy, radiculopathy, or plexopathy. Gerszten et al. (15) treated numerous patients with single-fraction therapy with similar tumor control and limited toxicity.

Recurrent spine tumors after standard external-beam radiation have posed a significant clinical problem, because the therapeutic options for local tumor control are limited. Tumors that recur, causing high-grade spinal cord compression, can be reoperated on, but the probability of achieving tumor control without meaningful adjuvant therapy is negligible. Many of these tumors will recur within a month or two of a major decompressive operation. The ability to decompress and safely reirradiate spinal cord lesions has given us the ability to control local tumor and thus maintain ambulation, bowel, and bladder, as well as biologic pain, for a prolonged period. In a review of 29 patients retreated with radiation to doses of 20 Gy in four or five fractions, 54% had durable tumor control at a median follow-up of 6.5 months (16). Twenty-four (92%) patients reported no pain or improved pain after treatment, and 19 (73%) patients had stable or improved performance status. No long-term toxicity has been observed to date.

Standard fraction sizes (1.8 to 2.0 Gy), to a total dose of 66 to 70 Gy and higher, have been used for primary radioresistant spine tumors, such as chordoma and chondrosarcoma, with proton-beam radiation (4,17). The question is whether proton-beam range dosing could safely be delivered by using IG-IMRT. The advantage of IG-IMRT may principally be one of availability, as a limited number of proton-beam facilities are in the United States.

SUMMARY

More than 175 patients have undergone spine IG-IMRT at MSKCC during the past 4 years without significant toxicity, including no myelopathy or radiculopathy. These patients appear to have excellent local control of treated disease. Although only half of the patients who have had repeated radiotherapy enjoyed durable local control, these patients had no other treatment options and would otherwise likely all have experienced local progression of disease. Dose escalation is currently ongoing in this cohort of patients.

Paraspinal IG-IMRT is proof of principle of the benefits of this paradigm of improved accuracy and treatment delivery of high-dose radiotherapy despite the presence of nearby spinal cord. Patients have experienced higher-than-expected rates of local control and durable palliation of symptoms. With image-guided techniques, setup errors have been minimized to allow the safe treatment of these otherwise clinically difficult tumors without an increased risk of significant toxicity. IG-IMRT therefore potentially represents an important new tool for the treatment of spinal tumors. As clinical experience matures, further refinements in technique and technology will allow dose escalation and continued improvements in outcomes.

REFERENCES

1. Patchell RA, Regine WF, Payne R, et al. Direct decompressive surgical resection in the treatment of spinal cord compression caused by metastatic cancer: a randomized trial. Lancet 2005;366: 643–68.
2. Katagiri H, Takahashi M, Inagaki J, et al. Clinical results of nonsurgical treatment for spinal metastases. Int J Radiat Oncol Biol Phys 1998;42:1127–1132.
3. Nutting CM, Cosgrove VP, Rowbottom C, et al. Improvements in target coverage and reduced spinal cord irradiation using intensity-modulated radiotherapy (IMRT) in patients with carcinoma of the thyroid gland. Radiother Oncol 2001;60:173–180.
4. Yamada Y, Lovelock DM, Yenice KM, et al. Multifractionated image-guided and stereotactic intensity-modulated radiotherapy of paraspinal tumors: a preliminary report. Int J Radiat Oncol Biol Phys 2005:62: 53–61.
5. Lovelock DM, Hua C, Wang P, et al. Accurate setup of paraspinal patients using a noninvasive patient immobilization cradle and portal imaging. Med Phys 2005;32:2606–2614.
6. ICRU 50. Prescribing, recording, and reporting photon beam therapy. Int Comm Radiat Units Measure 1993; 1–72.
7. Weber DC, Trofimov AV, Delaney TF, et al. A treatment planning comparison of intensity modulated photon and proton therapy for paraspinal sarcomas. Int J Radiat Oncol Biol Phys 2004;58:1596–1606.
8. Tong DGL, Hendrickson FR. The palliation of symptomatic osseous metastases: final results of the study by the Radiation Therapy Oncology Group. Cancer 1982;50:893–899.
9. Gerszten PC, Burton SA, Ozhasoglu C, et al. Stereotactic radiosurgery for spinal metastases from renal cell carcinoma. J Neurosurg Spine 2005;3:288–295.
10. Radiation Safety Committee, O.O.H.A.S. Radiation safety manual, U.D.O.H.A.H. services. Editor. 1999, Centers for Disease Control.
11. Bilsky MH, Lis E, Raizer J, et al. The diagnosis and treatment of metastatic spinal tumor. Oncologist 1999;4:459–469.
12. Noel G, Jarffret E, Crevoisier RD, et al. Radiation therapy for chordoma and chondrosarcoma of the skull base and the cervical spine: prognostic factors and patterns of failure. Strahlenther Onkol 2003;179:241–248.
13. Yenice KM, Lovelock DM, et al. CT image-guided intensity-modulated therapy for paraspinal tumors using stereotactic immobilization. Int J Radiat Oncol Biol Phys 2003;55:583–593.
14. Yamada Y, Bilsky LD, Zatcky MH, et al. Single fraction image guided intensity modulated radiotherapy (IG IMRT) for metastatic lesions of the spinal column. Int J Radiat Biol 2005;63:S155.
15. Gerszten PC, Welch WC. Cyberknife radiosurgery for metastatic spine tumors. Neurosurg Clin North Am 2004;15:491–501.
16. Wright JL, Lovelock DM, Bilsky MH, et al. Clinical outcomes after repeat irradiation of paraspinal tumors. Am J Clin Oncol 29(5): 495–502.
17. Hug E, Slater J Proton radiation therapy for chordomas and chondrosarcomas of the skull base. Neurosurg Clin North Am 2000;11:627–638.

Place of Bisphosphonates in Spinal Metastases

Jean-Jacques Body

7

CLINICAL CONSEQUENCES AND PATHOGENESIS OF BONE METASTASES: A BRIEF OVERVIEW

The skeleton is the most common site of metastatic disease in breast and prostate cancers, and tumor-induced bone destruction can complicate any neoplasm. The clinical consequences of cancer-mediated bone destruction are a source of misery for these patients. The term "skeletal-related events" (SREs) refers to the major complications of tumor bone disease: pathologic fractures, need for radiotherapy, need for bone surgery, spinal cord compression, and hypercalcemia. Across all tumor types, patients with breast cancer have the highest incidence of skeletal complications. Major complications will be observed in up to one third of patients whose first relapse is in bone (1,2). Taken from data in placebo groups of randomized bisphosphonates trials, the mean skeletal morbidity rate in breast cancer (i.e., the mean number of SREs per year) varies between 2.2 and 4.0 and is around 1.5 in advanced prostate cancer (2,3).

Bone destruction due to metastatic infiltration is essentially mediated by the osteoclasts. The propensity of cancer cells to proliferate in bone is best explained by a "seed and soil" concept (4). Breast cancer cells (the "seed") appear to secrete factors, such as parathyroid hormone–related protein (PTHrP), potentiating the development of metastases in the skeleton, which constitutes a fertile "soil" rich in cytokines and growth factors that stimulate cancer cells growth. Local production of PTHrP and of other osteolytic factors by cancer cells in bone stimulate osteoclastic bone resorption, essentially through the osteoblasts. Tumor factors thus alter the ratio between osteoprotegerin (OPG), whose production is decreased, and RANK ligand (receptor activator of NF-κB ligand), whose production is increased (5). The net result of such imbalance in these key regulatory factors of bone resorption is an increase in osteoclast proliferation and activity. In prostate cancer, histomorphometric analyses of bone biopsies and studies on biochemical markers of bone turnover demonstrated that enhanced bone formation in osteosclerotic lesions is accompanied by a marked increase in osteoclast-mediated bone resorption. These considerations explain why bisphosphonates have been so extensively used in oncology. These compounds are indeed able to interrupt the vicious circle between cancer cells, bone cells, and bone matrix by inducing osteoclast apoptosis. They also exert direct antitumoral effects whose clinical relevance remains unknown.

BISPHOSPHONATES FOR THE COMPLICATIONS OF TUMOR BONE DISEASE

Tumor-induced hypercalcemia was the first successful therapeutic application of bisphosphonates. Cancer hypercalcemia can now be successfully treated in at least 90% of the cases by rehydration and bisphosphonates (6).

Pain is the most frequent symptom of bone metastases. Bisphosphonates are useful co-analgesics for the treatment of moderate to severe metastatic bone pain. The current opinion is that the intravenous route has to be selected for the treatment of bone pain, but placebo-controlled trials have shown that all bisphosphonates can exert analgesic effects, whether they are given orally or intravenously. The analgesic effect of bisphosphonates in prostate cancer appears to be less than that in advanced breast cancer (3). The administration of a high "loading" dose of the bisphosphonate ibandronate could be especially useful in patients with severe bone pain, but this new concept must be further tested (7). Pain is now viewed more as a subjective SRE in long-term bisphosphonate trials, and the marked decrease in radiotherapy needs in these trials is a surrogate marker for clinically significant pain relief.

Placebo-controlled trials with oral or intravenous bisphosphonates have shown that their prolonged administration can reduce the frequency of SREs in patients with bone metastases from breast cancer (3). For patients with metastatic breast cancer demonstrated on plain films, computed tomography (CT) or magnetic resonance imaging (MRI), it is generally recommended to start bisphosphonates before the first bone complication occurs. Placebo-controlled trials have established that, when administered over a prolonged period by the oral route (clodronate and ibandronate) or by the intravenous route (pamidronate, ibandronate, and zoledronic acid), bisphosphonates reduce the skeletal morbidity rate by 25% to 40% in patients with breast cancer metastatic to the skeleton. Clodronate is now viewed as less effective than other bisphosphonates for the prevention of SREs. It has been shown in a large-scale controlled 2-year comparative trial between pamidronate and zoledronic acid that this latter compound has a superior efficacy, as the likelihood of getting an event during therapy is reduced by 20% in breast cancer, according to a multiple event analysis (8,9) (Fig. 7.1, upper panel). Zoledronic acid is also more convenient to administer than pamidronate (15-min vs. 2-hr infusion). However, zoledronic acid is not more efficient than pamidronate in myeloma patients (Fig. 7.1, upper panel). Importantly, the dose of 8 mg of zoledronic acid is not more effective than the 4-mg dose level, which probably indicates that we have reached the maximal efficacy of bisphosphonates in that setting. Rare cases of renal insufficiency have been reported in patients receiving zoledronic acid therapy. This has led to the recommendation that serum creatinine, and more recently creatinine clearance, be checked before each zoledronic acid infusion to adjust the dose. Conversely, ibandronate is well tolerated and, in phase III trials, this compound had a renal-safety profile similar to that of placebo. Repeated 6-mg monthly ibandronate infusions or oral ibandronate, 50 mg once daily, also constitute efficient strategies to reduce the morbidity rate of bone metastases from breast cancer (10,11). Multiple event analysis showed that oral or intravenous ibandronate led to a statistically significant 38% to 40% reduction in the risk of SREs compared with placebo, which appears to be comparable to the effect of zoledronic acid (Fig. 7.1, middle and lower panels) (9).

In prostate cancer, monthly zoledronic acid infusions have been shown to reduce the skeletal morbidity rate by about one third in patients with hormone-refractory disease (12) (Fig. 7.1, middle panel). The efficacy of other bisphosphonates has not been demonstrated in that setting and no proof exists that bisphosphonates are useful in prostate cancer

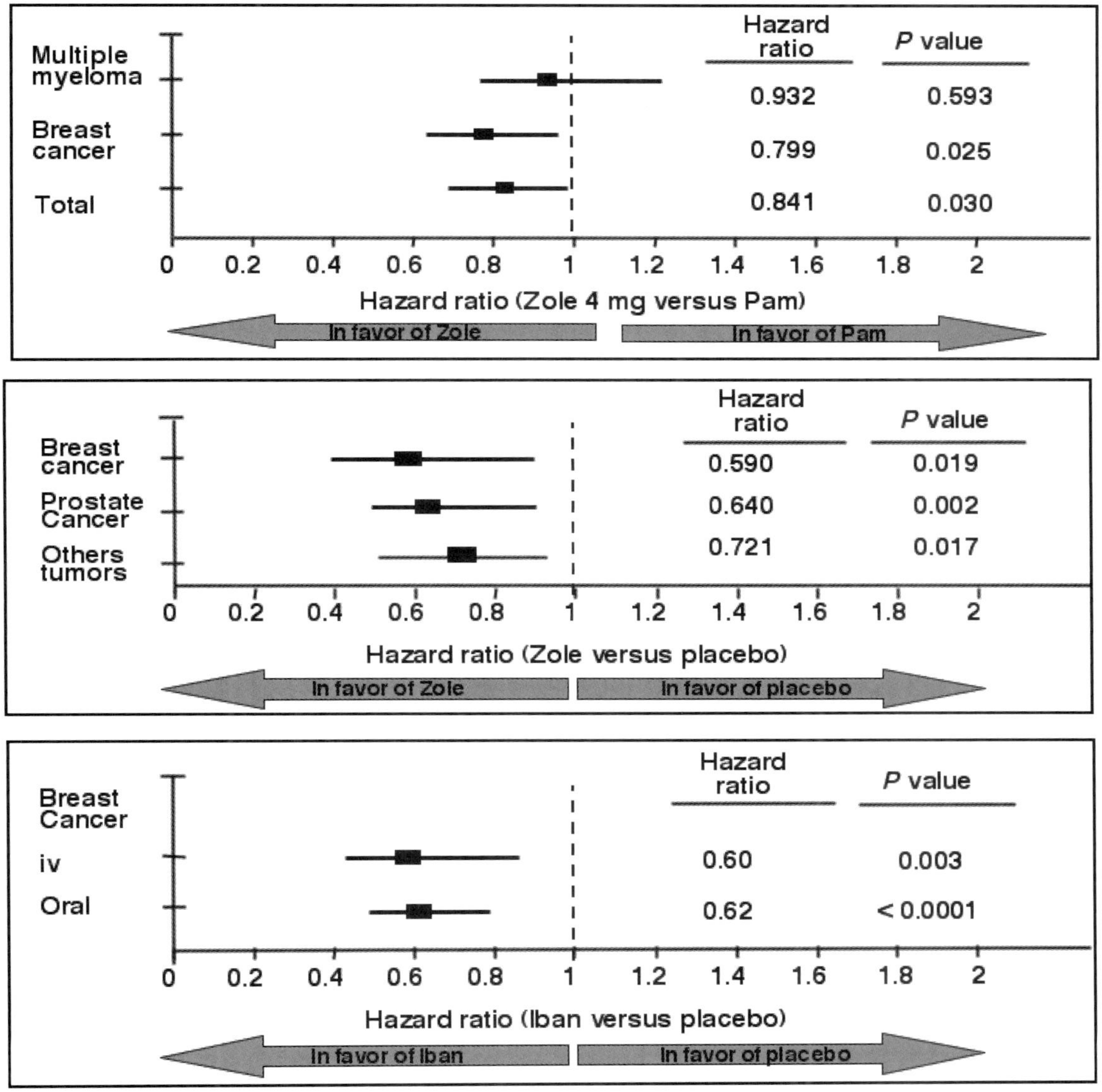

FIGURE 7.1 Effects of long-term therapy with bisphosphonates on the risk of developing a skeletal complication in patients with bone metastases. Data are summarized by multiple-event analyses (Andersen–Gill model for zoledronic acid and Poisson regression analysis for ibandronate). Hazard ratios (and 95% CI) are shown in the left part of each graph with corresponding *p* values indicated in the right parts. (Reproduced from Body JJ. Treatment and prevention of bone metastases and myeloma bone disease. In: Favus MJ, ed. Primer on the Metabolic Bone Diseases and Disorders of Mineral Metabolism, 6th ed. Washington: The American Society for Bone and Mineral Research, 2006:383–90, with permission.)

patients who are still sensitive to hormone manipulations. Zoledronic acid is also useful in patients with other solid tumors (Fig. 7.1, middle panel).

Recently, osteonecrosis of the jaw (ONJ) was reported to occur with prolonged bisphosphonate therapy, even if the exact pathogenesis requires further investigation (13). The prevalence of ONJ in cancer patients receiving bisphosphonate therapy appears to lie between 1% and 10% and is higher in myeloma patients than in patients with solid tumors. A greater risk may occur with zoledronic acid than with pamidronate that ONJ will develop sooner. Bisphosphonate-associated ONJ notably results from marked suppression of bone turnover, leading to accumulation of physiologic microdamage in the jawbones and compromising biomechanical properties. The antiangiogenic property of bisphosphonates and other medications and the presence of other comorbid factors may increase the risk. Length of exposure to bisphosphonates seems to be an essential risk factor for ONJ, and caution is required for use beyond 2 years. Clinicians must be vigilant and able to detect subtle changes that can precede ONJ, such as changes in the health of periodontal tissues, nonhealing mucosal ulcers, loose teeth, and unexplained soft tissue infection. Before commencing treatment with bisphosphonates in cancer patients, it is recommended that patients be seen by a dentist, and any oral disease should be stabilized (14).

BISPHOSPHONATES FOR SPINAL METASTASES

No specific trials exist for patients with vertebral metastases, and the effects of bisphosphonates on pathologic vertebral fractures rate are furthermore confounded by the efficacy of bisphosphonates to prevent osteoporotic fractures (15,16). Besides menopause, cancer treatment–induced bone loss indeed increases fracture rate (16). Moreover, in some studies, vertebral fractures have not been distinguished from peripheral fractures.

Data taken from placebo-controlled trials are shown in Table 7.1 (17–20). They are expressed as the percentages of patients who had at least one vertebral fracture during the trial. Pamidronate and zoledronic acid reduced the vertebral fracture rate as compared with that in patients receiving placebo infusions, but statistical significance is either not available (zoledronic acid) or not reached (pamidronate). This can be due to methodologic issues related to the number of patients with a fracture or to the lack of

TABLE 7.1 Effects of Bisphosphonates (BP) on Vertebral Fracture Rate —Placebo-controlled Trials

Tumor Type	BP	Nb of pts	Duration, yrs	% of patients BP	% of patients Placebo	P value	Ref
Breast	Pam (+Chemo)	382	2	25	26	NS	17
	Pam (+Horm)	372	2	28	31	NS	18
	Zole	228	1	25*	39*	?	19
Prostate	Zole	422	1	3.7	8.2	0.05	12
Other solid tumors	Zole	507	0.75	8	12	?	20

*No separation between vertebral and nonvertebral fractures

TABLE 7.2 Effects of Bisphosphonates (BP) on Spinal Cord Compression Rate—Placebo-controlled Trials

Tumor Type	BP	Nb of pts	Duration, yrs	Total nb of Events BP	Total nb of Events Placebo	Ref
Breast	Pam (+Ch)	382	2	4	7	17
	Pam (+H)	372	2	7	6	18
	Zole	228	1	4	13	19
Prostate	Zole	422	1	9	14	12
Other solid tumors	Zole	507	0.75	7	10	20

adequate criteria to define pathologic vertebral fractures. Conversely, intravenous ibandronate led to a significant reduction in the vertebral fracture rate (9), but the data were expressed as the "skeletal morbidity period rate" (number of 12-week periods with at least one event), preventing a direct comparison with the data summarized in Table 7.1. In the large controlled trial comparing zoledronic acid with pamidronate in breast cancer (8), the mean number of patients with a new vertebral fracture was similar in both groups (0.23 to 0.24 per year of treatment). In metastatic hormone-refractory prostate cancer, only zoledronic acid has been shown significantly to reduce the vertebral fracture rate (12). In other various solid tumors, mostly non–small cell lung cancers, zoledronic acid also reduced the vertebral fracture rate (Table 7.1).

Spinal cord compression is a classic and often serious complication of spinal metastases (1–3). The effects of prolonged bisphosphonate therapy on the incidence of spinal cord compression have not been systematically investigated. Data shown in Table 7.2 indicate the number of patients who were diagnosed with spinal cord compression during the previously mentioned placebo-controlled bisphosphonate trials. Caution is mandatory because of paucity of the data, but they generally indicate a reduction in the incidence of this dramatic complication under bisphosphonate therapy.

REFERENCES

1. Plunkett TA, Smith P, Rubens RD. Risk of complications from bone metastases in breast cancer: implications for management. Eur J Cancer 36: 476–482, 2000.
2. Body JJ. Metastatic bone disease. In: Seibel MJ, Robins SP, Bilezikian JP, eds. Dynamics of Bone and Cartilage Metabolism, 2nd ed. San Diego: Academic Press, 2006:793–810.
3. Body JJ. Breast cancer: bisphosphonate therapy for metastatic bone disease. Clin Cancer Res 12: 6258–6263, 2006.
4. Kakonen SM, Mundy GR. Mechanisms of osteolytic bone metastases in breast carcinoma. Cancer 97(3 suppl):834–839, 2003.
5. Dunstan CR. Osteoprotegerin and osteoprotegerin ligand mediate the local regulation of bone resorption. Endocrinologist 10:18–26, 2000.
6. Body JJ. Hypercalcemia of malignancy. Semin Nephrol 24:48–54, 2004.
7. Mancini I, Dumon JC, Body JJ. Efficacy and safety of ibandronate in the treatment of opioid-resistant bone pain associated with metastatic bone disease: a pilot study. J Clin Oncol 22:3587–3592, 2004.
8. Rosen LS, Gordon D, Kaminski M, et al. Long-term efficacy and safety of zoledronic acid compared with pamidronate disodium in the treatment of skeletal complications in patients with advanced multiple myeloma or breast carcinoma:

a randomized, double-blind, multicenter, comparative trial. Cancer 98:1735–1744, 2003.

9. Body JJ. Treatment and prevention of bone metastases and myeloma bone disease. In: Favus MJ, ed. Primer on the Metabolic Bone Diseases and Disorders of Mineral Metabolism, 6th ed. Washington: The American Society for Bone and Mineral Research, 2006:383–390.
10. Body JJ, Diel IJ, Lichinitser MR, et al., for the MF 4265 Study Group. Intravenous ibandronate reduces the incidence of skeletal complications in patients with breast cancer and bone metastases. Ann Oncol 14:1399–1405, 2003.
11. Body JJ, Diel IJ, Lichinitzer M, et al. Oral ibandronate reduces the risk of skeletal complications in breast cancer patients with metastatic bone disease: results from two randomized, placebo-controlled phase III studies. Br J Cancer 90: 1133–1137, 2004.
12. Saad F, Gleason DM, Murray R, et al., for the Zoledronic Acid Prostate Cancer Study Group. Zoledronic Acid Prostate Cancer Study Group: a randomized, placebo-controlled trial of zoledronic acid in patients with hormone-refractory metastatic prostate carcinoma. J Natl Cancer Inst 94: 1458–1468, 2002.
13. Woo SB, Hellstein JW, Kalmar JR. Bisphosphonates and osteonecrosis of the jaws. Ann Intern Med 144:753–761, 2006.
14. Migliorati C, Casiglia J, Epstein J, et al. Managing the care of patients with bisphosphonate-associated osteonecrosis. JADA 136:1658–1668, 2005.
15. Hillner BE, Ingle JN, Chlebowski RT et al., American Society of Clinical Oncology. American Society of Clinical Oncology 2003 update on the role of bisphosphonates and bone health issues in women with breast cancer. J Clin Oncol 21:4042–4057, 2003.
16. Body JJ, Bergmann P, Boonen S, et al. Management of cancer treatment-induced bone loss in early breast and prostate cancer: a consensus paper of the Belgian Bone Club. Osteop Int 2007 Aug 10; (Epub ahead of print) PMID 17690930.
17. Hortobagyi GN, Theriault RL, Lipton A, et al., on behalf of the Protocol 19 Aredia Breast Cancer Study Group. Long-term prevention of skeletal complications of metastatic breast cancer with pamidronate. J Clin Oncol 16:2038–2044, 1998.
18. Theriault RL, Lipton A, Hortobagyi GN, et al., on behalf of the Protocol 18 Aredia breast cancer study group. Pamidronate reduces skeletal morbidity in women with advanced breast cancer and lytic bone lesions: a randomized, placebo-controlled trial. J Clin Oncol 17:846–854, 1999.
19. Kohno N, Aogi K, Minami H, et al. Zoledronic acid significantly reduces skeletal complications compared with placebo in Japanese women with bone metastases from breast cancer: a randomized, placebo-controlled trial. J Clin Oncol 23: 3314–3321, 2005.
20. Rosen LS, Gordon D, Tchekmedyian S, et al. Zoledronic acid versus placebo in the treatment of skeletal metastases in patients with lung cancer and other solid tumors: a phase III, double-blind, randomized trial: the Zoledronic Acid Lung Cancer and Other Solid Tumors Study Group. J Clin Oncol 21:3150–3157, 2003.

The Role of Brachytherapy in the Management of Spinal Tumors

8

Yoshiya Yamada

ABSTRACT

Even with the most modern technology, radiation doses for spinal tumors are constrained by the relatively low tolerance of the spinal cord to the radiation. The use of brachytherapy (placing radioactive sources in very close proximity to tumors) has been described. The Inverse Square Law describes how a radiation dose is given from brachytherapy sources. As the distance increases away from the source, the dose fall-off can be described as the inverse square of the distance. Thus when brachytherapy sources are placed strategically in the tumor, the delivered dose to the nearby spinal cord can be much less. When radiation isotopes with low-energy photons, such as yttrium 90, are used, it is possible for the dose on the surface of the source to be 80% higher than a point 3 mm away. Brachytherapy in the spine is an attractive method of improving the therapeutic ratio in the radiotherapy of spine tumors by increasing the total dose delivered to a tumor without significantly increasing the dose delivered to the spinal cord or other nearby dose-sensitive structures.

INTRODUCTION

The goal of radiation therapy is to improve tumor control while minimizing the associated toxicity to normal tissues. The effects of radiation therapy on tumor and normal tissues are dependent on many factors, including the total dose of radiation, the dose per fraction, the radiosensitivity of tumor and normal tissues, and the volume of normal tissue irradiated. Of these factors, radiation dose is most likely the single most important determinant of the probability of both tumor control and normal tissue toxicity.

THE THERAPEUTIC RATIO

Radiation therapy is most effective when a high probability of tumor control and a low probability of normal tissue toxicity exist for any given dose of radiation. When these probabilities are plotted as a function of increasing radiation dose, they are typically described as S-shaped curves (Fig. 8.1). Between the low-dose area and the high-dose plateau, a region of rapid change exists, with a relatively small increase in dose. Ideally, for any given dose, the probability of toxicity should be low compared with the probability of tumor control. This difference is often referred to as the therapeutic ratio (Fig. 8.2)

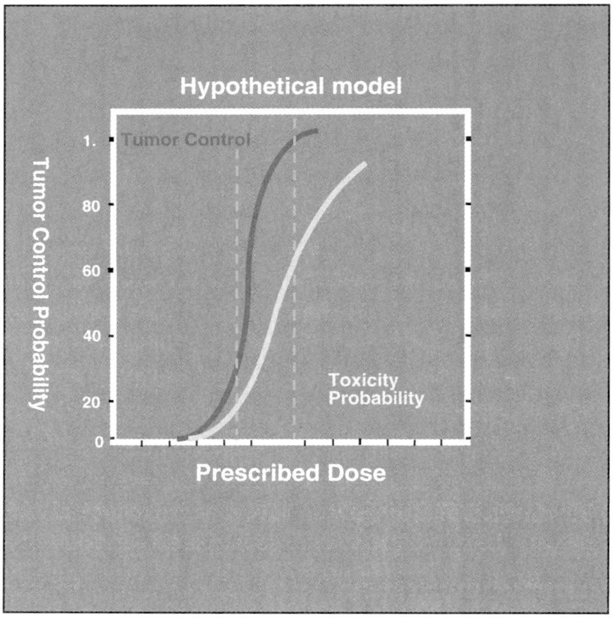

FIGURE 8.1 The therapeutic ratio is small. For a given dose, the difference between tumor control and toxicity probabilities is small.

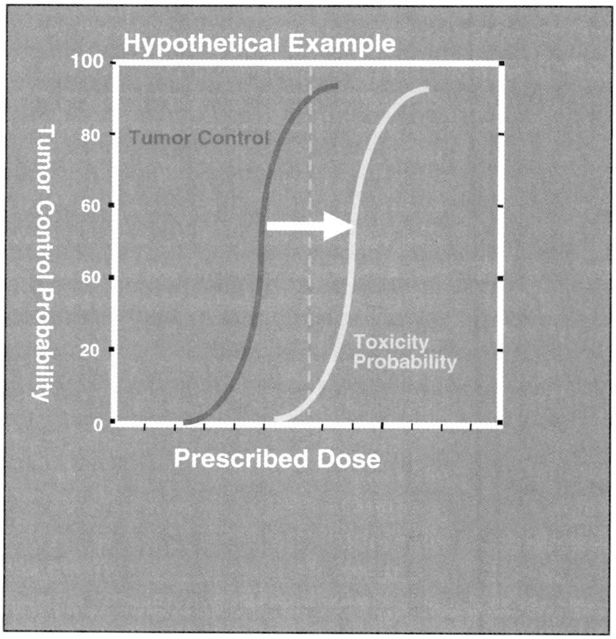

FIGURE 8.2 Idealized therapeutic ratio. The probability of tumor control is high, whereas the toxicity risk is low.

Radiation oncologists are constantly striving to improve the therapeutic ratio. Several commonly used strategies may improve the therapeutic ratio. Altering the dose-fractionation schedule can help improve the therapeutic ratio in many instances. Increasing the dose of radiation given per fraction will increase the biologic impact of radiation therapy. Unfortunately, this phenomenon is true for both normal tissues and tumor. Conversely, reducing the dose per fraction will result in less risk of toxicity but is also more likely to spare tumor cells. When a high dose gradient can be created, in which the tumor receives a significantly higher dose than the surrounding normal tissue, the therapeutic ratio improves.

ADVANTAGES OF BRACHYTHERAPY

Brachytherapy is an ideal way of delivering high doses to the tumor while sparing normal tissues. One of the major advantages of brachytherapy in this regard is that radiation-dose intensity falls off as a function of the square of the distance (1). For example, if a radioactive seed were placed in a tumor, the dose of radiation 2 cm from the source would be one fourth of the dose at 1 cm from the source (1 cm/2 cm)^2. When external-beam radiation is used, the tumor is typically 100 cm from the radiation source. Hence a minimal difference in the dose exists at 100 cm versus 101 cm (100 cm/101 cm)^2. Thus the inverse-square phenomenon is much more significant when brachytherapy is used, because doses for brachytherapy are calculated with relatively short distances. Isotopes that emit very weakly penetrating photons, such as yttrium 90 (2), can also be used in brachytherapy, because the sources are placed directly in the tumor, and the photons need not travel great distances. Thus the inverse-square law coupled with low-energy brachytherapy sources allows very high doses to be delivered to the tumor while allowing relative sparing of nearby and surrounding normal tissues (Fig. 8-3).

Another important advantage of brachytherapy is the lack of treatment error associated with patient positioning and movement. With external-beam radiotherapy, the positioning of the patient and the movement of the tumor during radiation therapy can add uncertainty and error to radiation treatment. Because of this, conventional radiation-treatment planning requires at least 1 to 2 cm of additional margin around a tumor to ensure that the tumor receives the intended dose (3). This extra volume of irradiated

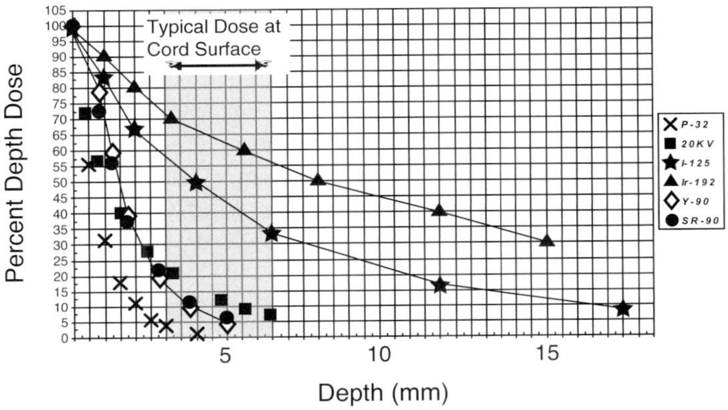

FIGURE 8.3 Percentage dose-depth comparisons of commonly used isotopes in brachytherapy. (Adapted from figure provided by Dr. T. Delaney.)

tissue may result in higher probabilities of toxicity because a greater volume of normal tissue must be treated to full dose. In the setting of spine tumors, in which the spinal cord and other dose-sensitive organs such as the kidneys, bowel, and esophagus are quite near, adding such a large margin may result in an excessive probability of serious radiation damage. When brachytherapy is used, radiation is applied directly to the volume in question, with no need to add extra margins for movement or set-up–related concerns.

One of the most feared complications of radiation therapy is radiation myelitis of the spinal cord. The spinal cord tolerance to radiation has traditionally been quoted to be between 45 and 50 Gy, in standard fractionation (4). This limit severely restricts the dose of radiation that can be given safely when using conventional radiotherapy techniques, as many tumors require significantly higher doses of radiation for a reasonable chance at tumor control. The advantages of brachytherapy make it a natural consideration for the treatment of paraspinal tumors.

REVIEW OF LITERATURE

Iodine 125 (^{125}I) has been the most widely reported isotope used in spinal brachytherapy. ^{125}I seeds are readily available and have been in clinical use for more than 40 years. Gutin et al. (5) reported the use of ^{125}I in 13 patients with recurrent primary axial paraspinal and base-of-skull tumors. All patients had undergone prior radiation therapy and multiple surgical interventions. These seeds were placed either as loose seeds via a Mick (Mick Radionuclear, Mount Vernon, NY) applicator or as seeds embedded in polyglactin suture and glued with biologic adhesive. Seeds were placed into circular or linear arrays by using stereotactic localization. Prescribed doses ranged from 70 to 150 Gy. Chordomas ($n = 5$) and malignant meningiomas ($n = 3$) were the most common histologies. Of the nine patients with at least 6 months of follow-up, six patients had experienced tumor progression. These results underscore the technical difficulty of implanting sources in these tumors. Even though ^{125}I emits a relatively low-energy photon (average energy, 28 keV), because of the proximity of the spinal cord, extreme care must be taken not to implant too close to the cord, because the dose given off by any one seed in very close proximity to the source is extremely high. Platinum foil was used to shield the spinal cord in one patient reported in this series. Although the use of foil is an excellent protection against radiation dose from ^{125}I, it has the disadvantage of shielding the dural surface, which in many tumors with epidural extension is at risk for tumor contamination.

Kumar et al. (6) reported the use of ^{125}I in the management of previously irradiated clival and sacral chordomas. The sacral chordoma showed an initial excellent response, but in the patient, who died 3 years after implant, meningeal carcinomatosis developed with chordoma cell contamination. A previously irradiated clival chordoma was implanted via the transnasal approach. This patient was reported to be well 19 months after the procedure.

At Memorial Sloan Kettering Cancer Center, 35 patients with paraspinal tumors underwent brachytherapy with low-dose iridium 192 (^{192}Ir) temporarily ($n = 21$) or permanent ^{125}I implantation ($n = 14$) (7). The median dose for patients receiving ^{192}Ir was 30 Gy, and 125 Gy with ^{125}I. The spinal cord dose was a median of 20 Gy for ^{192}Ir. Both metastatic disease and primary tumors were treated. All cases were incompletely resected at the time of treatment. Survival was limited in this cohort. Only 23 patients survived longer than 6 months, 16 lived more than 1 year, and 7 survived past 18 months. Dural tumor involvement was a poor prognostic sign. Overall, approximately 50% of patients were locally controlled, but only 22% of these patients were alive beyond the median time to local failure.

The use of gold foil to protect the spinal cord for brachytherapy has also been reported by Hamilton et al. (8). A 28-year-old had multiply recurrent chondrosarcoma at T-2 to T-4 causing epidural cord compression. After resection of the recurrent tumor, two layers of gold foil, 0.025 mm thick, were laid in place over the thecal sac. Sixty ^{125}I seeds were sutured into place in the resection cavity, to give 120 Gy at 5 mm. The cord dose with shielding was less than 5%. The patient was reported to be well without evidence of recurrence 18 months after the procedure.

The Barrows Neurologic Institute reported the use of ^{125}I brachytherapy in 30 consecutive patients; 25 brachytherapy procedures had adequate follow-up for reporting purposes (9). The ^{125}I seeds in vicryl suture were placed in the resection site. Gelfoam was placed around the dura, and seeds were placed over the Gelfoam to provide approximately 4 mm distance between the seed and the dural surface. The mean prescribed dose was 101 Gy (50–160 Gy). Most patients also had external-beam radiation (mean dose, 37.9; range, 12–50.4 Gy). With a mean follow-up of nearly 20 months, 87% and 73% actuarial survival was reported at 2 and 3 years, respectively. The mean calculated central spinal cord dose was found to be 33 Gy, giving a composite central spinal cord dose of 70 Gy when external-beam radiation was factored in. In those patients who had prior external-beam radiation and brachytherapy was the sole form of salvage, the mean central spinal cord dose was 67 Gy (22–167 Gy). No adverse sequelae, including no cases of myelitis, were noted.

Recent advances in image-guided technology have significantly improved the accuracy of delivery of very high dose radiation therapy to spinal tumors, making it safe to give very high doses of radiation within very close proximity to the spinal cord. However, even with proton beam radiation, the treatment of contaminated dura is problematic. Delaney et al. (10) reported the use of a Yttrium 90 (^{90}Yt) dural plaque to boost the dura with 10 to 20 Gy intraoperatively. ^{90}Yt is a beta particle–emitting isotope, which makes it particularly well suited for dural radiation. The dose fall-off is very steep. The plaque is placed directly on the region of interest. (Fig. 8.4). Whereas the dura receives

A

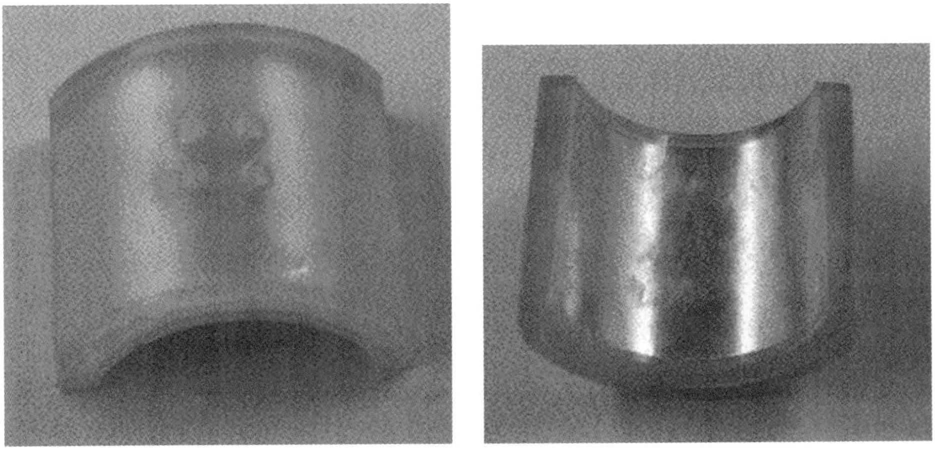

B

FIGURE 8.4 Yttrium dural plaque.

100% of the prescribed dose, the surface of the spinal cord typically receives less than 10% of the dural-surface dose. Because of its very low energy radiation, ^{90}Yt has the added advantage of posing few radiation safely risks to operating-room staff. With the use of intensity-modulated radiotherapy, a dose constraint on the dural surface can be applied at the time of postoperative radiation-treatment planning to account for the radiation given intraoperatively with the plaque. This allows the inverse treatment-planning algorithm to deliver a higher and more homogeneous dose to the rest of the tumor-resection cavity. The use of ^{90}Yt is currently part of the protocol used to treat primary spine tumors at the Northeast Proton Beam Center at the Massachusetts General Hospital (T. Delaney, personal communication).

SUMMARY

Brachytherapy is an attractive way to deliver tumoricidal doses of radiation to spinal tumors while minimizing the dose to the spinal cord. However, only limited data have been reported in the literature on the use of brachytherapy for spinal tumors. Although a paucity of published experience is specific to spine tumors, in small series, brachytherapy has not been associated with a risk of increased complications, including surgical complications or radiation myelopathy. Even in the era of image-guided intensity-modulated radiotherapy and increasing availability of proton-beam facilities, a role exists for the use of brachytherapy to increase the dose of radiation near the spinal cord.

REFERENCES

1. Anderson LL. A "natural" volume-dose histogram for brachytherapy. Med Phys 1986;13: 898–903.
2. DeLaney TF, Chen GT, Mauceri TC, et al. Intraoperative dural irradiation by customized 192iridium and 90yttrium brachytherapy plaques. Int J Radiat Oncol Biol Phys 2003;57:239–45.
3. ICRU submits new radiation unit system and reports. Radiol Technol 1978;50:50–51.
4. Emani BLJ, Brown A. Tolerance of normal tissue to therapeutic radiation. Int J Radiat Oncol Biol Phys 1991;21:109–122.
5. Gutin PH, Leibel SA, Hosobuchi Y, et al. Brachytherapy of recurrent tumors of the skull base and spine with iodine-125 sources. Neurosurgery 1987;20:938–945.
6. Kumar PP, Good RR, Skulety FM, et al. Local control of recurrent clival and sacral chordoma after interstitial irradiation with iodine-125: new techniques for treatment of recurrent or unresectable chordomas. Neurosurgery 1988;22:479–483.
7. Armstrong JG, Fass DE, Bains M, et al. Paraspinal tumors: techniques and results of brachytherapy. Int J Radiat Oncol Biol Phys 1991;20:787–790.
8. Hamilton A-J, Lulu B, Stea B, et al. The use of gold foil wrapping for radiation protection of the spinal cord for recurrent tumor therapy. Int J Radiat Oncol Biol Phys 1995;32:507–511.
9. Rogers CL, Theodore N, Dickman CA, et al. Surgery and permanent 125I seed paraspinal brachytherapy for malignant tumors with spinal cord compression. Int J Radiat Oncol Biol Phys 2002;54:505–513.
10. DeLaney TF, Trofimov A-V, Engelsman M, et al. Advanced-technology radiation therapy in the management of bone and soft tissue sarcomas. Cancer Control 2005; 12:27–35.

Biomechanics of Cement Augmentation in Tumor Treatment

Michael A.K. Liebschner and Tony S. Keller

9

ABSTRACT

This chapter provides a general overview of current practice in using cement augmentation in tumor treatment, particularly in the spine. Clinical challenges as well as biomechanical mechanisms that compete between long-term and short-term outcomes are discussed. Trends in the development of novel biomaterials for the augmentation in tumor treatment also are presented.

INTRODUCTION

Percutaneous vertebroplasty is a minimally invasive, fluoroscopically guided procedure wherein bone cement, typically polymethylmethacrylate (PMMA), is augmented into structurally weakened vertebrae (30,37). Indications include vertebral hemangioma, osteoporotic compression fractures, and other weakening lesions, such as vertebral myeloma or metastatic vertebral lesions. Unlike in Europe, where vertebroplasty is performed mainly to manage pain due to tumor-related bone diseases (25,26,52,71,94), the focus in North America has been on the relief of pain associated with osteoporotic vertebral fractures that have failed to respond to conservative therapy (40,57,73,75). The clinical success of this procedure is evidenced by the more than 500,000 procedures performed each year in the United States alone (40).

Besides providing additional biomechanical stability, this technique is also performed to alleviate pain by stabilizing metastatically compromised vertebrae that are at risk of pathologic burst fracture (19,67). The antalgic effect is excellent in more than 80% of cases and is very rapid, because a resumption of the support is often possible within 48 hours (39). Optimal cement-distribution patterns to improve biomechanical stability of metastatically involved vertebral bodies, however, remain unknown. The objective of this chapter is to elaborate on the biomechanical effects of cement augmentation in metastatically compromised spinal segments. Specifically, differences between fracture treatment (repair) and preventive treatment (reinforcement) are discussed, as well as variations in the procedure.

GOAL OF CEMENT AUGMENTATION IN THE METASTATIC SPINE

Various cancers exhibit the tendency to metastasize to bone, and the thoracolumbar spine is the most frequent site for this complication (3,22,34,36). Osseous metastatic disease in the spine results in the onset of severe bone pain and structural deficiency, leading to vertebral body fractures and neural deficits (3,34,55,96). Improving the patient's quality of life depends on achieving spinal stability to reduce pain and prevent neurologic deterioration (56). Conventional surgical decompression and stabilization is a major intervention requiring significant postoperative recovery, but few metastatic cancer patients are good candidates for such a surgery because of their health conditions (18,36,72).

Vertebroplasty for the palliative treatment of malignant spinal tumors has two goals: (a) vertebral stabilization when the lesion threatens the stability of the vertebrae, and (b) analgesic effect. Spinal pain, experienced in more than 70% of affected patients (33), is caused by mechanical micromotion within the osteolytic vertebrae (32). The *in situ* polymerization of PMMA immobilizes the vertebral body fractured fragments, contributing to the analgesic effect (64). More than 80% of vertebroplasty cases demonstrated significant rapid pain relief and improvement in mobility 24 to 48 hours after the procedure, and in two thirds of cases, prolonged pain relief was observed (7,35,40). Sufficient vertebral stabilization and strengthening require bone-cement filling of both the osteolytic area of the lesion and the surrounding regions of the vertebral body that seem structurally normal (2,32). However, injection of excess bone cement into the lesion must be avoided for fear of complications due to cement leakages (see page 75).

Much of the abstruseness of the ultimate biomechanical goal of vertebroplasty stems from the highly debated issue of what composes fracture risk. Previous biomechanical studies considered the repair of a collapsed vertebra successful when vertebral stiffness or strength was restored to prefracture values (13,68). By increasing vertebral strengths to almost prefracture levels, additional fractures could, theoretically, be prevented if the spine were loaded to the same magnitude that caused the initial fracture. This criterion was used as a basis to provide guidance as to the volume of cement needed for vertebroplasty to minimize risk of extravasations (13,68). Unfortunately, because 58% of vertebral fractures occur spontaneously during routine activities (24), the loads experienced in subsequent fractures can easily equal or exceed those of the initial collapse. As a result, the fractured vertebrae must be strengthened to levels that allow sufficient support of normal weight-bearing dynamics (87). The aim of vertebral repair and reinforcement therefore should be geared toward secondary fracture prevention through enhancement of the mechanical integrity of the compromised vertebrae to low-fracture-risk levels. A possible definition of "low fracture risk" could be adapted from the vertebral-strength prediction model developed by Biggemann et al. (16). He noted 100% fracture risk for strengths less than 3 kN (high risk) and no risk for strengths greater than 5 kN (low risk). Strengths between 3 and 5 kN were at an intermediate-risk group. As such, the "normal" or low-fracture-risk level for the L3 vertebra is when its compressive strength is at least 5 kN. Therefore the biomechanical goal of vertebroplasty for both fracture repair and prevention is to increase compressive ultimate stress of the vertebral body to beyond fracture-risk levels (>3.6 MPa) to prevent further fractures.

EFFECT OF BONE-CEMENT PROPERTIES IN VERTEBRAL REPAIR OR REINFORCEMENT

Since its introduction more than 20 years ago, multiple unanswered questions still remain concerning the biomechanics of vertebroplasty. These include (a) the optimal volume of material to be used, (b) the attributes of the ideal bone cement, and (c) its ideal placement within the vertebral body. Tohmeh et al. (87) performed a cadaveric study on the biomechanics of isolated osteoporotic vertebral bodies fractured and subsequently treated with unipedicular or bipedicular vertebroplasty. Their results demonstrated that both approaches successfully increased strength and stiffness of the vertebral bodies, even beyond the predamage values. Note that predamage values still present a significant fracture risk. However, experimental limitations (uniaxial loading) were later questioned by a numeric study performed by Liebschner et al. (68). By applying more physiologic loading conditions, vertebral endplate toggle was identified as a significant fracture risk factor in unipedicular vertebroplasty. In a series of studies, Belkoff et al. (9,11) investigated the stabilizing role of different types of bone cement on individual vertebral bodies. After fracturing each vertebral body mechanically and then filling (8 ml of bone cement) through a bipedicular approach, they found that all types of cement increased vertebral strength beyond predamage values, but that some cements did not restore stiffness. The reason for the latter finding was not understood, but it was mentioned that a sensitivity of the procedure to bone mineral density might be important, thus indicating that the procedure would be more effective in lower-density bone. This issue highlights the need for more detailed and extensive biomechanical studies of vertebroplasty.

Effect of Volume

The effect of cement volume was first determined by Belkoff et al. (13), who had recommended PMMA (Simplex P) and Orthocomp volumes needed to restore strength and stiffness for thoracic and lumbar vertebrae. Because the size of vertebral bodies varies greatly from patient to patient, the study was revisited by the same research group to determine the cement-volume effects based on percentage of vertebral body fill (74). They reported weak correlations between strength and stiffness restoration and percentage of volume fill. The poor correlations were due to wide scatter of the data, which is a result of bone-density variability in vertebral specimens manifested by pooling data from different donor spines of different bone density, as each specimen can be destructively tested only once. This biologic variability problem is eliminated when computer models are used. In the study by Liebschner et al. (68), a finite-element model of an L1 vertebral body was used to simulate vertebroplasty by using different volumes of PMMA (68). To replicate damage of the vertebral body model caused by fracture, the elastic modulus of the trabecular bone were reduced based on initial strain during reloading. The properties of the trabecular bone elements were replaced with those of PMMA at specific locations within the vertebral body to duplicate the shape of the PMMA bolus after vertebroplasty. The predicted vertebral stiffness from the uniaxial compression of the repaired model was found to increase with PMMA volume fill.

In general, vertebral stiffness and strength augmentation after PMMA cement augmentation is influenced strongly by volume fraction of the implanted cement and bone density, but least affected by the surgical approach (Fig. 9.1). Cement distribution typically varies with the surgical approach, where the posterolateral approach places the cement centrally, the bipedicular approach symmetrically along the sagittal plane, and the unipedicular approach asymmetric to the right or left side within a vertebra.

Stiffness and strength increases are directly proportional to PMMA filler volume, with greater stiffening and strengthening effects for the bipedicular approach versus posterolateral for PMMA volumes higher than 20%. In a numeric study, Sun et al. (82) reported no significant differences between two investigated fill approaches (bipedicular and posterolateral) for lower cement volumes ($p > 0.1$). Greater augmentation effects were observed for vertebral bodies with average QCT densities less than 0.1 g/cc, with even more

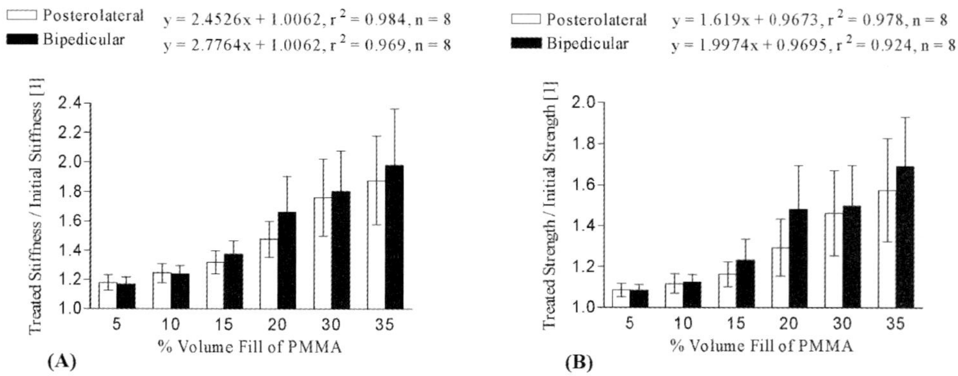

FIGURE 9.1 Effect of posterolateral and bipedicular placement and volume fill of PMMA on the **(A)** average normalized compressive stiffness increase, and **(B)** average normalized compressive strength increase of reinforced vertebral bodies. Stiffness and strength augmentations were linearly proportional to the PMMA volume fill for both approaches (82).

pronounced effects as the bone densities decreased, whereas for densities greater than 0.1 g/cc, the mechanical augmentations were less dependent on bone density. These results agree closely with previous *in vitro* vertebral augmentation studies on single vertebral bodies, which were mechanically tested under uniaxial compression after injection with calcium phosphate (31), PMMA, or experimental brushite cement (29). In those studies, greater augmentation effect at lower initial bone mineral density was also observed.

Based on the reported results of experimental and numeric studies, the minimal volumes of PMMA bone cement needed to improve the mechanical integrity of vertebral bodies at risk for fracture to low-fracture-risk levels were identified. Vertebral bodies at high risk of fracture required at least 20% volume fill of PMMA for preventive augmentation, whereas between 5% and 15% and 20% to 30% fill was successful in achieving the desired strength improvements for vertebral bodies in the low and high spectrum of the medium-risk range, respectively (Fig. 9.2) (83). However, with any volume fill higher than 20%, the typical amount used clinically, the risk of cement leakage will be greater than that for current vertebroplasty procedure for fracture repair (50). Therefore alternative materials must be investigated for use on vertebral bodies at high risk of fracture.

With regard to cement placement, bipedicular vertebroplasty might be biomechanically more efficient because of its higher strengthening effect and easier surgical access than the posterolateral case.

Effect of Material Properties

The inherent limitations of acrylic bone cement (PMMA), including nonbiodegradability, barrier to bone remodeling, damage to neighboring tissue due to drastic temperature increase from polymerization (23,51), and possible provocation of fractures in the adjacent vertebrae (4,8,26,46,57), make the acrylic cement not ideal for use in vertebroplasty, especially as a preventive treatment. As a result, alternative bone substitutes with the desired material properties to replace PMMA must be investigated.

The biomechanically optimal bone cement mechanical properties for vertebral reinforcement have not been identified. However, parameter studies executed on numeric models can indicate the effects of varying the cement compressive elastic modulus and strength on the overall structural behavior of the treated vertebrae (63,83). In simulating

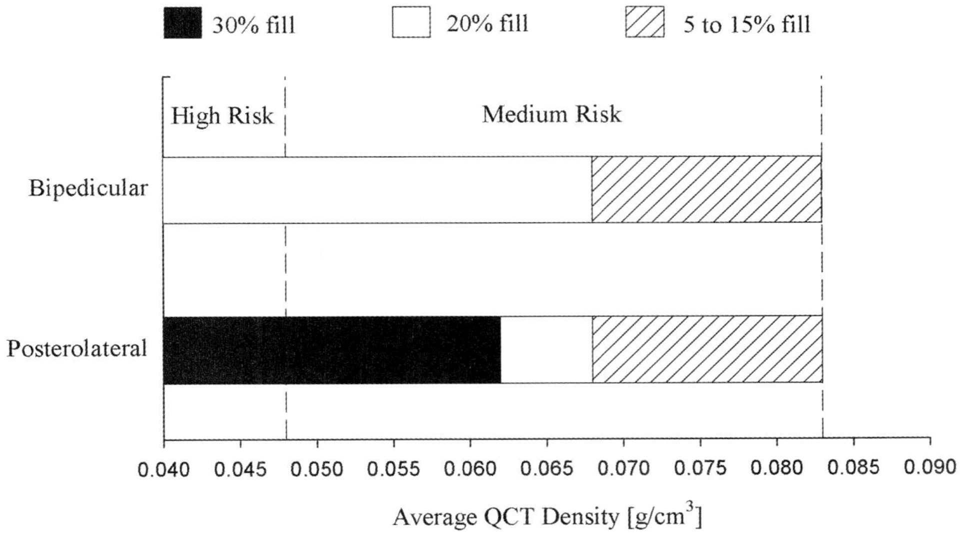

FIGURE 9.2 Biomechanically optimal poly(methyl-lmethacrylate) (PMMA) volume fill relative to vertebral body volume required to reduce fracture risk to low levels for bipedicular and posterolateral prophylactic vertebroplasty (n = 8) (83).

bipedicular vertebroplasty with a 20% cement volume fill, various bone-cement properties were investigated. Optimal cement properties were determined when the reinforcement goal of maximal strength increase and minimal stiffness increase was reached. Strength of bone cement was noted to have no influence on vertebral stiffness, but it did have an augmenting effect on vertebral fracture load (Fig. 9.3). Both vertebral stiffness and fracture load were affected by the elastic modulus of the implanted bone cement (Fig. 9.4). The biomechanical goal of maximal vertebral strength increase with minimal vertebral stiffness augmentation was achieved with cement modulus of 1,300 MPa and strength of at least 30 MPa. Repeating the analysis by using the optimal cement properties (modulus, 1,300 MPa; strength, 30 MPa) resulted in an average increase of 40.5% in vertebral strength

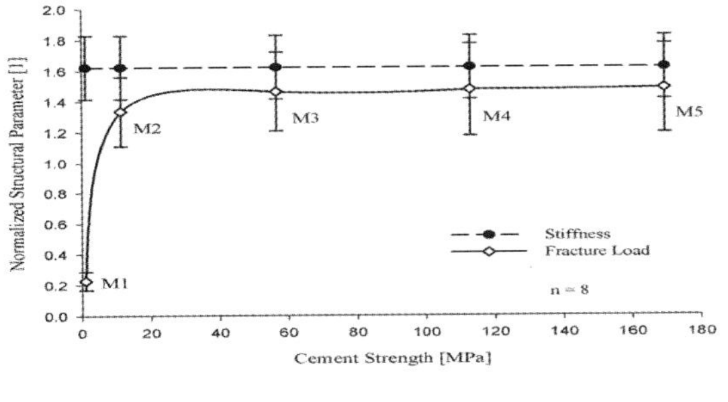

FIGURE 9.3 Effect of bone-cement compressive strength on the average normalized compressive vertebral stiffness increase (treated stiffness/initial stiffness) and fracture-load increase (treated fracture load/initial fracture load).

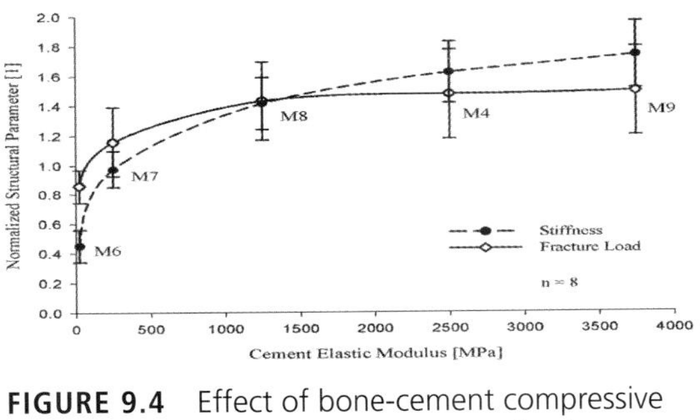

FIGURE 9.4 Effect of bone-cement compressive elastic modulus on the average normalized compressive vertebral stiffness increase (treated stiffness/initial stiffness) and fracture-load increase (treated fracture load/initial fracture load).

and a 45.9% average increase in vertebral stiffness. As a result, a material with 50% less stiffness than PMMA could still achieve the same level of reinforcement.

Although cadaveric studies must follow for verification purposes, future research can now be centered on injectable bone substitutes possessing these lower material properties. Most of the *in vitro* studies evaluated the biomechanical efficacies of different bone cements, such as hydroxyapatite (HA) (12,14,69), Orthocomp (10), calcium phosphate (CaP) (6), and different types of PMMA (9), on single vertebral bodies. All these bone cements were able to either increase or restore vertebral strength, but only Orthocomp and CaP were able also to restore vertebral stiffness. Multileveled vertebrae have also been used to show reduction of compliance in flexion–extension after repair with PMMA (97), and similar flexibility with PMMA and HA cements (51).

Effect of Distribution Patterns

The compact distribution of PMMA within the vertebrae has been shown to cause stress concentrations in the bone tissue directly above and below the PMMA, which can lead to additional fractures of the already treated vertebrae and adjacent untreated ones (see later) (8,61,77). Conversely, a more dispersed filling of the vertebral body with cement is thought to be able to provide a more uniform structural reinforcement, alleviating the high-stress concentrations and their consequences. A recently introduced bone cement, CORTOSS (Orthovita, Inc., Malvern, PA), engineered specifically to mimic the strength characteristics of human cortical bone, demonstrated greater dispersed fill within the vertebral body than that with PMMA (Fig. 9.5). It is believed that the high affinity of the cement to bone is due to its synthetic combeite glass–ceramic particle composition, which makes the cement "spread itself out" to attain maximal contact with bone tissue. Similar to PMMA, CORTOSS is viscous and self-setting. However, unlike PMMA, CORTOSS allows direct bone apposition at the cement–bone interface, cures at temperatures 27°C lower than that for PMMA and is twice as strong and twice as stiff as PMMA (76).

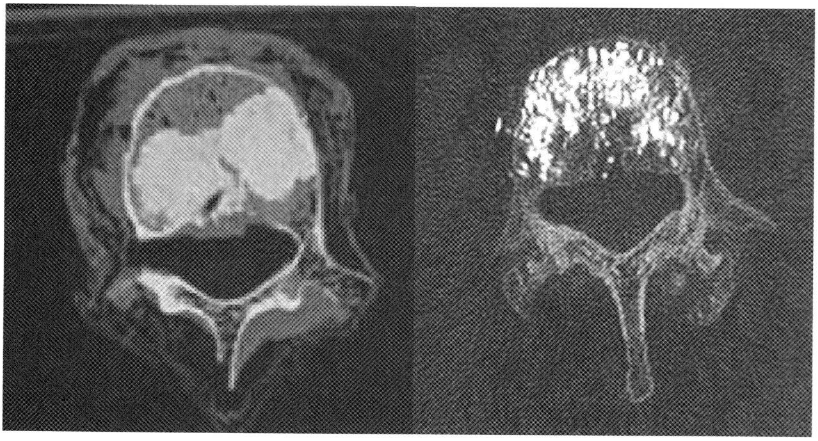

FIGURE 9.5 Quantitative computed tomography scans of vertebrae treated with PMMA and CORTOSS. The compact distribution of PMMA (10-cc fill) within vertebra (left) is distinctly different from the more dispersed distribution of CORTOSS with 3-cc fill (right).

In a biomechanical study on the effect of filling pattern on the biomechanics of vertebroplasty, patient-specific data after compact fill with PMMA and dispersed fill with CORTOSS were used (84). The results indicated that the CORTOSS-treated (dispersed fill) and PMMA-treated (compact fill) vertebral body models showed significant differences in both the extra- and intravertebral biomechanics. The accumulation of PMMA at one locale focuses the shift in the applied load to that area, causing the bone above and below the PMMA to experience high axial stress. The CORTOSS material dispersed throughout the vertebral body was unable to cause such major shifts in the applied load, and thus no additional high axial stresses were present. Additionally, the spatially distributed reinforcement of small areas of trabecular bone within the entire vertebral body with CORTOSS enabled the whole cross-sectional area of the vertebral body to bear the applied load, resulting in a higher increase in vertebral stiffness than that with PMMA, whose compact fill forces the applied load to act on a smaller area because of load transfer.

When the cement properties of CORTOSS and PMMA were equalized, thereby neutralizing the effect of cement properties, the dispersed cement-fill pattern with CORTOSS produced higher vertebral stiffness than with a compact cement-fill pattern with PMMA with the same volume of cement (Fig. 9.6) (81,84). The greater augmentation of the vertebral stiffness with a dispersed cement filling of the vertebral body means that a smaller volume of the filler material will still produce the same amount of stiffness augmentation achieved with a compact fill. The dispersed cement distribution also avoids intravertebral axial stress concentrations that are generated as a consequence of load transfer and may lead to future fractures of the adjacent untreated vertebrae. As a result, a dispersed cement-distribution pattern may result in a lower risk of complications because of cement leakages, because smaller cement volume would be just as biomechanically effective as well as prevent subsequent fractures in the adjacent untreated vertebrae, as intravertebral stress-risers are minimal (84).

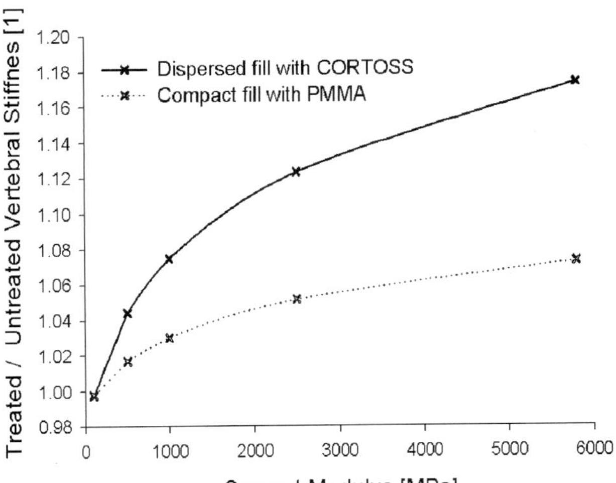

FIGURE 9.6 The effect of cement-distribution patterns on the biomechanics of vertebroplasty. The dispersed fill seems biomechanically more efficient than the compact fill.

COMPETING MECHANISM: INTERNAL AND EXTERNAL LOADING MECHANISM

The strength of vertebroplasty is its simplicity and good clinical success in terms of pain relief in the repair of fractured vertebrae. However, it has been demonstrated through both finite-element analyses and biomechanical studies of vertebroplasty that it is very challenging to restore the biomechanical properties of fractured vertebrae to low-fracture-risk levels without risking complications arising from, for example, cement leakages. This goal can be more effectively achieved by applying vertebroplasty preventatively on vertebrae that have yet to fracture but are at risk to do so. Because approximately half the cement volume is required to gain the sufficient augmentation to prevent further fractures for vertebral reinforcement compared with fracture repair, the risk of cement extravasation and its related complications is significantly reduced. As a result, preventive vertebroplasty may have a higher chance of success in fracture prevention. Furthermore, the surgical feasibility and safety of the preventive treatment for multilevel spinal reinforcement has already been demonstrated clinically (28,48).

The caveat for preventive surgery is that we must better understand the underlying mechanism of complications, such as secondary tissue damage and adjacent bone fracture. Moreover, because PMMA for use in vertebroplasty has numerous adverse side effects (4,8,23,26,46,51,58), the cement may soon be replaced with more suitable biocompatible substitutes. Unfortunately, evaluation guidelines, such as what are ideal properties of a bone cement in vertebroplasty, have not been established. Mitigation strategies to prevent secondary tissue damage have not been developed.

Based on the previously mentioned effects of bone-cement volume and distribution pattern on the biomechanics of vertebroplasty, it is evident that at least two competing mechanisms are at work, operating at two different structural levels of the vertebra. The extravertebral level represents the structural level of the whole bone, whereas the intravertebral level is at the microarchitectural level of the trabecular bone tissue. From numeric models, we know that both the extravertebral mechanical properties and the intravertebral bone-stress levels increase with increasing cement-augmentation volume. However, whereas an increase in extravertebral properties after vertebroplasty is the goal of fracture repair and reinforcement, the increased intravertebral stress levels are thought to be the cause of secondary tissue damage.

The biomechanical goal of maximal vertebral strength increase with minimal vertebral-stiffness augmentation cannot necessarily be achieved by just substituting the bone cement with another material that has inherent mechanical properties similar to those of bone tissue. The load-transfer mechanism, or stiff-riser effect, will still remain the same, thereby overloading the tissue directly underneath the augmented material (see page 82). Alleviation of the stiff-riser effect could be achieved by increasing the effective cross-sectional area of the vertebral body used for load bearing after vertebroplasty. However, such a goal would require a radical change in bone-cement properties in terms of viscosity, shear stress, affinity to bone tissue, and hydrophobicity.

In an investigative study, Sun and colleagues (84) compared the extravertebral biomechanical properties with the intravertebral stress levels for a dispersed fill– and a compact fill–treated vertebral body. In the compact-fill case, the applied load was shifted toward the augmented area, causing the bone tissue above and below the bone cement to experience high axial stress. In the dispersed-fill case, throughout the vertebral body, it was unable to cause such major shifts in the applied load, and thus no additional high-axial stresses were present. Additionally, the spatially distributed reinforcement of small areas of trabecular bone within the entire vertebral body with dispersed fill enabled the whole cross-sectional area of the vertebral body to bear the applied load, resulting in a higher increase in vertebral stiffness than with the compact fill, which forces the applied load to act on a smaller area because of load transfer (Fig. 9.5).

When the cement properties for the compact- and dispersed-fill cases were equalized, thereby neutralizing the effects of cement properties, the dispersed cement–fill pattern produced higher vertebral stiffness than with a compact cement–fill pattern with the same volume of cement (Fig. 9.6). The greater augmentation of the vertebral stiffness with a dispersed cement filling of the vertebral body means that a smaller volume of the filler material will still produce the same amount of stiffness augmentation achieved with a compact fill. The dispersed cement distribution also avoids intravertebral axial stress concentrations that are generated as a consequence of load transfer and may lead to future fractures of the adjacent untreated vertebrae. As a result, a dispersed cement-distribution pattern may result in a lower risk of complications due to cement leakages, because smaller cement volume would be just as biomechanically effective as well as prevent subsequent fractures in the adjacent untreated vertebrae, as intravertebral stress-risers are minimal.

RISK OF COMPLICATIONS: SECONDARY TISSUE DAMAGE

Percutaneous vertebroplasty has been shown to be effective in reducing pain and improving daily function in the treatment of osteolytic tumors (5,18,22,26,34,39,56,66,98). The most prevalent reported complication of vertebroplasty is cement extravasation, but few adverse effects on the functional status of patients have been reported as a result (3,5,22,34,36,39,49,66,95,98). The nerve root foramen is where cement extravasations is most likely to be hazardous (44,49). Resulting symptoms may range from transient radiculopathy to significant neurologic deficits (40,49,94). In addition, aggressive vertebroplasty may provoke fat embolism (1,47,65,86), mainly caused by the displacement of the bone marrow during the bone-cement injection into the treated vertebrae. It has been shown that the risks of cement extravasation can be mitigated by increasing the duration of time between cement polymerization and injection (increased cement viscosity), and by decreasing cement injection volume (36). The complication rates are low, ranging from 1% to 10%, with different frequencies depending on the initial indications of percutaneous vertebroplasty (93). For osteoporotic vertebral collapse and vertebral angioma, complications are uncommon, with rates of only 1% to 3% and 2% to 5%, respectively (75). The complication rates are much higher for malignant spinal tumors, up to 10%, because of the higher risk of cement extravasations resulting from vertebral cortex destruction associated with the osteolytic processes (21,31). The most common causes for the complications have been reported as (a) inappropriate patient selection; (b) poor visualization due to inadequate fluoroscopic equipment, poor patient cooperation, or unsatisfactory cement opacification; (c) operator error, such as lack of knowledge of the radiographic spinal anatomy and poor fluoroscopic triangulation skills; (d) lack of patient monitoring; and (e) improper aseptic technique (78).

The increased risk of additional fractures in adjacent nontreated levels after augmentation with bone cement is a topic that continues to be of intense interest to the clinical community. In the context of osteoporosis, review of the clinical sequelae of patients with at least one vertebral compression fracture suggests that these patients have 5 times the risk of subsequent fracture (79,88,92), most of which may be adjacent and some of which may be remote to the index fracture. It remains unclear whether adjacent vertebral body fractures are related to the natural progression of osteoporosis (20,70,80,91), or if the fractures are a consequence of augmentation with bone cement (38,43,45,88,90). Therefore it is of utmost importance to obtain a better understanding of the immediate biomechanical effects of vertebroplasty (even if done preventatively) on adjacent vertebral bodies, and how this biomechanical state compares with that already present due to the natural progression of osteoporosis or the effects of a cancer.

One way to improve the safety of vertebroplasty is to minimize cement leakage by using less cement, because complication rates due to cement extravasations are directly related to the amount of cement injected. A study by Cotton et al. (27) has shown that pain relief is not dependent on the percentage volume of cement used, but rather on the distribution of cement within the vertebral body, specifically within the fracture planes. Therefore adequate pain relief with minimal cement fill might best be attained through the strategic placement of cement at fracture locations and intraoperative evaluation of the vertebroplasty biomechanics (Templeton A, Sun K, Fukshansky M, et al. Intraoperative inferior-superior visualization of PMMA bolus in vertebroplasty. Transcript, Orthopaedic Research Society, Chicago, IL, March 19–22, 2006).

Secondary Tissue Damage in Vertebroplasty-treated Vertebrae

Introduction of bone cement into the vertebral body results in an increase in overall strength of the vertebra. However, in the area peripheral to the injection point, the trabecular bone may actually be weakened over time due to stress shielding by the stronger, injected material (63). With more of the load applied to the treated vertebra transferred to the stiffer cement, the uneven load distribution causes bone resorption in the peripheral trabecular bone. The trabecular bone now, with reduced bone mass, becomes more fragile and more susceptible to fractures. As a result of stress-shielding, new fractures may occur in untreated areas within an already repaired vertebra (93). Ikeuchi et al. (53) compared the effects of vertebral augmentation at different locations by injecting CaP cement at the cranial half of the vertebra and through the entire vertebra. When compression tests were performed, two peaks were seen in the load-deformation curve for the vertebra with the top half reinforced. The first peak corresponded to failure of the caudal side of the vertebra, and the second, higher peak corresponded to failure of the CaP-bone composite, which was of the same magnitude as the ultimate load for the vertebra completely filled with CaP. These results were further corroborated with sagittal CT scans and morphology of the fractured vertebrae.

A recent biomechanical investigation on the failure of adjacent vertebrae by Berlemann et al. (15) showed a 19% lower ultimate failure load for treated intact vertebrae compared with the untreated control. The caudal vertebrae of osteoporotic two-vertebrae functional spine units (FSUs) were augmented with PMMA and were subjected to cyclic sinusoidal dynamic compression at a constant displacement rate of 0.5 mm/sec. The untreated FSUs acted as a control. The geometric mean treated-to-untreated ratio of the failure load was 0.81 (95% CI, 0.70–0.92). No significant difference was found in overall FSU stiffness. In the treated FSUs, failure always occurred in the nonaugmented, cranial vertebral body, whereas in the untreated control FSUs, both cranial and caudal vertebrae sustained fractures. The authors suggested that the mechanism for such failure may be due to the alteration of the biomechanics of load transfer to the adjacent vertebrae caused by the increase in stiffness of the augmented fractured vertebrae. The early failure of the adjacent, nonaugmented level may be a result of a "stress-riser" effect (87) and a significant disparity in biomechanical properties between the two involved vertebral bodies.

As mentioned previously, fractures may also occur in areas above and below that of the cement. This phenomenon can be illustrated with a simple calculation by using a series of springs representing the regions of bone and cement (Fig. 9.7) and can show the effect of

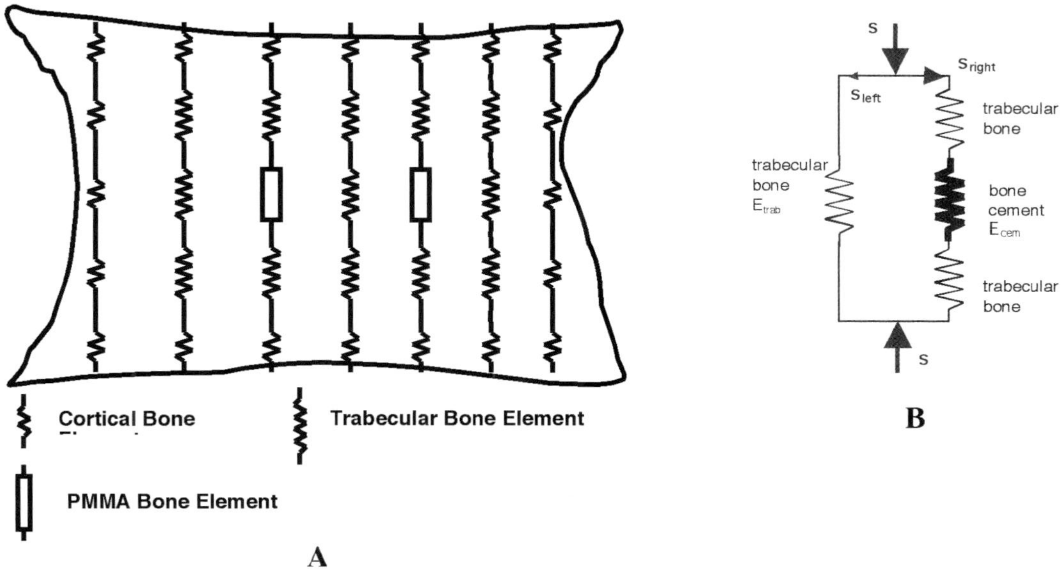

FIGURE 9.7 Modeling of the vertebral stiffness resulting from vertebroplasty. **A:** Cross section of a vertebral body represented as a conglomeration of springs in series and parallel. **B:** Simplification of the model of a vertebral cross section.

vertebroplasty on the strain experienced by surrounding bone. The range of possible strain values from a single applied load can be attained by examining an isostress condition (Voight model with minimized potential energy) and the isostrain condition (Reuss model with minimized work). Assuming a 5-kN load (3.5 kN of which is experienced by the anterior portion of the vertebral body and 1.5 kN by the posterior elements) and a fill volume of 30%, the strain experienced by trabecular bone above the cement (S_{right} in Fig. 9.7B) in the isostress condition can be calculated as 0.0177, the same as that experienced under nonfractured, intact condition (assuming elastic moduli of 600 MPa for vertebral cortex and endplate, 200 MPa for vertebral trabecular bone, and 800 MPa for PMMA). In the isostrain condition, this strain is increased to 0.025. The true increased strain lies between the two numbers, depending on the type of loading conditions, and is affected by several parameters, such as, for example, the shape of the injected PMMA. It is indisputable that PMMA, with higher stiffness than the surrounding bone, will cause an increased strain in the areas directly above and below the filled regions, possibly promoting fractures.

Adjacent Bone Fracture after Vertebroplasty

Vertebroplasty may have the ability to prevent fractures in the augmented vertebrae, but it also has the potential to promote fractures in the adjacent vertebrae. As many as 20% of patients with repaired vertebrae are expected to sustain further fractures (42,59,62,88), and a majority of the new fractures (67%) are estimated to happen within just 30 days of the procedure, with approximately 67% of the new fractures occurring in the vertebrae adjacent to the one that was treated (39,59). The increased risk of collapse in the neighboring vertebrae after fracture repair has been demonstrated in both retrospective reviews of vertebroplasty clinical studies (17,26,57,61,62) and in the *in vitro* biomechanical and numerical studies (8,83), and has been attributed to the altered distribution of forces to the nearby vertebrae caused by the shift in load or the "stress-riser" effect within the treated vertebra (54).

The results of mainly three numeric studies [Baroud et al. (8), Polikeit et al. (77), and Sun et al. (83)] showed a change in deformation pattern within the intervertebral disc after augmentation with PMMA cement, which led to a large deflection of the endplate into the adjacent vertebrae (12% to 20%). The results were verified in an experimental study by Kayanja and colleagues (60) in a cadaver model by using strain-gauges to measure cortical bone biomechanical changes after augmentation. Because fractures had been observed to occur preferentially at trabecular areas close to the endplate and at the endplate itself (41), the resultant increase in endplate deflection from prophylactic vertebroplasty may consequently lead to fractures in the adjacent vertebrae. It is hypothesized that drastic changes in the mechanical dynamics and kinematics of the vertebral column lead to an increase in mechanical demands on the neighboring vertebrae, thereby increasing the risk of fracture. A similar phenomenon is observed with regard to spinal fusion, in which increased risk for disc degeneration in vertebrae adjacent to a fusion is observed. However, limited information exists on this phenomenon.

Retrospective reviews of vertebroplasty clinical studies are inconclusive. A retrospective review of 109 patients with 174 fractures by Jenson and Dion (58) demonstrated no statistical difference in the rate of adjacent-level fractures between patients who returned with new fractures after vertebroplasty ($n = 19$; fractures, 27) and a control group consisting of patients who had multiple fractures of the same acuteness ($n = 21$; fractures, 43). This suggests that the vertebrae adjacent to the site of cement injection are at no higher risk of fracture than any other vertebrae (79). Conversely, in a retrospective study of 25 (67%) of 40 patients with symptomatic osteoporotic vertebral compression fracture, the odds ratio (OR) of a vertebral compression fracture adjacent to a cemented vertebra was higher, at 2.27 (95% CI, 1.11–4.56) compared with 1.44 (95% CI, 0.82–2.55) for a compression fracture adjacent to an uncemented vertebral collapse (mean duration of follow-up was 48 months; range, 12–84 months) (38). In another follow-up observational study of clinical vertebroplasty cases, 12.4% of patients with repaired vertebrae sustained further fractures, and 67% of the new fractures happened within just 30 days of the procedure, with approximately 67% of the new fractures occurring in the vertebrae adjacent to the one that was treated (90).

Experimental studies under ideal laboratory conditions are just now starting to become available. In a recent study, Sun et al. (85) investigated whether vertebroplasty contributed to the reduction in fracture strength of adjacent untreated vertebrae under physiologic loading conditions. A unique "worse-case scenario" vertebroplasty case was generated by treating the top and bottom vertebrae of a three-vertebral-level segment, while leaving the middle vertebra untreated. This so-called "pincher effect" is expected to have the greatest affect on the adjacent vertebra. Five of the six spinal segments demonstrated reductions in fracture strengths after vertebroplasty. Additionally, the untreated segments experienced mainly wedge fractures with some biconcave and crush fractures, whereas only biconcave fractures were observed in the treated segments. Wedge, biconcave, and crush fractures occur in all levels of the vertebral column, with wedge fractures being the most common, and crush, the least (54). Therefore the exclusivity of biconcave fractures in the treated segments and the more common wedge-type fractures in only the untreated segments are indicative of the effect of vertebroplasty. This change in fracture pattern concurs with the endplate-deflection fracture mechanism proposed by Baroud et al. (8) and Polikeit et al. (77). Because of the use of a 6-DOF robotic arm by Sun et al. (85) to apply unconstrained axial compression that closely duplicates physiologic loading on the main loading axis of the vertebrae, the results are therefore the most realistic that can be obtained from an *in vitro* cadaveric study. It must be noted that even though the risk of fracture to the untreated adjacent vertebrae after vertebroplasty is higher, the amount it has increased depends on other factors like bone density, intervertebral disc quality, distribution and volume of the bone cement, and vertebral levels treated. How these parameters interplay has to be shown.

The success of the bone-strengthening technique relies heavily on the mechanical properties of the augmentation material. The injected cement must have sufficient strengthening effect to increase the strength of the augmented vertebrae to low-fracture-risk levels to prevent future fractures in the treated vertebrae. For the adjacent vertebrae, fracture prevention would require a minimal effect of augmentation on load distribution. Because the premise behind the load-transfer mechanism is based on structural stiffness, to minimize changes in load distribution would mean that vertebral-stiffness augmentations must also be kept to a minimum. Therefore the aim of vertebral reinforcement for fracture prevention should be to attain maximal strength augmentation, while maintaining the smallest stiffness changes on the treated vertebrae.

Asymmetric Bolus Distribution

One important biomechanical issue for vertebroplasty is to minimize the amount of bone cement used and yet to improve stiffness of the damaged vertebral body in a biomechanically significant manner; another issue is whether the spatial distribution of the introduced cement is an important consideration (89). Little information is available on the biomechanical efficacy of unipedicular versus bipedicular vertebroplasty. Tohmeh et al. (87) performed a cadaveric study on the biomechanics of osteoporotic fractured vertebral bodies treated with unipedicular vertebroplasty (6 cc of bone cement) or bipedicular vertebroplasty (5 cc of bone cement through each pedicle). Their results demonstrated that unipedicular and bipedicular vertebroplasty increased strength and restored stiffness of vertebral bodies with compression fractures. The experimental approach taken by Tohmeh et al. (87), however, did not address the effects of distribution or volume fraction of the filling material. Furthermore, the experimental limitations, including the constraint on specimen motion, did not allow thorough investigation of the deformation behavior on the noninjected side for the unipedicular vertebroplasty cases (50). No information is available on the optimal protocols for such procedures, including the biomechanically optimal volume and placement of the filler material. An interesting finding of the study was that no significant loss of height occurred on either side of the vertebral bodies that received unilateral treatment resulting in toggle. Toggle occurs when the treated side of the vertebral body becomes significantly stronger than the untreated side of the vertebral body. Under loading, this could lead to failure on the untreated aspect of the vertebral body, leading to a loss of height skewed to one side of the vertebral body and ultimately scoliosis (68).

To investigate the possible occurrence of toggle, Liebschner et al. (68) used computer simulations to apply a pressure load to a fracture-repaired vertebral body. Pressure-loading conditions are believed to be the load-transfer mechanism between intervertebral discs and the underlying vertebral bone. Anatomically detailed finite-element models, generated from CT scans and calibrated to mechanical testing results, were used to simulate bipedicular, posterolateral, unipedicular vertebroplasty on the right and left side by virtually implanting the PMMA cement into the respective locations. The virtually treated specimens were loaded with a pressure boundary condition, which allowed the deformation of the vertebral body without a fixed center of rotation outside of the vertebral body. The study observed a medial–lateral bending motion or toggle toward the untreated side of vertebral body that underwent unipedicular vertebroplasty when

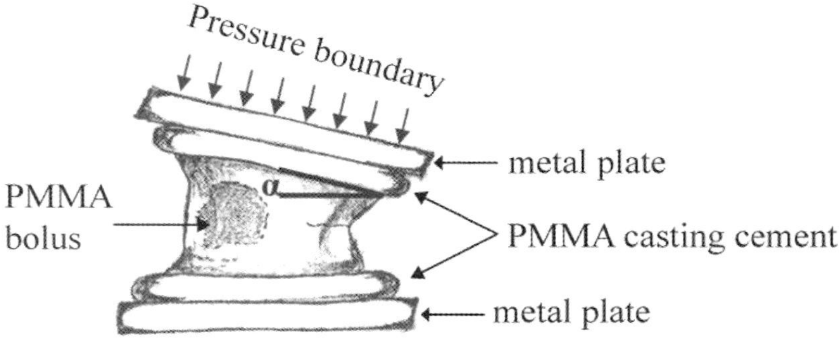

FIGURE 9.8 High angle of rotation in the sagittal plane of the vertebral body after unipedicular vertebroplasty when loaded under pressure-boundary conditions brings instability to the treated vertebra.

the uniform compressive load was applied, which was absent in the bipedicular and posterolateral approaches (Fig. 9.8) The asymmetric distribution of cement promotes single-sided load transfer and thus instability. This instability was proportional to filler volume, with greater degree of toggle as the amount of cement fill increased.

SUMMARY

The percutaneous application of an acrylic bone cement, polymethylmethacrylate, to vertebral defects associated with vertebral compression fracture, vertebral angioma, and osteolytic metastasis and myeloma has proven successful in alleviating back pain. However, because fractures often occurred during daily activities, mechanical support offered through this procedure could be insufficient. Strength of the vertebral body must be increased beyond fracture-risk levels (>3.6 MPa) to prevent further fractures. Unfortunately, to attain such strength levels by using PMMA, the volume of bone cement needed would be much higher than currently used. Large cement fills increase the risk of extravasations and, subsequently, complications that threaten the health and life of the patient. Another risk associated with vertebroplasty is the adjacent vertebral-body fracture. The heightened risk has been attributed to the increased stiffness or rigidness of the treated vertebral body that leads to a "stress-riser" effect, altering the biomechanics of load transfer to the adjacent vertebrae. This effect may be avoided with the use of alternative filler materials to increase strength while the increase in stiffness is kept minimal. The distribution pattern as well as affinity to bone tissue may play a far more significant role in the biomechanics of vertebroplasty than initially thought.

Vertebroplasty has also taken a turn, from repair of fractured vertebrae to preventive vertebral reinforcement of intact vertebrae, especially in patients who have previously sustained fractures and are at a high risk for subsequent fractures resulting from other treatment modalities (e.g., radiation or chemotheraphy). However, the numerous disadvantages of PMMA make it a nonideal candidate for this procedure. Instead of injecting with a permanent material, biodegradable filler materials may be more suitable. The biodegradable material provides a temporary scaffold onto which new bone can grow. As the degradable material starts to be resorbed by the body, new bone growth replaces the resorbed material. Bone mass and strength will increase, thereby reducing the risk of fracture for vertebral reinforcement and remodeling the damaged site for vertebral repair. This new approach for vertebroplasty also faces the same complication risks associated with leakage of filler material. The risk of extravasations can be minimized by optimizing the amount of filler material needed for biomechanical efficacy through the strategic placement of the material at either high risk of fracture regions within the vertebral body for vertebral reinforcement or fracture sites for vertebral repair. As a result, by focusing research on the optimization of filler material, volume, and placement for vertebral repair and reinforcement, vertebroplasty will enjoy success in achieving pain relief and biomechanical enhancements with minimal risk of complications. Vertebroplasty for vertebral reinforcement may even help in reversing the effects of bone loss when combined with other pharmacologic therapy.

REFERENCES

1. Aebli N, Krebs J, Davis G, et al. Fat embolism and acute hypotension during vertebroplasty: an experimental study in sheep. Spine 2002;27:460–466.
2. Ahn H, Mousavi P, Roth S, et al. Stability of the metastatic spine pre and post vertebroplasty. J Spinal Disord Tech 2006;19:178–182.
3. Alvarez L, Perez-Higueras A, Quinones D, et al. Vertebroplasty in the treatment of vertebral tumors: postprocedural outcome and quality of life. Eur Spine J 2003;12:356–360.
4. Ananthakrishnan D, Berven S, Deviren V, et al. The effect on anterior column loading due to different vertebral augmentation techniques. Clin Biomech (Bristol, Avon) 2005;20:25–31.
5. Atalay B, Caner H, Gokce C, et al. Kyphoplasty: 2 years of experience in a neurosurgery department. Surg Neurol 2005;64(suppl 2): S72–S76.
6. Bai B, Jazrawi LM, Kummer FJ, et al. The use of an injectable, biodegradable calcium phosphate bone substitute for the prophylactic augmentation of osteoporotic vertebrae and the management of vertebral compression fractures. Spine 1999;24: 1521–1526.
7. Barath K, Martin JB, Fasel HJ, et al. [Percutaneous vertebroplasty: methods, indications, results]. Orv Hetil 2002;143:2469–2477.
8. Baroud G, Nemes J, Heini P. Load shift of the intervertebral disc after a vertebroplasty: a finite-element study. Eur Spine J 2003;12:421–426.
9. Belkoff SM, Maroney M, Fenton DC. An in vitro biomechanical evaluation of bone cements used in percutaneous vertebroplasty. Bone 1999;25(2 suppl):23S–26S.
10. Belkoff SM, Mathis JM, Deramond H, et al. An ex vivo biomechanical evaluation of a hydroxyapatite cement for use with kyphoplasty. AJNR Am J Neuroradiol 2001;22: 1212–1216.
11. Belkoff SM, Mathis JM, Erbe EM. Biomechanical evaluation of a new bone cement for use in vertebroplasty. Spine 2000;25:1061–1064.
12. Belkoff SM, Mathis JM, Jasper LE. Ex vivo biomechanical comparison of hydroxyapatite and polymethylmethacrylate cements for use with vertebroplasty. AJNR Am J Neuroradiol 2002; 23:1647–1651.
13. Belkoff SM, Mathis JM, Jasper LE. The biomechanics of vertebroplasty: the effect of cement volume on mechanical behavior. Spine 2001;26: 1537–1541.
14. Belkoff SM, Mathis JM, Jasper LE, et al. An ex vivo biomechanical evaluation of a hydroxyapatite cement for use with vertebroplasty. Spine 2001;26:1542–1546.
15. Berlemann U, Ferguson SJ, Nolte LP, et al. Adjacent vertebral failure after vertebroplasty: a biomechanical investigation. J Bone Joint Surg Br 2002;84:748–752.
16. Biggemann M, Hilweg D, Seidel S, et al. Risk of vertebral insufficiency fractures in relation to compressive strength predicted by quantitative computed tomography. Eur J Radiol 1991;13: 6–10.
17. Bostrom MP, Lane JM. Future directions: augmentation of osteoporotic vertebral bodies. Spine 1997;22(24 suppl):38S–42S.
18. Burton AW, Reddy SK, Shah HN, et al. Percutaneous vertebroplasty: a technique to treat refractory spinal pain in the setting of advanced metastatic cancer: a case series. J Pain Symptom Manage 2005;30:87–95.
19. Burton AW, Rhines LD, Mendel E. Vertebroplasty and kyphoplasty: a comprehensive review. Neurosurg Focus 2005;18:e1.
20. Cher D, Talmadge K, Edidin A. Risk of subsequent vertebral body compression fractures after

balloon kyphoplasty. In: Advances in Minimally Invasive Spine Therapies. Sunnyvale, CA: White Paper, Kyphon Inc., 2005.

21. Chiras J, Depriester C, Weill A, et al. [Percutaneous vertebral surgery: technics and indications]. J Neuroradiol 1997;24:45–59.
22. Chow E, Holden L, Danjoux C, et al. Successful salvage using percutaneous vertebroplasty in cancer patients with painful spinal metastases or osteoporotic compression fractures. Radiother Oncol 2004;70:265–267.
23. Christiansen C. Osteoporosis: diagnosis and management today and tomorrow. Bone 1995;17:S513–S16.
24. Cooper C, Atkinson EJ, O'Fallon WM. Incidence of clinically diagnosed vertebral fractures: a population-based study in Rochester, Minnesota, 1985–1989. J Bone Miner Res 1992;7:221–227.
25. Cortet B, Cotten A, Boutry N, et al. Percutaneous vertebroplasty in patients with osteolytic metastases or multiple myeloma. Rev Rheum Engl Ed 1997;64:177–183.
26. Cotten A, Boutry N, Cortet B, et al. Percutaneous vertebroplasty: state of the art. Radiographics 1998;18:311–320.
27. Cotten A, Dewatre F, Cortet B, et al. Percutaneous vertebroplasty for osteolytic metastases and myeloma: effects of the percentage of lesion filling and the leakage of methyl methacrylate at clinical follow-up. Radiology 1996;200:525–530.
28. Cyteval C, Sarrabere MP, Roux CP, et al. Acute osteoporotic vertebral collapse: open study on percutaneous injection of acrylic surgical cement in 20 patients. AJR Am J Roentgenol 1999;173:1685–1690.
29. Dahl OE, Garvik LJ, Lyberg T, et al. Methylmethacrylate monomer on leukocytes and endothelial cells in vitro. Acta Orthop Scand 1994;65:147–153.
30. Debussche-Depriester C. Percutaneous vertebroplasty with acrylic cement in the treatment of osteoporotic vertebral crush fracture syndrome. Neuroradiology 1991;33(suppl):149–152.
31. Deramond H, Depriester C, Galibert P, et al. Percutaneous vertebroplasty with polymethylmethacrylate: technique, indications, and results. Radiol Clin North Am 1998:36:533–546.
32. Diamond TH, Bryant C, Browne L, et al. Clinical outcomes after acute osteoporotic vertebral fractures: a 2-year non-randomised trial comparing percutaneous vertebroplasty with conservative therapy. Med J Aust 2006;184:113–117.
33. Diamond TH, Champion B, Clark WA. Management of acute osteoporotic vertebral fractures: a nonrandomized trial comparing percutaneous vertebroplasty with conservative therapy. Am J Med 2003;114:257–265.
34. Diamond TH, Hartwell T, Clarke W, et al. Percutaneous vertebroplasty for acute vertebral body fracture and deformity in multiple myeloma: a short report. Br J Haematol 2004;124:485–487.
35. Ferretti JL, Cointry GR, Capozza RF. Bone mass, bone strength, muscle-bone interactions, osteopenias and osteoporoses. Mech Ageing Dev 2003;124:269–279.
36. Fourney DR, Schomer DF, Nader R. Percutaneous vertebroplasty and kyphoplasty for painful vertebral body fractures in cancer patients. J Neurosurg 2003;98(1 suppl):21–30.
37. Galibert P, Deramond H, Rosat P. [Preliminary note on the treatment of vertebral angioma by percutaneous acrylic vertebroplasty]. Neurochirurgie 1987;33:166–168.
38. Grados F, Depriester C, Cayrolle G, et al. Long-term observations of vertebral osteoporotic fractures treated by percutaneous vertebroplasty. Rheumatology (Oxford) 2000;39:1410–1414.
39. Hacein-Bey L, Baisden JL, Lemke DM, et al. Treating osteoporotic and neoplastic vertebral compression fractures with vertebroplasty and kyphoplasty. J Palliat Med 2005;8:931–938.
40. Hadjipavlou AG, Tzermiadianos NM, Katonis PG. Percutaneous vertebroplasty and balloon kyphoplasty for the treatment of osteoporotic vertebral compression fractures and osteolytic tumours. J Bone Joint Surg Br 2005;87:1595–1604.
41. Hansson T, Keller T, Jonson R. Fatigue fracture morphology in human lumbar motion segments. J Spinal Disord 1988;1:33–38.
42. Hansson T, Roos B. The relation between bone mineral content, experimental compression fractures, and disc degeneration in lumbar vertebrae. Spine 1981;6:147–153.
43. Hardouin P, Grados F, Cotten A. Should percutaneous vertebroplasty be used to treat osteoporotic fractures? An update. Joint Bone Spine 2001;68:216–221.
44. Harrington KD. Major neurological complications following percutaneous vertebroplasty with polymethylmethacrylate: a case report. J Bone Joint Surg Am 2001;83:1070–1073.
45. Harrop JS, Prpa B, Reinhardt MK, et al. Primary and secondary osteoporosis incidence of subse-

quent vertebral compression fractures after kyphoplasty. Spine 2004;29:2120–2125.
46. Heini PF, Berlemann U, Kaufmann M, et al. Augmentation of mechanical properties in osteoporotic vertebral bones: a biomechanical investigation of vertebroplasty efficacy with different bone cements. Eur Spine J 2001;10:164–171.
47. Heini PF, Orler R. [Vertebroplasty in severe osteoporosis: technique and experience with multisegment injection]. Orthopade 2004;33:22–30.
48. Heini PF, Walchli B, Berlemann U. Percutaneous transpedicular vertebroplasty with PMMA: operative technique and early results: a prospective study for the treatment of osteoporotic compression fractures. Eur Spine J 2000; 9:445–450.
49. Hentschel SJ, Burton AW, Fourney DR. Percutaneous vertebroplasty and kyphoplasty performed at a cancer center: refuting proposed contraindications. J Neurosurg Spine 2005;2:436–440.
50. Higgins KB, Harten RD, Langrana NA. Biomechanical effects of unipedicular vertebroplasty on intact vertebrae. Spine 2003;28:1540–1547; discussion 1548.
51. Hitchon PW, Goel V, Drake J, et al. Comparison of the biomechanics of hydroxyapatite and polymethylmethacrylate vertebroplasty in a cadaveric spinal compression fracture model. J Neurosurg 2001;95(2 suppl):215–220.
52. Ide C, Gangi A, Rimmelin A. Vertebral haemangiomas with spinal cord compression: the place of preoperative percutaneous vertebroplasty with methyl methacrylate. Neuroradiology 1996;38: 585–589.
53. Ikeuchi M, Yamamoto H, Shibata T, et al. Mechanical augmentation of the vertebral body by calcium phosphate cement injection. J Orthop Sci 2001;6:39–45.
54. Ismail AA, Cooper C, Felsenberg D, et al. Number and type of vertebral deformities: epidemiological characteristics and relation to back pain and height loss: European Vertebral Osteoporosis Study Group. Osteoporos Int 1999;9:206–213.
55. Jacofsky DJ, Papagelopoulos PJ, Sim FH. Advances and challenges in the surgical treatment of metastatic bone disease. Clin Orthop Relat Res 2003;(415 suppl):S14–S8.
56. Jang JS, Lee SH. Efficacy of percutaneous vertebroplasty combined with radiotherapy in osteolytic metastatic spinal tumors. J Neurosurg Spine 2005;2:243–248.
57. Jensen ME, Dion JE. Vertebroplasty relieves osteoporosis pain. Diagn Imaging (San Franc) 1997;19:68, 71–72.
58. Jensen, ME, Dion JE. Percutaneous vertebroplasty in the treatment of osteoporotic compression fractures. Neuroimaging Clin North Am 2000;10:547–568.
59. Jensen ME, Evans AJ, Mathis JM, et al. Percutaneous polymethylmethacrylate vertebroplasty in the treatment of osteoporotic vertebral body compression fractures: technical aspects. AJNR Am J Neuroradiol 1997;18:1897–1904.
60. Kayanja MM, Togawa D, Lieberman IJ. Biomechanical changes after the augmentation of experimental osteoporotic vertebral compression fractures in the cadaveric thoracic spine. Spine J 2005;5:55–63.
61. Keller TS, Kosmopoulos V, Lieberman IH. Vertebroplasty and kyphoplasty affect vertebral motion segment stiffness and stress distributions: a microstructural finite-element study. Spine 2005; 30:1258–1265.
62. Kim SH, Kang HS, Choi JA, et al. Risk factors of new compression fractures in adjacent vertebrae after percutaneous vertebroplasty. Acta Radiol 2004;45:440–445.
63. Kosmopoulos V, Keller TS. Damage-based finite-element vertebroplasty simulations. Eur Spine J 2004;13:617–625.
64. Lane JM, Hong R, Koob J, et al. Kyphoplasty enhances function and structural alignment in multiple myeloma. Clin Orthop Relat Res 2004; 426:49–53.
65. Laredo JD, Hamze B. Complications of percutaneous vertebroplasty and their prevention. Semin Ultrasound CT MR 2005;26:65–80.
66. Levine SA, Perin LA, Hayes D, et al. An evidence-based evaluation of percutaneous vertebroplasty. Manag Care 2000;9:56–60, 63.
67. Lieberman I, Reinhardt MK. Vertebroplasty and kyphoplasty for osteolytic vertebral collapse. Clin Orthop Relat Res 2003;415 (suppl):S176–S186.
68. Liebschner MA, Rosenberg WS, Keaveny TM. Effects of bone cement volume and distribution on vertebral stiffness after vertebroplasty. Spine 2001;26:1547–1554.
69. Lim TH, Brebach GT, Renner SM, et al. A Biomechanical evaluation of an injectable calcium phosphate cement for vertebroplasty. Spine 2002;27: 1297–1302.
70. Lindsay R, Silverman SL, Cooper C, et al. Risk of new vertebral fracture in the year following a fracture. JAMA 2001;285:320–323.
71. Martin JB Jean B, Sugiu KD, et al. Vertebroplasty: clinical experience and follow-up results. Bone 1999;25(2 suppl):11S–15S.

72. Masala S, Roselli M, Massari F, et al. Radiofrequency heat ablation and vertebroplasty in the treatment of neoplastic vertebral body fractures. Anticancer Res 2004;24:3129–3133.
73. McGraw JK, Lippert JA, Minkus KD, et al. Prospective evaluation of pain relief in 100 patients undergoing percutaneous vertebroplasty: results and follow-up. J Vasc Interv Radiol 2002; 13:883–886.
74. Molloy S, Mathis JM, Belkoff SM. The effect of vertebral body percentage fill on mechanical behavior during percutaneous vertebroplasty. Spine 2003;28:1549–1554.
75. Murphy KJ, Deramond H. Percutaneous vertebroplasty in benign and malignant disease. Neuroimaging Clin North Am 2000;10:535–545.
76. Orthovita, www.orthovita.com. 2006.
77. Polikeit A, Nolte LP, Ferguson SJ, et al. The effect of cement augmentation on the load transfer in an osteoporotic functional spinal unit: finite-element analysis. Spine 2003;28:991–996.
78. Rapado A. General management of vertebral fractures. Bone 1996;18(3 suppl):191S–196S.
79. Ross PD, Davis JW, Epstein RS. Pre-existing fractures and bone mass predict vertebral fracture incidence in women. Ann Intern Med 1991;114: 919–923.
80. Ross PD, Ettinger B, Davis JW, et al. Evaluation of adverse health outcomes associated withvertebral fractures. Osteoporos Int 1991;1:134–140.
81. Sun K. A finite element approach towards biomechanical optimization of prophylactic vertebroplasty. Thesis, Department of Bioengineering, Houston: Rice University 2006.
82. Sun K, Liebschner MA. Biomechanics of prophylactic vertebral reinforcement. Spine 2004;29: 1428–1435; discussion, 1435.
83. Sun K, Liebschner MA. Evolution of vertebroplasty: a biomechanical perspective. Ann Biomed Eng 2004;32:77–91.
84. Sun K, Tawackoli W, Fukshansky M, et al. Disperse cement filling is more important than cement material properties in biomechanics of vertebroplasty. 21st Annual Meeting of the North American Spine Society, NASS 2006, Seattle, WA, July 23–27, 2006.
85. Liebschner M, Sun K, Tawackoli W, et al. Aggressive vertebroplasty reduces adjacent strength and may lead to premature vertebral bone failure. Bone Innovation Summit, 2006, Cleveland, OH, May 3–5, 2006.
86. Syed MI, Jan S, Patel NA, et al. Fatal fat embolism after vertebroplasty: identification of the high-risk patient. AJNR Am J Neuroradiol 2006;27:343–345.
87. Tohmeh AG, Mathis JM, Fenton DC, et al. Biomechanical efficacy of unipedicular versus bipedicular vertebroplasty for the management of osteoporotic compression fractures. Spine 1999; 24:1772–1776.
88. Trout AT, Kallmes DF, Kaufmann TJ. New fractures after vertebroplasty: adjacent fractures occur significantly sooner. AJNR Am J Neuroradiol 2006;27:217–223.
89. Tschirhart CE, Roth SE, Whyne CM. Biomechanical assessment of stability in the metastatic spine following percutaneous vertebroplasty: effects of cement distribution patterns and volume. J Biomech 2005;38:1582–1590.
90. Uppin AA, Hirsch JA, Centenera LV, et al. Occurrence of new vertebral body fracture after percutaneous vertebroplasty in patients with osteoporosis. Radiology 2003;226:119–124.
91. Villarraga ML, Bellezza AJ, Harrigan TP, et al. The biomechanical effects of kyphoplasty on treated and adjacent nontreated vertebral bodies. J Spinal Disord Tech 2005;18:84–91.
92. Wasnich RD. Vertebral fracture epidemiology. Bone 1996;18(3 suppl):179S–183S.
93. Watts NB, Harris ST, Genant HK, et al. Treatment of painful osteoporotic vertebral fractures with percutaneous vertebroplasty or kyphoplasty. Osteoporos Int 2001;12:429–437.
94. Weill A, Chiras J, Simon JM, et al. Spinal metastases: indications for and results of percutaneous injection of acrylic surgical cement. Radiology 1996;199:241–247.
95. Wenger M, Markwalder TM. Surgically controlled, transpedicular methyl methacrylate vertebroplasty with fluoroscopic guidance. Acta Neurochir (Wien) 1999;141:625–631.
96. Whyne CM, Hu SS, Lotz JC. Parametric finite element analysis of vertebral bodies affected by tumors. J Biomech 2001;34:1317–1324.
97. Wilson DR, Myers ER, Mathis JM, et al. Effect of augmentation on the mechanics of vertebral wedge fractures. Spine 2000;25:158–165.
98. Winking M, Stahl JP, Oertel M, et al. [Polymethylmethacrylate-vertebroplasty: a new and effective method of pain treatment in vertebral compression]. Dtsch Med Wochenschr 2003;128: 2525–2530.

Advances in the Management of Hypervascular Tumors of the Spine

A. Hadjipavlou, K. Kakavelakis, E. Pateromichelakis, P. Katonis

10

INTRODUCTION

Tumors of the spine are more difficult to manage than their counterparts in the appendicular skeleton, mostly because they are located in areas that are difficult to access, often in close proximity to vital neurovascular elements.

Optimal surgical management of spinal tumors consists of decompression of neural elements with wide excision of the tumor mass, reconstruction of spinal structures, and stabilization with instrumentation.

The most commonly encountered hypervascular tumors in the spine are (a) primary tumors, which include hemangiomas, aneurysmal bone cysts, osteoblastomas, and hemangioendotheliosarcomas; and (b) metastatic tumors, which include renal cell carcinomas, hepatoma, hypervascular pheochromocytomas, and infrequently, certain types of adenocarcinomas, multiple myelomas, and cancers of the thyroid.

Hypervascular tumors of the spine are extremely challenging. Profuse intraoperative bleeding usually interferes with radical excision of the tumor; surgery may even have to be aborted. This in turn potentially results in compromised outcomes with high morbidity and mortality. For this reason, several modalities have been suggested as an adjunct or as an alternative to surgery. These procedures include cell saver, radiation therapy, transarterial embolization, intralesional injections of various substances, vertebral cement augmentation through vertebroplasty or kyphoplasty techniques, thermal ablation (cryotherapy, etc.), and combinations of various modalities. Each of these procedures has its advantages and its disadvantages.

Cell Saver

Cell saver can be helpful in some cases but is not optimal in patients with malignant tumors to save blood and minimize transfusions. Reinfusion of irradiated red blood cells is a possible solution (40). However, this does not prevent intraoperative bleeding that interferes with surgery.

Radiation Therapy

According to Tong et al. (89) and Ratanatharatorn et al. (72), who reviewed the existing literature on the outcomes of radiation, the reports are not satisfactory. The overall effectiveness rates were 54% for complete response and was obtained in only 50% of patients. The relapse rate of the patients who survived at least 12 weeks was 30%.

Radiation therapy can reduce the vascularity of hypervascular tumors, but it is not an ideal alternative in their management; the response is often neither immediate nor effective. Furthermore, healing can be compromised, predisposing to infections. Treating benign lesions with radiotherapy is controversial because of the unacceptable risk of severe complications. Reported complications include postradiation myelopathy, radiation-induced sarcoma, and possible growth disturbance in children (30,51,52,69,76,83). Papagelopoulos et al. (69) reported a case of postradiation osteosarcoma that occurred 7 years after radiation for a spinal aneurysmal bone cyst and that resulted in death of the patient.

Some promote radiation therapy as the treatment of choice for vertebral hemangiomas, particularly for multiple spinal involvement (10,23). Vertebral hemangiomas are sensitive to radiation and respond to doses of 2,000 to 4,000 cGy (37,57). However, the recommended dose of 2 Gy per day for several weeks precludes the immediate effectiveness of radiation therapy; therefore, radiation is not recommended in acute situations. Furthermore, no clear dose–response relation has been reported, and complete pain relief after irradiation ranges from 37% to 87.5% (4,93). Radiographic regression of the lesion is often minimal. A review article that included 21 reports of 63 cases of vertebral hemangiomas demonstrated that, overall, radiotherapy resulted in a complete remission of symptoms in 57% of cases, partial remission in 32%, and no response in 11% of cases (45). Radiation also has the potential risk of radionecrosis (37,62) and may induce sarcoma (54,67).

Transarterial Embolization

Transarterial embolization of spinal hypervascular tumors has been described as both a primary therapeutic measure (22,48) and an adjunct to surgical resection (12,28,61,68).

The goal of preoperative transarterial embolization is to improve perioperative blood loss to facilitate more-radical resectability of the tumor. Transarterial embolization has been promoted as a safe and effective procedure for treating hypervascular spinal tumors (Fig. 10.1). The most commonly used embolic materials are polyvinyl alcohol foam, gelfoam particles, absolute alcohol sponges, and metallic coils, as well combinations of these materials. Results of embolization largely depend on the materials used. Gelfoam particles have been used in early studies. Proximal gelfoam occlusion may augment the distal thrombosis within the tumor and produce a transient devascularization of the region adjacent to the tumor. However, proximal occlusion of large vessels without penetration into the tumor architecture results in ineffective embolization with very early recanalization through enzymatic resorption of the material. Rapid revascularization of the tumor was observed within 3 days from adjacent collaterals, resulting in considerable intraoperative bleeding (34). For this reason, surgery should be undertaken within 24 hours after gelfoam particle embolization. Polyvinyl alcohol, composed of nonresorbable particles of 150- to 250-mm, diameter allows relatively distal embolization at the capillary level (68). After polyvinyl alcohol particle embolization, the same arteries can be occluded proximally by using gelfoam. Absolute ethanol has also been successfully used for preoperative embolization of spinal metastases from renal cancer because of its deep penetration and intimal sclerosis with inflammatory reaction (85). However, the use of liquid embolization agents for spinal metastases has been associated with a high rate of neurologic complications (8,75). Additional use of coils after polyvinyl alcohol particle embolization has been reported to provide no further benefit (9).

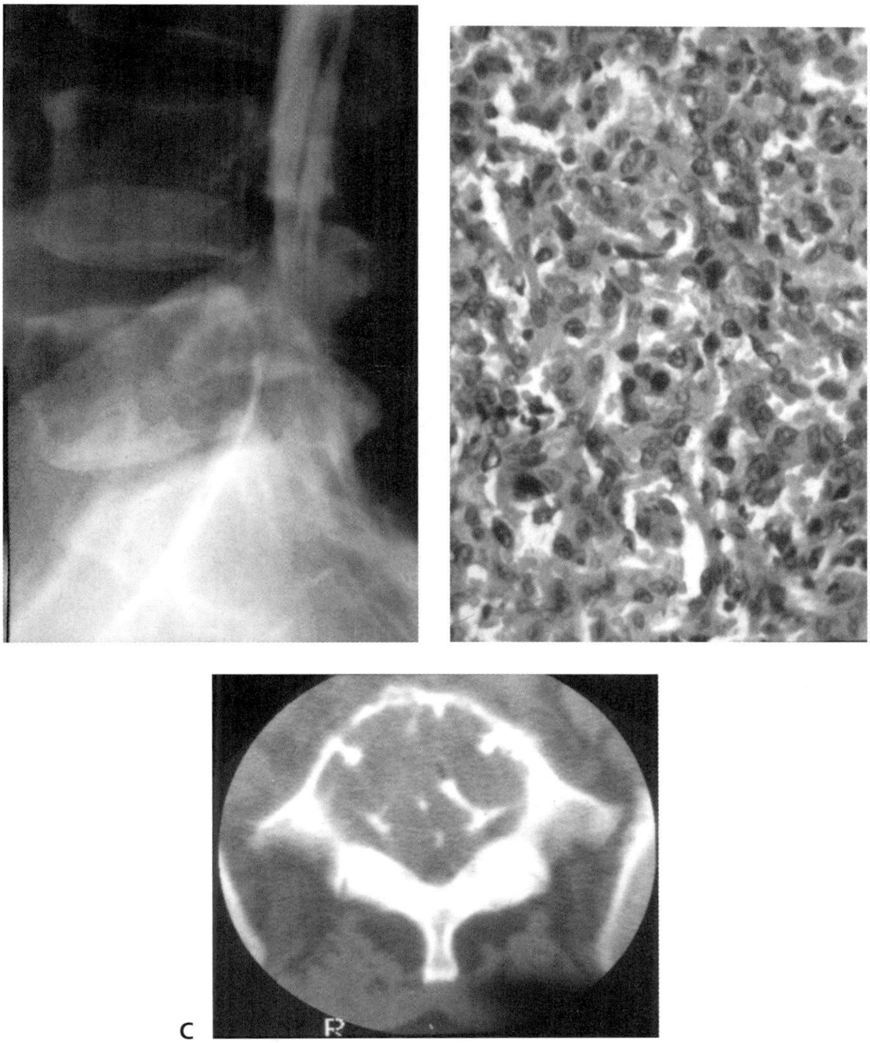

FIGURE 10.1 A 45-year-old male patient with severe back pain and weakness in the legs. Myelogram demonstrates complete block at L4–L5 level (**A**). Profuse bleeding was encountered during biopsy (estimated blood loss, 4,000 ml), which demonstrated aggressive hemangioendotheliosarcoma (**B**). Axial CT scan demonstrated a destructive osteolytic lesion caused. (**C**)The patient scored 9 on the Tokuhashi scale (From Tokuhashi Y, Matsuzaki H, Toriyama S, et al. Scoring system for the preoperative evaluation of metastatic spine tumor prognosis. Spine 1990;15:1110–3, with permission.) which is an evaluation system for the prognosis of metastatic spine tumors. It is a useful guideline for selecting the appropriate surgical approach. *(Continued)*

hemangioendotheliosarcoma

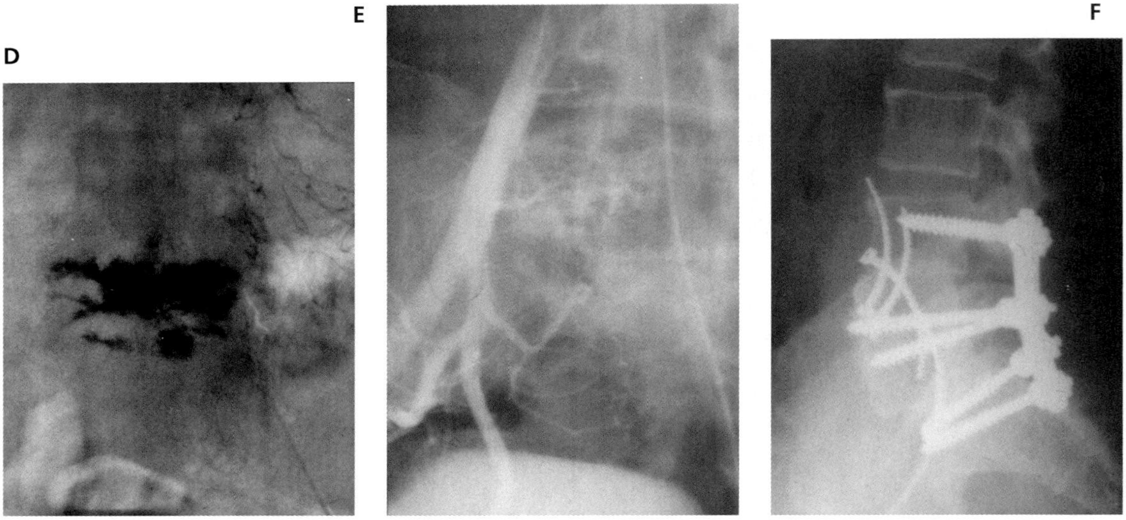

FIGURE 10.1 *(Continued)* The patient underwent three repeated successful transarterial embolizations (**D**) that dramatically reduced the vascularity (**E**) of the lesion that allowed successful radical anterior and posterior excision of the whole L5 vertebra. Reconstruction was achieved by means of allograft and transpedicular posterior instrumentation. (**F**) Radical surgery resulted in an excellent outcome. At last follow-up 15 years after surgery, the patient was free of tumor.

After transarterial embolization, the expected average perioperative blood loss may range from 1.5 to 2.2 L in the lumbar and thoracic spine (11,34,53,68,73,82,84,85), as opposed to 5 to 15 L blood loss when preoperative embolization is not used (34,53,73).

In our series of 10 cases, in which a preoperative embolization alone was conducted, intraoperative estimated blood loss in excess of 3 L occurred in five cases. Mean estimated blood loss was 2.8 L. In one of our patients, bleeding was profuse (>8 L), and surgery was prematurely terminated, resulting in suboptimal tumor resection (61). The mean intraoperative blood loss after preoperative embolization in the cervical spine is 2.4 L (90). However, transarterial embolization of tumors in the cervical spine is technically more difficult and involves a higher risk of neurologic complications (18,23,27,47,73). Frequent anastomoses between the carotid, vertebral, and subclavian artery branches increase the risk of cerebral or spinal cord embolization, although ring anastomoses at the base of the brain allow occlusion of one of the main arteries entering the neurocranium (8,35,58,88). In several situations, successful embolization may not be possible. Embolization may be incomplete because of peculiarities of vascular anatomy or because embolization into vessels feeding the tumor may potentially compromise the vascularity of the spinal cord. The presence of an anterior spinal artery at the same pedicle is a contraindication for embolization (84). The untoward embolization of an anterior spinal artery may injure the pyramidal tracts and cause severe motor deficits (15). Although partial embolization seems to reduce blood loss in most patients, this may not be sufficient to prevent profuse bleeding during the procedure (53,73). Angiography may also fail to encounter feeding vessels that could be embolized (3). Finally, the watershed area of the mid-thoracic spine embolization may well be too dangerous in which to perform (86).

Surgical techniques for decreasing blood loss in tumors that are incompletely embolized involve adjacent-level segmental artery ligation and the use of *en bloc* rather than piecemeal resection.

Preoperative coil embolization has failed to show any significant effect on intraoperative blood loss in hypervascular spinal metastases (9), especially in metastases from renal cell carcinoma that may open collateral channels within hours.

Even technically successful and subjectively complete transarterial embolization may fail to eliminate intraoperative bleeding satisfactorily. Complete devascularization of a hypervascular tumor requires that precapillaries, capillaries, and even the proximal parts of the draining veins are occluded by depositing the embolic agents as deeply into the tumor as possible (55). Distribution of embolizing particles can be less than optimal when multiple feeders supply the microvascular tumor bed. Furthermore, tumors like metastatic renal cell carcinoma have irregular arterial feeders, widespread networks of arteriovenous shunts, and dilated capillaries, resulting in rapid circulation with early venous drainage (49,55). Furthermore after successful transarterial embolization, the remaining central tumor core can recruit previously minor arterial supply in response to the occlusion of its primary arterial feeders (79).

In conclusion, the overall reported outcomes of preoperative transarterial embolization are suboptimal. This has led to the use of alternative techniques such as intralesional injection of various agents, cryotherapy, and vertebral-body cement augmentation. These therapeutic interventions can be used as adjuncts to surgery or as stand-alone procedures.

Intralesional Injection of *N*-butyl cyanoacrylate or sclerosing agents [ethanol alcohol, bleomycin, OK-432 (Picibanil), Ethiblock]

Direct intralesional injection can be useful in tumors with a peculiar vascular anatomy or when embolization into the feeding vessels is not recommended (e.g., in watershed areas of the mid-thoracic spine, or failure to encounter the feeding vessels). Direct intralesional injection of a sclerosing agent has several advantages. The procedure is minimally invasive, can be performed under local anesthesia and intravenous sedation, and usually does not entail significant blood loss. Herbreteau et al. (44) reported a case of a metastasis located in the fourth cervical vertebra, and Chiras et al. (17) reported on a hypervascular pheochromocytoma metastasis of the sixth cervical vertebral body that were both successfully managed preoperatively by a direct intravertebral injection of an alcoholic embolizing emulsion. Cotten et al. (20) reported intralesional percutaneous injection of *N*-butyl cyanoacrylate, a rapidly polymerizing cyanoacrylate plastic, into the posterior arch to minimize blood loss during decompressive laminectomy in four patients with vertebral hemangiomas with neurologic compression. More recently, Schirmer et al. (79) reported five cases with metastatic renal cell carcinoma to the spine treated with a combination of transarterial embolization and direct percutaneous injection of *N*-butyl cyanoacrylate. They theorize that direct intralesional injection achieves closer to a true end-organ embolization at the level of the capillary bed than does the more proximal occlusion of the blood supply at the level of small arterioles that is usually achieved by transarterial embolization. The injected material assumes the form of the entire tumor, including a portion of the epidural component, without changing its volume, thus minimizing the risk of neurologic deficit. The embolized tumor maintains a soft consistency and can be readily removed in a piecemeal fashion. Intralesional embolization can effectively reduce tumor vascularity and result in decreased blood loss compared with preoperative transarterial embolization. The estimated blood loss during surgery reported in the series of Schirmer ranged from 300 to 800 ml. However, a possible drawback to this technique is the risk of retrograde flow of embolic material through a feeder artery. Casasco et al. (14) described this complication when treating juvenile nasopharyngeal angiofibromas at the cranial base in two patients. They encountered a fatal polymerization of *N*-butyl cyanoacrylate in the middle cerebral artery in one patient, and embolization of a collateral of the ophthalmic artery in another patient, resulting in vision loss. For this reason, direct *N*-butyl cyanoacrylate injection should be avoided into any tumor receiving arterial supply from a vessel leading to a spinal or cerebral artery.

Sclerosing agents are substances that cause marked tissue irritation and thrombosis with subsequent local inflammation and tissue necrosis. This inflammation and tissue necrosis result in fibrosis and tissue contraction. The most popular sclerosing agents are Ethibloc alcohol, bleomycin, and OK-432 (Picibanil).

Ethibloc is a sclerosing agent that has been used in the treatment of hypervascular tumors of the spine. It is an emulsion of zein, alcohol, oleum papaveris, propylene glycol, and a contrast medium that thickens immediately when in contact with aqueous solution (2,50). Ethibloc injection in an aneurysmal bone cyst of C2 in a 4-year-old boy resulted in embolization of the material to the vertebrobasilar system, with subsequent fatal brainstem and cerebellar infarctions (70).

Alcohol has been used in treating varicose veins for more than a century. It is the most potent sclerosant, quickly diluted, inexpensive, and readily available. Its mode of action involves injuring the vascular endothelium and denaturing blood protein, which results in an intense thrombosis. Alcohol is typically used in the venous type of malformation and has been mainly applied in the management of spinal hemangiomas.

Intralesional alcohol injection is an effective procedure for the management of vascular vertebral hemangiomas associated with pain, neurologic compromise, or both (38). Successful intralesional ethanol alcohol injection for the treatment of vertebral hemangiomas with spinal cord compression was first described by Heiss et al. (41), and subsequently reported by others either as a stand-alone procedure (7,24,36,59) or in combination surgery (59). However, serious complications have been reported after treatment with alcohol injection, including Brown-Sequard syndrome (one case report) (65), cardiac arrest (patient recovered after intravenous administration of atropine) (51), and pathologic fractures caused by osteonecrosis (1,24). The incidence of pathologic fractures ranges from 21% to 28.5% (24,36). To prevent these potential complications, in our series of 10 vertebral hemangiomas, we treated three hypervascular hemangiomas combining intralesional alcohol injection with balloon kyphoplasty by using PMMA bone cement. Transient deterioration of neurologic status after intralesional alcohol injection has also been reported as another potential side effect of this treatment (36). Neurologic complications were not encountered in our series. We injected 15 ml of absolute alcohol at a rate of 2 ml per 10 minutes, as suggested in the literature (41,65). Alcohol can be made radioopaque by mixing it with metrizamide powder to allow a more precise administration. By injecting the ethanol at a very slow rate, one may prevent retrograde flow from the hemangiomas through the capillary leading to the feeding arteries. Unlike transarterial embolization, which cannot be used more than once because it occludes the feeding arteries, and unlike radiation, which is limited by constraints on dosage, intralesional ethanol alcohol injection can be repeated as needed to obliterate residual hemangiomas. Local anesthesia and mild sensation allow neurologic monitoring during the procedure (41).

The success rate of intralesional alcohol injection alone ranges from 75% to 100% (7,24,36,59).

Percutaneous Cement Augmentation

We are familiar with two techniques of percutaneous vertebral body (VB) cement augmentation: vertebroplasty (VP) and balloon kyphoplasty (BK). The technique of VP was first conceived and performed by Deramond and Galibert (21,31) for an aggressive hemangioma of the cervical spine in 1984, and subsequently reported in 1987. VB cement augmentation has become a popular technique for the treatment of benign or malignant osteolytic bone tumors (hemangiomas, myelomas, lymphomas, and various metastatic tumors) that predispose to pathologic fracture. Many osteolytic metastatic lesions often become refractory to chemotherapy and radiation therapy, and patients are often too moribund to undergo palliative major reconstructive surgery. In these situations, an ideal solution is a minimally invasive surgery such as percutaneous BK or percutaneous VP, which addresses both vertebral body stability and pain. For the management of hypervascular tumors, whether primary or metastatic, VB cement-augmentation techniques can be used either alone or as adjuncts to other surgical procedures such as laminectomy, instrumentation, cryotherapy, intralesional sclerotic agents, and radiofrequency ablation. We describe the application of BK alone or in combination with other modalities for the management of hemangiomas and malignant hypervascular tumors.

Vertebral Hemangiomas

Vertebral hemangiomas are usually asymptomatic and discovered incidentally during imaging investigations. A small proportion, however, may develop symptoms related to variable degrees of pain and neurologic deficit. Vertebral hemangiomas can compromise the neural tissue and cause neurologic deficit by several mechanisms involving concentric narrowing of the spinal canal, bone intrusion into the canal after fracture, vertebral enlargement with ballooning of the posterior vertebral wall into the spinal canal, soft tissue extension of the lesion into the spinal canal, and spontaneous or traumatic bleeding of the tumor into the epidural space (3,37). Pregnancy, particularly during the last 3 months of gestation, can precipitate neurologic complications in 10% of patients (16,62).

Several options are available for the management of symptomatic vertebral hemangiomas, including surgical resection and spinal stabilization (29,61), transarterial embolization (43), intralesional alcohol injection (41), radiotherapy (26), vertebroplasty (21,63), and kyphopasty (5,66).

Each of these procedures has its advantages and disadvantages. An open surgical approach is a major procedure. The hypervascularity of the lesions may provoke serious complications such as profuse bleeding (61) and consumptive coagulopathy (Kassabach–Merritt syndrome) (78,80). Embolization of the feeding artery is not always useful, because it may not reduce intraoperative bleeding (61). Radiation therapy is not the ideal treatment (see Radiation Therapy). Translesional embolization, although beneficial in the presence of neurologic deficit (42) by devascularizing the tumor, is not as effective in controlling vertebral pain as are other treatments. The overall success rate of intralesional injection of pure alcohol is reported to range from 75% (1) to 85% (36), with 72% in the presence of paraplegia (91) (see Translesional Embolization of Sclerosing Substances).

The success rate for the management of VH with VP is reported to range from 71.4% to 91.6% (19,32,33,36,60,87). Only two case reports exist using BK; one of these reports involved the management of a painful sacral hemangioma (5), and the other, a T-12 hemangioma (66).

Cement leakage is less likely to occur during BK than during VP (39). For this reason, we decided to use BK with polymethylmethacrylate bone cement (PMMA) for the management of symptomatic VH.

Ten of our patients underwent 12 surgical procedures on 15 VBs (lumbar: 10; thoracic: 5). The indications were (a) painful hemangiomas (eight patients had 13 BKs alone); (b) severe back pain with Frankel C paraplegia from cord compression caused by soft tissue extension from a thoracic vertebral hemangioma (one patient: underwent BK and intralesional alcohol injection); (c) acute bleeding causing Frankel B paraplegia from asymptomatic vascular hemangioma (one patient: underwent laminectomy and BK). Seven patients exhibited features of vascular (aggressive) hemagiomas, and three exhibited lipomatous (nonaggressive) hemagiomas. One patient who underwent a unilateral BK had recurrence of symptoms from the nontreated side of the VB hemangioma, which was also subsequently treated successfully with BK. BK was carried out successfully and safely in all 10 patients, with excellent outcomes at follow-up periods ranging from 6 to 48 months.

Epidural bleeding from vertebral hemangioma either can be precipitated by trauma or can occur spontaneously (16). Strong evidence in the literature recommends treating spinal cord compression with surgical decompression alone, or combining treatment with surgical decompression and either vertebroplasty, arterial embolization, or intralesional alcohol injection (21,46,61). Spinal decompression is usually highly effective (1), but nevertheless may not always provide the expected results. Not all patients in whom neurologic deficits develop from compression and who are treated by combining laminectomy and vertebroplasty are expected to regain complete neurologic function (13). Furthemore, Purkayashda et al. (71) observed only a mild to moderate regression of epidural extension of hemangioma after embolization or intralesional alcohol injection. Surgical decompression should be entertained for severe paraparesis (Frankel B or C) or for failure of other procedures (6,29,56) (Figs. 10.2 and 10.3)

According to Brunot (13), repeated vertebroplasty for recurrent symptoms was reported in 19% of patients in their series. We also encountered this in the patient mentioned earlier in whom partial recurrence of symptoms developed, necessitating BK in the opposite side. We therefore infer that to prevent similar events, a complete obliteration of vertebral hemangioma through a biportal BK may be appropriate.

From our data and review of the literature, the following conclusions can be drawn. Aggressive vascular hemangiomas usually manifest with pain, whereas nonaggressive lipomatous hemangiomas are asymptomatic. Moreover, aggressive vascular hemangiomas may remain asymptomatic until the occurrence of serious complications, such as paraplegia. However, lipid-filled hemangiomas, particularly those that are large, may occasionally become symptomatic (38).

Because intralesional alcohol injection is frequently associated with avascular necrosis and pathologic fractures, it is reasonable to stabilize the vertebrae with cement augmentation. An extensive review of the literature (39) revealed that BK is associated with less cement leakage compared with VP. For this reason, we prefer BK for vertebral-body cement augmentation. If a unilateral approach does not obliterate the hemangiomatous lesion, then a bilateral approach is recommended to prevent a recurrence of symptoms.

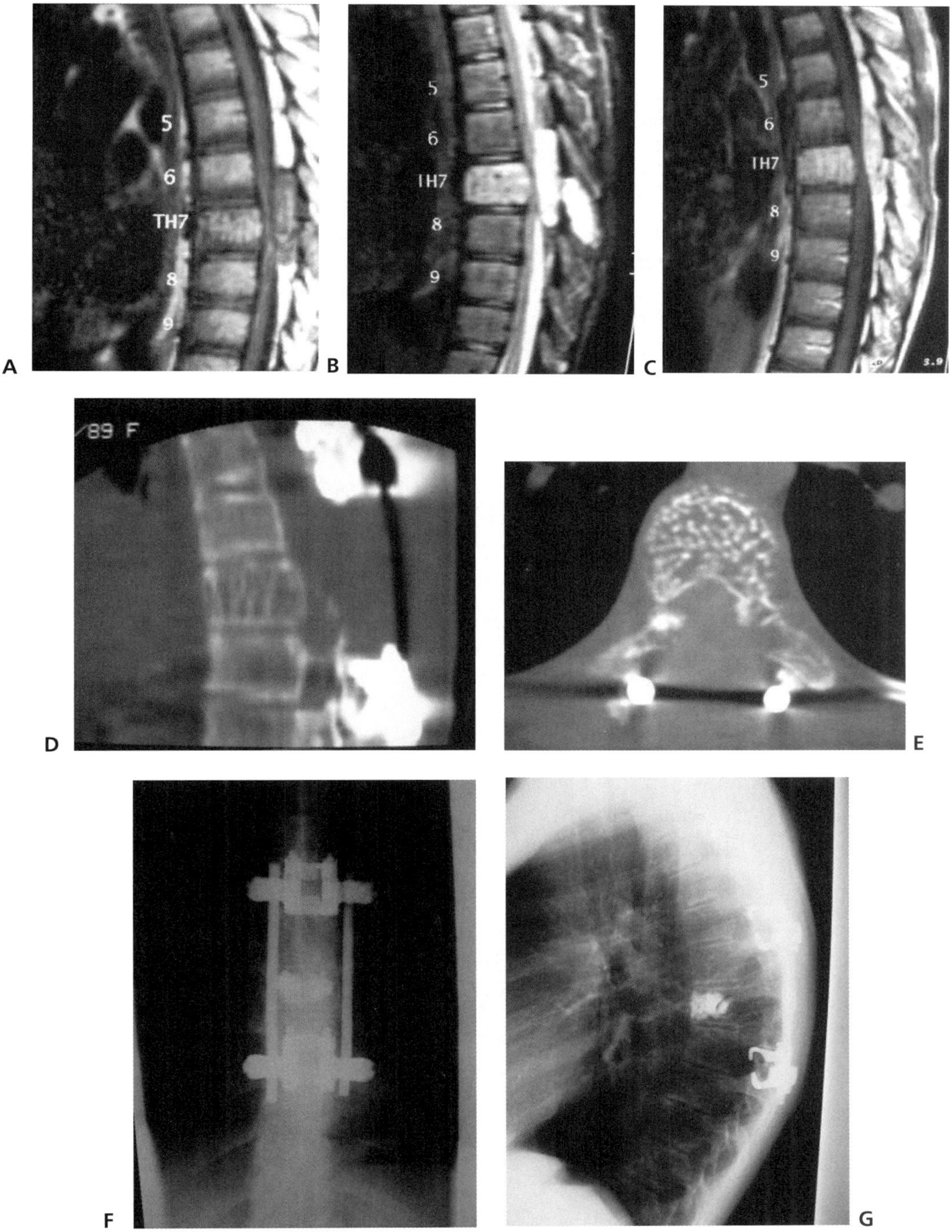

FIGURE 10.2 Images demonstrating the appearance of an aggressive vertebral body hemangioma with epidural bleeding. There is a hypointense signal on T_1-weighted image (A), hyperintense on T_2-weighted image (**B**), and hyperintense on gadolinium-enhanced T1-weighted image of the 7th thoracic vertebra (**C**). Sagittal view of postoperative CT scan demonstrates successful decompression of an aggressive lesion (ballooning of the vertebral body with expansion of the posterior wall into the spinal canal) (**D**). Axial CT view shows the typical polka-dot appearance and extension of the lesion into the pedicles and transverse processes. Successful balloon kyphoplasty and posterior instrumentation, as seen on plain radiographs (**E**). Anteroposterior (**F**) and lateral (**G**) views. [From Hadjipavlou A, et al. J Bone Joint Surgery [Br] 2007;89:495–502 with permission.]

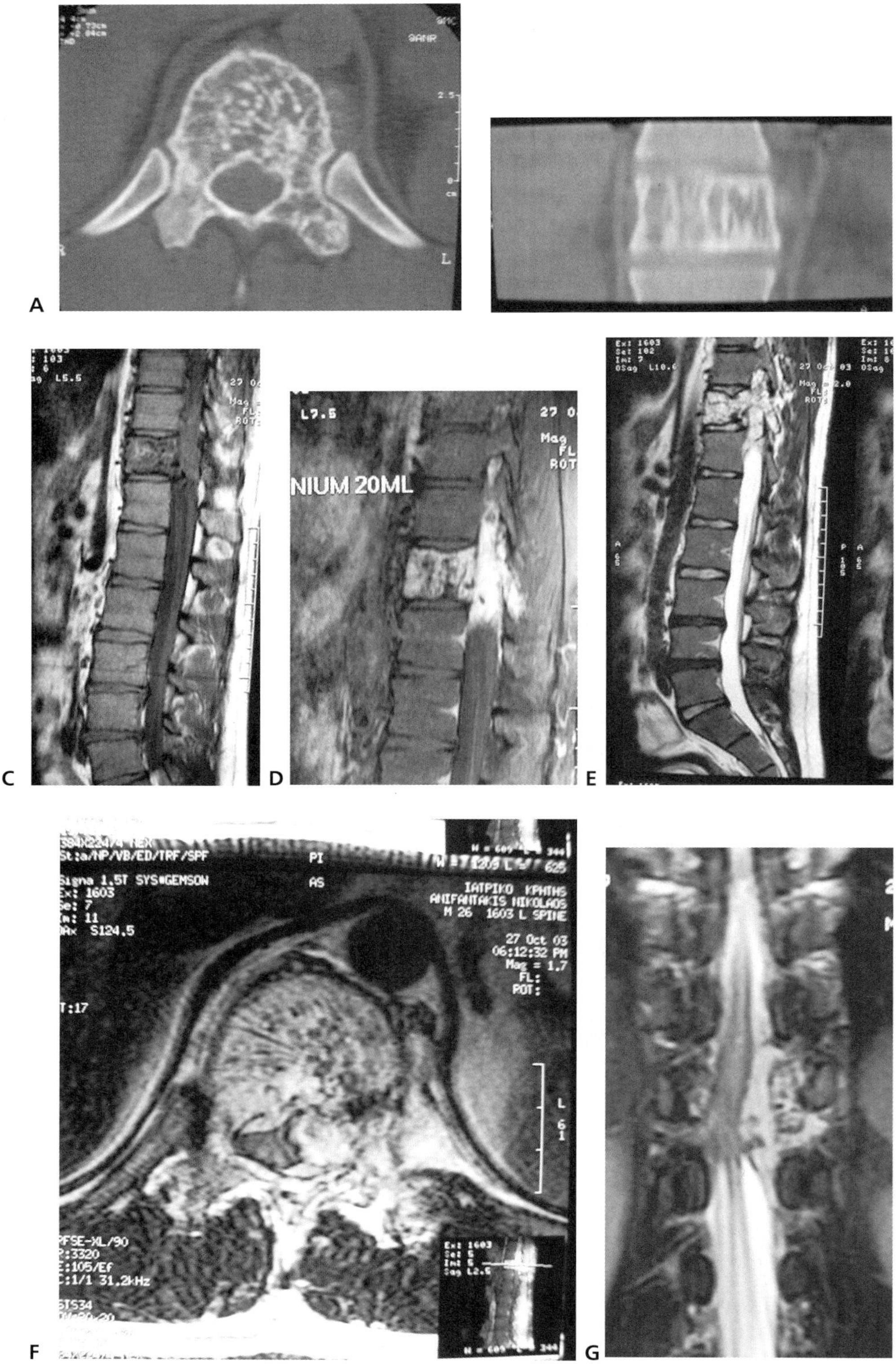
A
B
C
D
NIUM 20ML
E
27 Oct 03
F
G

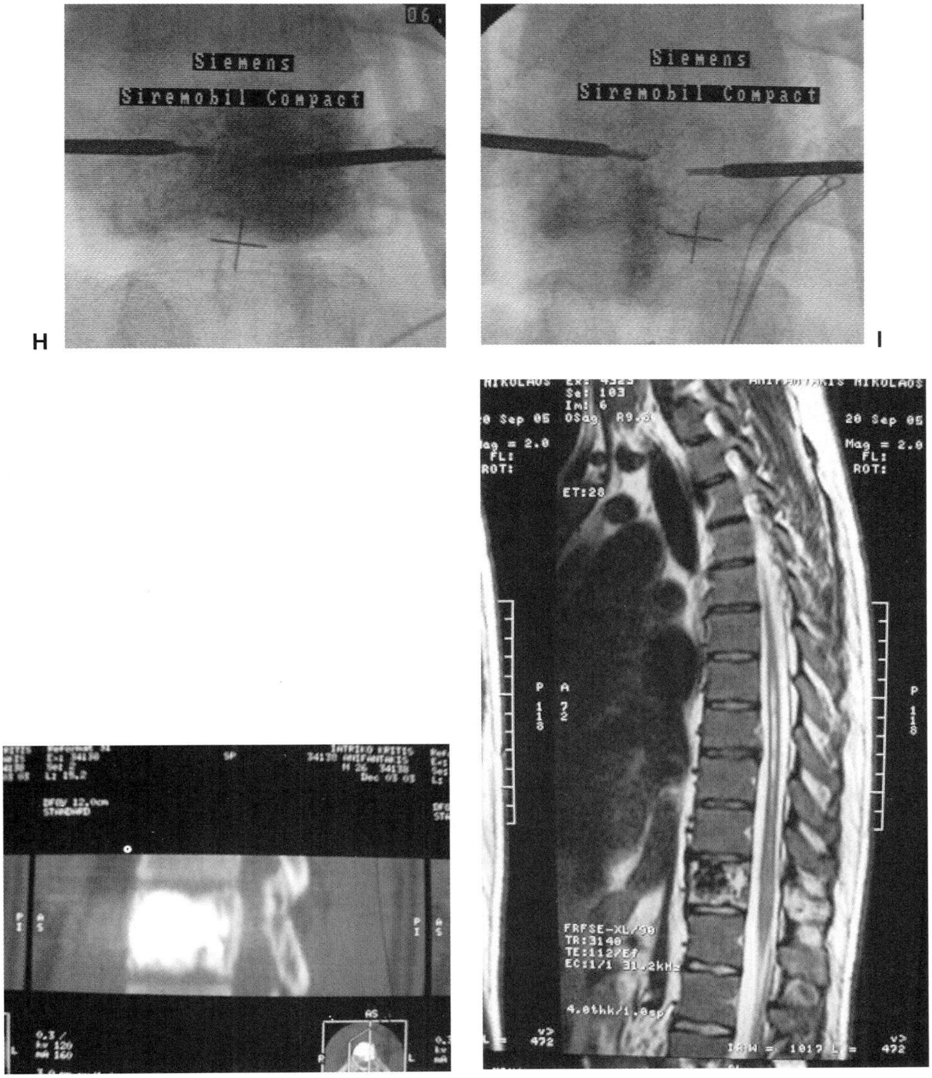

H I J K

FIGURE 10.3 Axial CT views demonstrating "polka-dot" appearance of thickened trabeculae (**A**), sagittal CT reformating images demonstrating cavernous hemangioma with thickened trabeculae simulating "corduroy-cloth" pattern (**B**). Sagittal T1-weighted MRI demonstrates mottled low signal intensity of T-11 vertebral body and soft tissue extension into the spinal canal (**C**). Gadolinium-enhanced T_1-weighted image demonstrates hypervascularity of the whole vertebral body with soft tissue extension into the spinal canal, compromising the spinal cord (**D**). Extension of the lesion posteriorly into the pedicle neural arch and facet are seen on T_2-weighted MRI. These findings indicate an aggressive vascular hemangioma (**E**). Axial (**F**) and frontal (**G**) views of gadolinium-enhanced T_1-weighted MRI, demonstrating a soft tissue hemangioma occupying the lateral one half of the spinal canal, displacing the spinal cord to the right. [From Hadjipavlou et al. J Bone Joint Surg [Br] 2007;89:495–502, with permission]. Direct transosseous (Ultravist 300, Schering AG, Germany) venography of T-11 vertebral body through a transpedicular approach (anteroposterior view) before intraosseous alcohol injection (**H**) and after intraosseous alcohol injection (**I**). Midsagittal CT scan view showing a successful postoperative bone-cement enhancement after balloon kyphoplasty. (**J**) Twelve months postoperative T_2-weighted MRI sequence demonstrating complete resolution of the soft tissue hemangioma in the spinal canal (**K**).

For the management of painful vertebral hemangiomas, we suggest the following flow chart (38):

1. Hemangiomas limited to the vertebral body can be treated with BK alone.
2. Hemangiomas complicated with paraplegia caused by acute bleeding can be addressed with spinal decompression with or without instrumentation and BK to stabilize VBs and prevent further bleeding.
3. Hemangiomas that extend posteriorly into the neural arch can be managed with BK for the VB hemangioma and intralesional ethanol alcohol injection into the posterior arch.
4. For the treatment of hemangioma with extension into the spinal canal with or without neurologic compromise, intraosseous venography and subsequent intralesional injection of ethanol alcohol should be followed by BK.

Hypervascular Tumors

We have also applied VB cement augmentation for the management of hypervascular hepatoma and two cases of renal cell carcinomas. The latter are notoriously the most hypervascular malignant tumor and refractory to radiation therapy and chemotherapy. One patient with renal cell carcinoma underwent VPs in the cervical spine and BKs in the thoracic and lumbar spine with spinal instrumentation (Fig. 10.4). Two other patients underwent minimally invasive surgery with maximized effects. One patient with hepatoma underwent BK and laminectomy, and one patient with renal cell carcinoma, BK and spinal stabilization through minimally invasive transpedicular instrumentation (Pathfinder; Abbot Co., Austin, TX).

The tumor is so vascular that patients may exsanguinate during surgery. Transarterial embolization as an adjunct to conventional surgery is not always successful (61). VB cement augmentation has the advantage of creating a permanent incompressible cast within the lytic lesion that provides structural support at the site of the osseous defect. Balloon expansion within the lytic lesion compresses the vascular structure of the tumor and temporarily controls the bleeding until the cement is injected to provide a more permanent effect.

In a study by San Millan Ruiz et al. (77), polymethylmethacrylate (PMMA) exhibited a macroscopic and microscopic rim of tumor necrosis 6 months after implantation. This effect of PMMA may be caused by the variable toxicity of acrylic implants, including the different degrees of the exothermic reaction during polymerization.

The combination of intralesional alcohol injection with PMMA cement augmentation most likely has an additive effect. The effectiveness of BK can be also enhanced when combined with cryotherapy and spinal instrumentation (see Thermal Ablation).

Thermal Ablation

Percutaneous image-guided ablation with the use of radiofrequency (RF) or often thermal energy sources, such as microwave, high-intensity focused ultrasonography or cryotherapy and laser, have been applied for soft tissue tumor surgery (25) and particularly for hepatic lesions. More recently, radiofrequency ablation and cryotherapy have been successfully used for musculoskeletal malignant and benign lesions (25,39,61,74). Cryoablation surgery has been successfully used for metastatic tumors in the liver, for cancer of the prostate, and for induction of cryogenic injury to the thal-

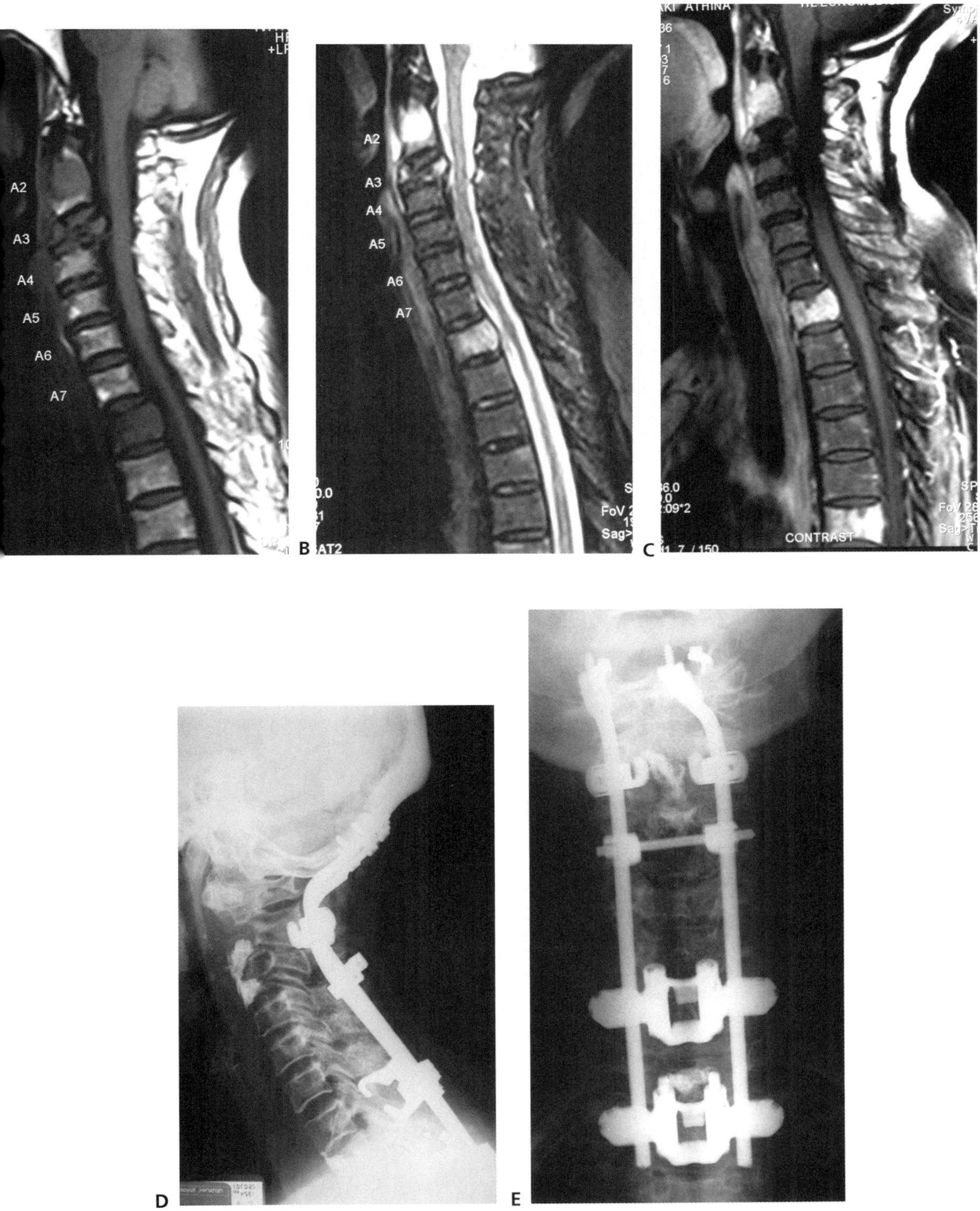

FIGURE 10.4 A 56-year-old patient with metastatic renal cell cancer involving the C-2, C-3, T-1, T-6, and L-4 vertebrae, as seen on T_1-weighted MRI (**A**), T_2-weighted MRI (**B**), and vascularity demonstrated on gadolinium-enhanced T_1-weighted MRI (**C**). The patient complained of severe pain for which radiation therapy failed (inappropriate treatment). Pain and disability responded to cervical vertebroplasty and occipitocervical instrumentation. (**D**) Lateral view. (**E**) Frontal view. *(Continued)*

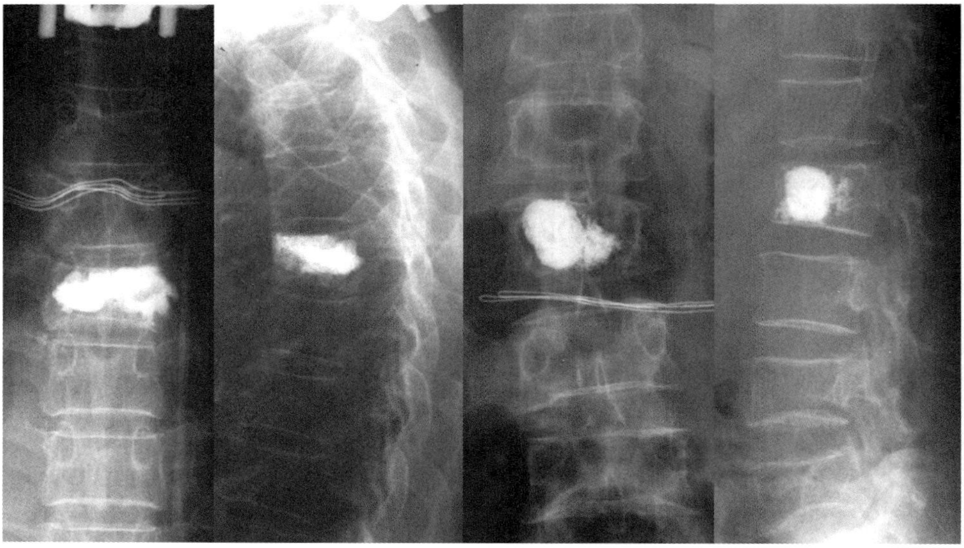

F G H I

FIGURE 10.4 *(Continued)* Demonstration of successful balloon kyphoplasty in the thoracic and lumbar vertebrae. Thoracic, one (**F**); thoracic, six (**G**); and lumbar, two (**H**) and (**I**).

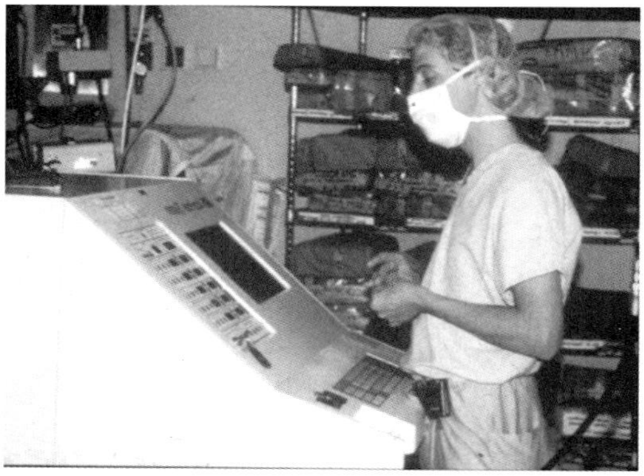

A

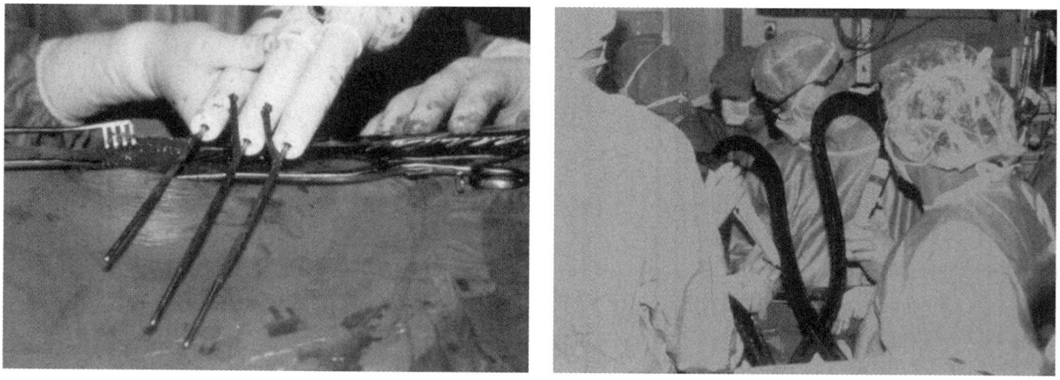

B

FIGURE 10.5 Demonstration of cryocoagulation device (**A**), cryoablation probes, 3 and 5 mm (**B**).

amus in parkinsonism. Cryocoagulation is achieved by means of liquid nitrogen delivered through 3- to 5-mm diameter probes introduced into the lesion. The cryogenic effect is produced by −180°C temperature for 5 to 10 minutes (Fig. 10.5). The effectiveness of cryoablation surgery to promote rapid avascularity is reproducible. The cryogenic lesion kills malignant and benign lesions and is characterized by sharply delimitating borders. However, the experience with cryocoagulation in the treatment of hypervascular tumors of the spine is limited. Its use, whether alone or in conjunction with embolization, may be helpful in reducing estimated blood loss beyond what can be achieved with embolization alone (Fig. 10.6). Cryocoagulation may also assist

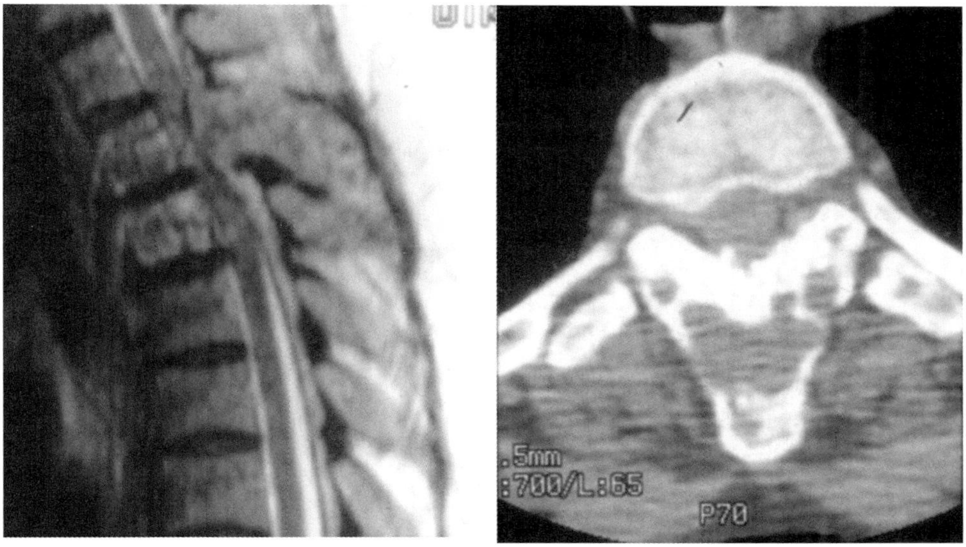

A

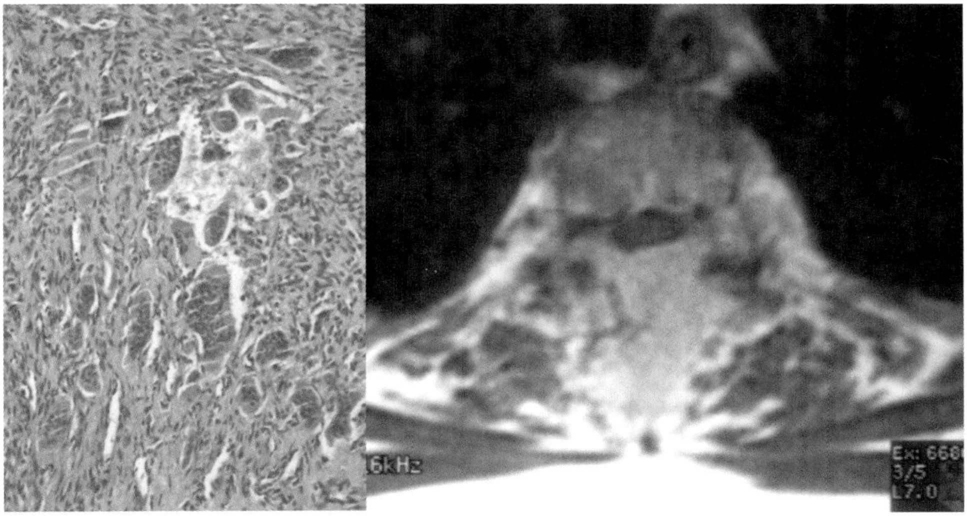

B

FIGURE 10.6 **A:** T_1-weighted MRI image demonstrating a vascular hemangioma compromising spinal cord, producing Frankel D paraplegia. Axial CT scan typical of cavernous vascular hemangioma. **B:** Histologic picture typical of hemangioma. (A) Axial CT scan after laminectomy demonstrating cord compression from hematoma. Frankel B paraplegia developed. *(Continued)*

C

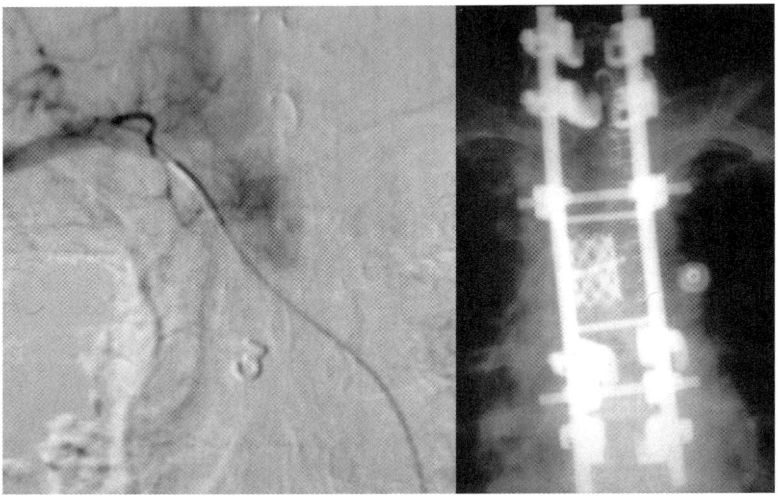

FIGURE 10.6 *(Continued)* **C:** A successful preoperative transarterial embolization. Corpectomy with excision of hemangioma and reconstruction with cage filled with autograft and posterior stabilization with spinal instrumentation. This procedure was combined with cryotherapy. The patient regained his neurologic function completely.

resection by preventing spillage of tumor contents, allowing more radical excision, and facilitating better spinal reconstruction (Fig. 10.7). Freezing damage to the cord and nerve roots remains a concern, and therefore monitoring is recommended. The extent of cryocoagulation could be adequately controlled by using ultrasonography or by establishing physical separation between the tumor and spinal cord. The changes in echogenicity on ultrasound allow monitoring of the extent of the freezing process (61). Additionally, somatosensory evoked potential monitoring may provide early warning of spinal cord cooling (61).

Nader et al. (61) compared preoperative embolization alone with intraoperative cryotherapy alone, or cryotherapy in conjunction with embolization to minimize the estimated blood loss. In 10 cases, embolization alone resulted in blood loss (EBL) in excess of 3 L in 50% of 10 treated patients. Mean blood loss was of 2.8 L per patient. In one patient, who underwent only embolization, excessive bleeding (>8 L) required premature termination of surgery and resulted in suboptimal tumor resection. Intraoperative cryocoagulation alone or in combination with preoperative embolization resulted in a mean blood loss of only 500 ml per patient. Initially cryocoagulation was successfully used in five hypervascular tumors (renal cell carcinoma: four; aneurysmal bone cyst: one). As an adjunct procedure, it allowed radical excision of the tumor with minimal morbidity and excellent outcomes. Subsequently, cryocoagulation was successfully used as an adjunct procedure to minimally invasive tumor surgery in the treatment of four cases of metastatic hypervascular tumors (renal cell carcinoma: 2, follicular thyroid adenocarcinoma: 1). The cryoablation probe was introduced percutaneously through the pedicle. Minimally invasive procedure consisted of combining balloon kyphoplasty with percutaneous transpedicular instrumentation.

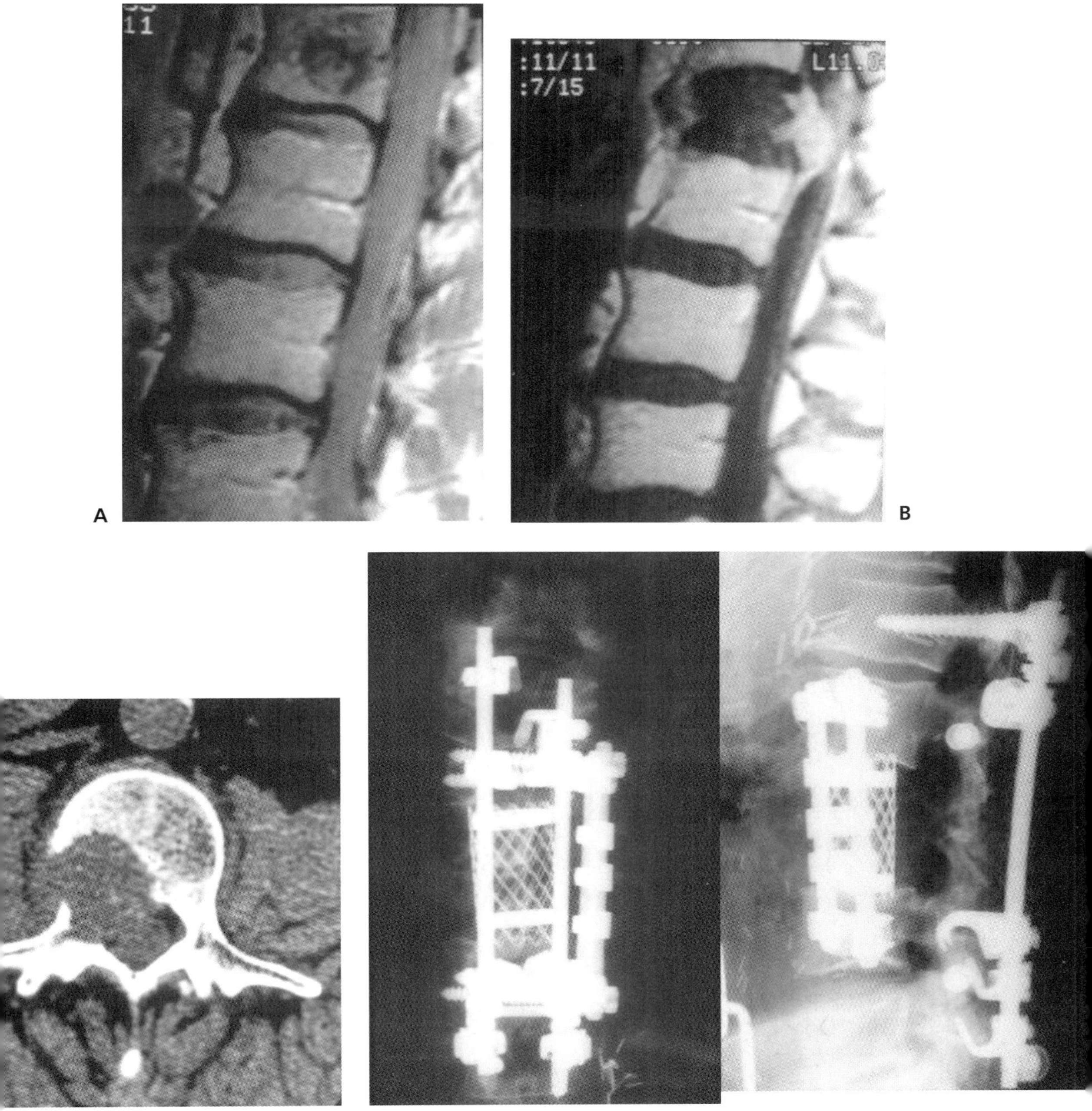

A B C D E

FIGURE 10.7 Metastatic renal cell carcinoma, misconstrued as a metastatic cancer of the colon (5 years before the patient was treated for cancer of the colon) in a 61-year-old patient. (**A**). Radiation failed, and the tumor expanded posteriorly to produce serious neurologic deficit (**B**). CT axial cuts demonstrated the lytic lesion (**C**), The patient underwent radical excision of the tumor and reconstruction anteriorly with cages and Kaneda plating system. Posterior was stabilized with screws-and-hooks instrumentation (**D**) and (**E**). The patient survived more than 4 years at last follow-up. Apparently radical surgery, controlled bleeding, and prevention of tumor spillage resulted in patient's increased survival. The reported survival of renal cell metastatic cancer to the spine according to King GJ, et al, is 8 ± 1.5 months. (King GJ, Kostuik JP, McBroom RJ, et al. Surgical management of metastatic renal carcinoma of the spine. Spine 1991;16:265–71.)

CONCLUSION

Radiation therapy is not the optimal treatment for hypervascular tumors. Preoperative transarterial embolization alone may not always be effective in minimizing blood loss during surgery for hypervascular tumors of the spine. Cryocoagulation by freezing and delineating tissue planes allows easier tumor respectability, without spillage of tumor tissues, and kills tumor cells that infiltrate surrounding tissues. This modality is also effective in decreasing blood loss, which in turn allows more radical tumor excision and better spinal reconstruction with less morbidity and mortality. Finally, it may potentially improve longevity after tumor surgery. Because freezing damage to the cord or nerve roots remains of some concern during cryocoagulation, somatosensory evoked potential and ultrasound imaging are recommended for monitoring the neural elements. When our guidelines are followed, balloon kyphoplasty as a single or adjunct procedure to intralesional alcohol injection is a safe and effective procedure for the management of vertebral hemangiomas and vascular tumors.

REFERENCES

1. Acosta FL Jr, Dowd CF, Chin C, et al. Current treatment strategies and outcomes in the management of symptomatic vertebral hemangiomas. Neurosurgery 2006;58:287–295.
2. Adamsbaum C, Leclet H, Kalifa G. Intralesional Ethibloc injections in bone cysts. Semin Musculoskel Radiol 1997;1:301–304.
3. Ahn H, Haveri S, Yee A, et al. Lumbar vertebral hemangioma causing cauda equina syndrome: a case report. Spine 2005;30:E662–E664.
4. Asthana AK, Tandon SC, Pant GC, et al. Radiation therapy for symptomatic vertebral haemangioma. Clin Oncol (R Coll Radiol) 1990;2: 159–162.
5. Atalay B, Caner H, Yilmaz C, et al. Sacral kyphoplasty for relieving pain caused by sacral hemangioma. Spinal Cord 2006;44:196–199.
6. Bandiera S, Gasbarrini A, De Iure F, et al. Symptomatic vertebral hemangioma: the treatment of 23 cases and a review of the literature. Chir Organ Mov 2002;87:1–15.
7. Bas T, Aparisi F, Bas JL. Efficacy and safety of ethanol injections in 18 cases of vertebral hemangioma: a mean follow-up of 2 years. Spine 2001; 26:1577–1582.
8. Berenstein A, Young W, Ransohoff J, et al. Somatosensory evoked potentials during spinal angiography and therapeutic transvascular embolization. J Neurosurg 1984;60:777–785.
9. Berkefeld J, Scale D, Kirchner J, et al. Hypervascular spinal tumors: influence of the embolization technique on perioperative hemorrhage. AJNR Am J Neuroradiol 1999;20:757–763.
10. Bremnes RM, Hauge HN, Sagsveen R. Radiotherapy in the treatment of symptomatic vertebral hemangiomas: technical case report. Neurosurgery 1996;39:1054–1058.
11. Breslau J, Eskridge JM. Preoperative embolization of spinal tumors. J Vasc Interv Radiol 1995; 6:871–875.
12. Broaddus WC, Grady MS, Delashaw JB Jr, et al. Preoperative superselective arteriolar embolization: anew approach to enhance resectability of spinal tumors. Neurosurgery 1990;27:755–759.
13. Brunot S, Berge J, Barreau X, et al. Long term clinical follow up of vertebral hemangiomas treated by percutaneous vertebroplasty. J Radiol 2005;86: 41–47.
14. Casasco A, Houdart E, Biondi A, et al. Major complications of percutaneous embolization of skull-base tumors. AJNR Am J Neuroradiol 1999; 20:179–181.
15. Casasco AE, Houdart E, Gobin YP, et al. Embolization of spinal vascular malformations. Neuroimaging Clin North Am 1992;2:337–358.
16. Castel E, Lazennec JY, Chiras J, et al. Acute spinal cord compression due to intraspinal bleeding from a vertebral hemangioma: two case-reports. Eur Spine J 1999;8:244–248.
17. Chiras J, Cognard C, Rose M, et al. Percutaneous injection of an alcoholic embolizing emulsion as an alternative preoperative embolization for spine

tumor. AJNR Am J Neuroradiol 1993;14:-1113–1117.
18. Choi IS, Berenstein A. Surgical neuroangiography of the spine and spinal cord. Radiol Clin North Am 1998;29:1131–1141.
19. Cohen JE, Lylyk P, Ceratto R, et al. Percutaneous vertebroplasty: technique and results in 192 procedures. Neurol Res 2004;26:41–49.
20. Cotten A, Deramond H, Cortet B, et al. Preoperative percutaneous injection of methyl methacrylate and n-butyl cyanoacrylate in vertebral hemangiomas AJNR Am J Neuroradiol 1996;17:137–142.
21. Deramond H, Depriester C, Galibert P, et al. Percutaneous vertebroplasty with polymethylmethacrylate: technique, indications, and results. Radiol Clin North Am. 1998;36:533–546.
22. DeRosa GP, Graziano GP, Scott J. Arterial embolization of aneurysmal bone cyst of the lumbar spine: a report of two cases. J Bone Joint Surg Am 1990;72:777–780.
23. Djindjian R, Cophignon J, Theron J, et al. Embolization by superselective arteriography from the femoral route in neuroradiology, I and II. Neuroradiology 1973;6:20–26.
24. Doppman JL, Oldfield EH, Heiss JD. Symptomatic vertebral hemangiomas: treatment by means of direct intralesional injection of ethanol. Radiology 2000;214:341–348.
25. Dupuy De, Goldberg SN. Image-guided radiofrequency tumor ablation: challenges and opportunities: Part II. J Vasc Interv Radiol 2001;12: 1135–1148.
26. Eisenstein S, Spiro F, Browde S, et al. The treatment of a symptomatic vertebral hemangioma by radiotherapy. Spine 1986;11:640–642.
27. Eskridge J. Interventional neuroradiology. Radiology 1989;172:991–1006.
28. Esparza J, Castro S, Portillo JM, et al. Vertebral hemangiomas: spinal angiography and preoperative embolization. Surg Neurol 1978;10:171–173.
29. Fox MW, Onofrio BM. The natural history and management of symptomatic and asymptomatic vertebral hemangiomas. J Neurosurg 1993;78: 36–45.
30. Frassica FJ, Frassica DA, Wold LE, et al. Postradiation sarcoma of bone. Orthopedics 1993;16: 105–106.
31. Galibert P, Deramond H, Rosat P, et al. Preliminary note on the treatment of vertebral angioma by percutaneous acrylic vertebroplasty. Neurochirurgie 1987;33:166–168.
32. Gangi A, Dietemann JL, Schultz A, et al. Interventional radiologic procedures with CT guidance in cancer pain management. Radiographics 1996;16:1289–1306.
33. Gangi A, Guth S, Imbert JP, Marin H, et al. Percutaneous vertebroplasty: indications, technique, and results. Radiographics 2003;23:e10.
34. Gellad FE, Sadato N, Numaguchi Y, et al. Vascular metastatic lesions of the spine: preoperative embolization. Radiology 1990;176:683–686.
35. Gonzales CF, Moret J. Balloon occlusion of the carotid artery prior to surgery for neck tumors. AJNR Am J Neuroradiol 1990;11:649–652.
36. Goyal M, Mishra NK, Sharma A, et al. Alcohol ablation of symptomatic vertebral hemangiomas. AJNR Am J Neuroradiol 1999;20:1091–1096.
37. Guedea F, Majo J, Guardia E, et al. The role of radiation therapy in vertebral hemangiomas without neurological signs. Int Orthop 1994;18:77–79.
38. Hadjipavlou AG, Tosounidis TI, Gaitanis IN, et al. Balloon kyphoplasty as a single or as an adjunct procedure for the management of symptomatic vertebral hemangiomas. J Bone Joint Surg (in press)[2].
39. Hadjipavlou AG, Tzermiadianos MN, Katonis PG, et al. Percutaneous vertebroplasty and balloon kyphoplasty for the treatment of osteoporotic vertebral compression fractures and osteolytic tumours. J Bone Joint Surg Br 2005;87:1595–1604
40. Hansen E, Altmeppen J, Targer K. Practicability and safety of intra-operative autotransfusion with irradiated blood. Anaesthesia 1998;53(suppl 2): 42–3.
41. Heiss JD, Doppman JL, Oldfield EH. Brief report: relief of spinal cord compression from vertebral hemangioma by intralesional injection of absolute alcohol. N Engl Med 1994;331: 508–511.
42. Heiss JD, Doppman JL, Oldfield EH. Treatment of vertebral hemangioma by intralesional injection of absolute alcohol [Letter]. N Engl J Med 1996;13:336–1340.
43. Hekster REM, Luyendijk W, Tan TI. Spinal-cord compression caused by vertebral hemangioma relieved by percutaneous catheter embolisation. Neuroradiology 1972;3:160–164.
44. Herbreteau D, Guichard JP, Reizine D, et al. [Preoperative embolization of cervical bone metastasis with radio-controlled direct puncture] Rev Chir Orthop Reparatrice Appar Mot 1992;78:480–484. [Article in French].

45. Heyd R, Strassmann G, Filipowicz I, et al. Radiotherapy in vertebral hemangioma. Rontgenpraxis 2001;53:208–220.

46. Ide C, Gangi A, Rimmelin A, et al. Vertebral haemangiomas with spinal cord compression: the place of preoperative percutaneous vertebroplasty with methyl methacrylate. Neuroradiology 1996; 38:585–589.

47. Kagetsu NJ, Berenstein A, Choi IS. Interventional radiology of the extracranial head and neck. Cardiovasc Intervent Radiol 1991;14:325–333.

48. Konya A, Szendroi M. Aneurysmal bone cysts treated by superselective embolization. Skeletal Radiol 1992;21:167–172.

49. Kuether TA, Nesbit GM, Barnwell SL. Embolization as treatment for spinal cord compression from renal cell carcinoma: case report. Neurosurgery 1996;39:1260–1262.

50. Leclet H, Adamsbaum C. Intraosseous cyst injection. Radiol Clin North Am 1998;36:581–587.

51. Lichtenstein L. Aneurysmal bone cyst: observations on fifty cases. J Bone Joint Surg Am 1957; 39:873–882.

52. MacCarty CS, Dahlin DC, Doyle JB Jr, et al. Aneurysmal bone cysts of the neural axis. J Neurosurg 1961;18:671–677.

53. Manke C, Bretschneider T, Lenhart M, et al. Spinal metastases from renal cell carcinoma: effect of preoperative particle embolization on intraoperative blood loss. AJNR Am J Neuroradiol 2001;22:997–1003.

54. Marcove RC, Sheth DS, Takemoto S, et al. The treatment of aneurysmal bone cyst. Clin Orthop Relat Res 1999;311:157–163.

55. Mariani L, Haldemann AR, Schroth G. Arteriovenous shunt measurement during endovascular therapy for cerebrospinal lesions. AJNR Am J Neuroradiol 1997;18:1679–1689.

56. McAllister VL, Kendall BE, Bull JW. Symptomatic vertebral haemangiomas. Brain 1975;98:71–80.

57. Miszczyk L, Ficek K, Trela K, et al. The efficacy of radiotherapy for vertebral hemangiomas. Neoplasma 2001;48:82–84.

58. Moody EB, Dawson RC III, Sandler MP. 99m-Tc-HMPAO SPECT imaging in interventional neuroradiology: validation of balloon test occlusion. AJNR Am J Neuroradiol 1991;12:1043–1044.

59. Murugan L, Samson RS, Chandy MJ. Management of symptomatic vertebral hemangiomas: review of 13 patients. Neurol India 2002;50: 300–305.

60. Muto M, Muto E, Izzo R, et al. Vertebroplasty in the treatment of back pain. Radiol Med (Torino). 2005;109:208–219.

61. Nader R, Alford BT, Nauta HJ, et al. Preoperative embolization and intraoperative cryocoagulation as adjuncts in resection of hypervascular lesions of the thoracolumbar spine. J Neurosurg. 2002;97(3 suppl):294–300.

62. Nguyen JP, Djindjian M, Gaston A, et al. Vertebral hemangiomas presenting with neurologic symptoms. Surg Neurol 1987;27:391–397.

63. Nicola N, Lins E. Vertebral hemangioma: late results of retrograde embolization stabilization with methyl methacrylate in two cases. Surg Neurol 1993;40:491–494.

64. Nickolisen R, Fallon B. Locally recurrent hypernephroma treated by radiation therapy and embolization: a report of two cases. Cancer 1985; 56:1049–1051.

65. Niemeyer T, McClellan J, Webb J, et al. Brown-Sequard syndrome after management of vertebral hemangioma with intralesional alcohol: a case report. Spine 1999;24:1845–1847.

66. Noez, CollignonL, Bex V, et al. Kyphoplasty for the treatment of painful vertebral hemangioma. Rev Med Liege 2006;61:91–96.

67. Obana Y, Tanji K, Furuta I, et al. A case of malignant transformation in thoracic vertebral hemangioma following repetitive irradiation and extraction. Pathol Int 1996;46:71–78.

68. Olerud C, Jonsson H, Lofberg AM, et al. Embolization of spinal metastases reduces preoperative blood loss. Acta Orthop Scand 1993;64: 9–12.

69. Papagelopoulos PJ, Currier BL, Shaughnessy WJ, et al. Aneurysmal bone cyst of the spine: management and outcome. Spine 1998;23: 621–628.

70. Peraud A, Drake JM, Armstrong D, et al. Fatal Ethibloc embolization of vertebrobasilar system following percutaneous injection into aneurysmal bone cyst of the second cervical vertebra. AJNR Am J Neuroradiol 2004;25:1116–1120.

71. Purkayastha S, Gupta AK, Kapilamoorthy TR, et al. Percutaneous vertebroplasty in the management of vertebral lesions. Neurol India 2005;53: 167–172.

72. Ratanatharathorn V, Powers WE, Moss WT, et al. Bone metastasis: review and critical analysis of random allocation trials of local field treatment. Int J Radiat Oncol Biol Phys 1999;44:1–18.

73. Roscoe MW, McBroom RJ, Louis EST, et al. Preoperative embolization in the treatment of osseous metastases from renal cell carcinoma. Clin Orthop Rel Res 1989;238:302–307.
74. Rosenthal DI, Hornicek FJ, Wolfe MW, et al. Percutaneous radiofrequency coagulation of osteoid osteoma compared with operative treatment. J Bone Joint Surg Am 1998;80:815–821.
75. Rossi C, Ricci S, Boriani S, et al. Percutaneous transcatheter arterial embolization of bone and soft tissue tumors. Skeletal Radiol 1990;19:555–560.
76. Sabanas AO, Dahlin DC, Childs DS Jr, et al. Postradiation sarcoma of bone. Cancer 1956;9: 528–542.
77. San Millan Ruiz D, Burkhardt K, Jean B, et al. Pathology findings with acrylic implants. Bone 1999;25:85S–90S.
78. Schild SE, Buskirk SJ, Frick LM, et al. Radiotherapy for large symptomatic hemangiomas. Int J Radiat Oncol Biol Phys 1991;21:729–735.
79. Schirmer CM, Malek AM, Kwan ES, et al. Preoperative embolization of hypervascular spinal metastases using percutaneous direct injection with n-butyl cyanoacrylate: technical case report. Neurosurgery 2006;59:431–432.
80. Scott DL, Pedlow FX, Hecht AC, et al. Primary Benign and Malignant Extradural Spine Tumors, 3rd ed. Philadelphia: Lippincott Williams & Wilkins, 2004:207–210.
81. Sharma D, Jain V, Rath GP. Asystole during percutaneous ethanol injection of symptomatic vertebral haemangioma. Anaesth Intensive Care 2006; 34:656–658.
82. Shi HB, Suh DC, Lee HK, et al. Preoperative transarterial embolization of spinal tumor: embolization techniques and results. AJNR Am J Neuroradiol 1999;20:2009–2015.
83. Sim FH, Cupps RE, Dahlin DC, et al. Postradiation sarcoma of bone. J Bone Joint Surg Am 1972; 54:1479–1489.
84. Smith TP, Gray L, Weinstein JN, et al. Preoperative transarterial embolization of spinal column neoplasms. J Vasc Interv Radiol 1995;6: 863–869.
85. Sundaresan N, Choi IS, Hughes JEO, et al. Treatment of spinal metastases from kidney cancer by presurgical embolization and resection. J Neurosurg 1990;73:548–554.
86. Templin CR, Stambough JB, Stambough JL. Acute spinal cord compression caused by vertebral hemangioma. Spine J 2004;4:595–600.
87. Teng GJ, He SC, Deng G, et al. A simplified method of opacifying and mixing acrylic cement for percutaneous vertebroplasty: a clinical and in vitro study. Cardiovasc Intervent Radiol 2005;28: 570–577.
88. Theron J, Cosgrove R, Melanson D, et al. Embolization with temporary balloon occlusion of the internal carotid or vertebral arteries. Neuroradiology 1986;28:246–253.
89. Tong D, Gillick L, Hendrickson FR. The palliation of symptomatic osseous metastases: final results of the study by the radiation therapy oncology group. Cancer 1982;50:893–899.
90. Vetter SC, Strecker EP, Ackermann LW, et al. Preoperative embolization of cervical spine tumors. Cardiovasc Intervent Radiol 1997;20:343–347.
91. Yang Z-Y, Zhang L-J, Chen Z-X, et al. Hemangioma of the vertebral column: a report on twenty-three patients with special reference to functional recovery after radiation therapy. Acta Radiol Oncol 1985;24:129–132.
92. Yang XJ, Wu ZX, Zhao JF, et al. Treatment of vertebral hemangioma with percutaneous vertebroplasty. Zhongguo Yi Xue Ke Xue Yuan Xue Bao 2004;26:643–646.
93. Winkler C, Dornfeld S, Baumann M, et al. [The efficacy of radiotherapy in vertebral hemangiomas] Strahlenther Onkol 1996;172:681–684. [Article in German]

A Randomized Trial of Decompressive Surgery in Metastatic Epidural Spinal Cord Compression

11

Roy A. Patchell

The role of surgery in the management of metastatic epidural spinal cord compression (MESCC) has been controversial. Before radiation therapy (RT) became available, surgery (simple laminectomy) was the only treatment. With the introduction of RT, the results with laminectomy plus RT did not appear to be different from the results with radiation alone. Surgical treatment was largely abandoned when several retrospective studies and one small randomized trial failed to find any benefit for laminectomy alone or in combination with RT. However, laminectomy was not the best operation for MESCC. The majority of spinal metastases that cause MESCC are located in the vertebral body, anterior to the spinal cord. A laminectomy (removal of the posterior elements of the spinal column) does not remove tumor and often does not result in immediate decompression. A laminectomy also may cause destabilization of the spine because it is often only the posterior elements that are intact, and removal of these causes instability.

In the 1980s, another type of surgical procedure was developed for the treatment of MESCC. The tumor was removed, and immediate circumferential decompression was achieved, usually through an anterior approach. It was possible also to reconstruct the spine intraoperatively and provide immediate stabilization. A randomized trial comparing direct decompressive surgery plus postoperative RT with RT alone was recently completed. The study population consisted of patients with known cancer in whom symptoms of MESCC developed. These patients had magnetic resonance imaging (MRI) scans to confirm the presence of a true MESCC. Patients were started on dexamethasone, 100 mg, initially, followed by 24 mg every 6 hours until they began treatment. After that, steroids were decreased but continued until the completion of RT. After stratification for primary tumor type, ambulatory status, and presence or absence of spinal stability, patients were randomly assigned to one of two treatment groups. Patients in the radiation-alone group began RT within 24 hours after study entry and received 3,000 cGy (300 cGy $\times$ 10 fractions). Patients in the surgery-plus-radiation group were operated on within 24 hours after study entry and received radiation within 2 weeks after surgery.

The intent of surgery in all cases was to remove as much tumor as possible and provide immediate decompression and intraoperative spinal stabilization (when needed). The major end point of the study was the ability to walk after treatment. The immediate success of treatment was determined by comparing the proportion of patients in each group who were able to walk after treatment. The long-term success of treatment was measured by comparing the length of time patients maintained the ability to walk. Secondary end points were post-treatment continence rates, length of time patients maintained muscle strength and functional status, and survival time.

The original study design called for a sample size of 200 patients. However, after an interim analysis, the study was stopped because the criterion of a predetermined early stopping rule was met. One hundred and one patients were entered into the study. The percentage of patients able to walk after treatment was significantly (p = 0.001) higher in surgical patients (84%) than in the radiotherapy-alone patients (57%). Patients treated with surgery also retained the ability to walk significantly longer than did those with radiotherapy alone (median, 122 days vs. 13 days; p = 0.003). Thirty-two patients (16 in each treatment group) entered the study unable to walk; patients in the surgery group regained the ability to walk in a significantly greater proportion than did patients in the radiation-alone group [10 (62%) of 16 vs. three (19%) of 16; p = 0.01]. The need for corticosteroids and opioid analgesics was significantly lower in the surgical group, and muscle strength and functional status were also maintained for significantly longer in patients treated with surgery. Survival times were also significantly (p = 0.033) longer in the surgery group (median, 126 days in the surgery group vs. 100 days in the radiation-alone group). The randomized trial showed that patients with MESCC treated with direct decompressive surgery plus postoperative RT retain the ability to walk longer and regain it more often than patients treated with RT alone. Surgery permitted most patients to remain ambulatory for the remainder of their lives, whereas patients treated with radiation alone spent a large portion of their remaining time as paraplegics.

However, the results of this trial cannot be used to justify surgery in all patients with MESCC and apply only to those patients who were comparable to those included in the study. Even in this group of patients, reasonable clinical judgment must be used in the selection of patients for surgery.

Oncologically Appropriate Surgery in the Treatment of Primary Bone Tumors of the Spine: Correct Terminology, Planning and Results

Stefano Boriani, Stefania Paderni, Michele Cappuccio, Alessandro Gasbarrini, Luca Boriani, and Stefano Bandiera

12

ABSTRACT

Background

The so-called limb-salvage surgery based on the Enneking staging system allowed excellent results in the treatment of bone tumors of the limb.

Methods

We evaluated the possibility to extend to the spine the same oncologic criteria accepted for bone tumors of the limbs. A series of 125 *en bloc* resections for 467 primary tumors of the spine was reviewed to assess the relation among the tumor aggressiveness, the surgical margins, and the outcome

Results

The rate of local control after *en bloc* resection was 70.4% at 89 months' average follow-up, ranging from 90.7% in intact cases to 54.8% in previously treated cases. For a better assessment of the results, these were explored by diagnosis. Full local control was achieved in 11 *en bloc* resections performed in a series of 31 stage 3 giant cell tumors (GCTs) at 6 to 172 months' follow-up. In a series of 35 stage IA/B chondrosarcomas, full local control was achieved in 12 *en bloc* resections with appropriate margins at 6 to 168 months' follow-up, whereas in eight cases with tumor contamination (intralesional margin), the success rate was 62.5% at 30 to 165 months. In osteosarcoma (osteogenic sarcoma; OGS), the combination of appropriate margin and a full course of multiple-drug chemotherapy is critical (six cases: no local recurrences at 24 to 108 months), whereas inappropriate margins, incomplete chemotherapy, and chemotherapy alone were always followed by a local recurrence.

Conclusions

En bloc resection is the procedure of choice in the treatment of aggressive benign and low-grade malignancies in the spine. High-grade tumors like OGS and Ewing sarcoma (ES) require combination of chemotherapy (in OGS and ES) and radiation (in ES) with *en bloc* resection to obtain the best results

INTRODUCTION

According to the criteria proposed by Enneking (7) and widely accepted among oncologists, "radical" resection is a thigh amputation when the tumor is located in the tibia. Unfortunately, many surgeons define "radical" as the excision they believe to be appropriate. These are mostly intralesional excisions performed without any consideration for oncologic principles. This incorrect use of the terminology prevents us from comparing results and sharing experiences.

The role of a common nomenclature in sharing information is obvious. Our proposal is to adopt the terminology proposed by Enneking (7) to describe surgical tumor excision, based on the margin achieved. The margin is a shell of healthy tissue all around the tumor mass, the width of which (*marginal,* only the tumor pseudocapsule; *wide,* a coverage of healthy tissue, like muscle or fascia, or layer, like pleura) is requested according to the oncologic stage (7).

The term *radical* means the resection of the whole compartment of tumor origin. In the spine, this is virtually impossible, as it should mean to resect *en bloc* the full vertebra (content of the canal included), provided that the tumor does not grow outside. In our series, even a five-vertebrae resection, including the cord, was performed, but it should be considered wide or even marginal, as in a small area, the tumor is covered only by the pleura. Further, the epidural space being an extracompartmental area, the tumor invasion of that space immediately makes inappropriate the term *radical.*

A full preoperative workup is mandatory for diagnosis and staging purpose and must be completed with a careful collection of clinical data and laboratory tests to confirm the patient's suitability to major surgery. Advanced age and poor general conditions are relative contraindications and must be considered case by case with the anesthesiology team (6).

It is important to consider the role of magnetic resonance imaging (MRI) to evaluate the epidural extension and to find a cleavage between the tumor pseudocapsule and the dura. Some surgeons suggest (when needed) resection of the dura together with the tumor to enlarge the margins (1). The risk is to further increase the morbidity of such a long and difficult procedure, without absolute certainty of achieving an appropriate margin in case of epidural involvement of the tumor. Complications like cerebrospinal fluid (CSF) leakage, wound dehiscence, or infection may delay adjuvant treatments (like chemotherapy), which are mandatory in many conditions like ES or OGS.

The spillage of tumor in the tissues due to incisional biopsy may prevent adequate treatment, as it is seldom possible to resect the wound, especially the peridural scar. Previous surgery, as well as radioinduced fibrosis, increases the risk of intraoperative damage of structures in the perimeter of the tumor (ureter, vena cava, aorta, sympathetic chain).

The planning of the surgical treatment of a bone tumor of the spine must consider the extension of the tumor, the anatomic structures that cannot be resected or displaced, and the possibilities of different surgical approaches. Three surgical procedures have been identified and described according to an original surgical staging system (4), based on the division into 12 sectors and five layers of the transverse section of the vertebra, which should allow standardization of the approach to these tumors.

Vertebrectomy is a surgical procedure performed by double approach (first posterior, second posterior combined with anterior) (Fig. 12.1A and B), aiming to achieve *en bloc*

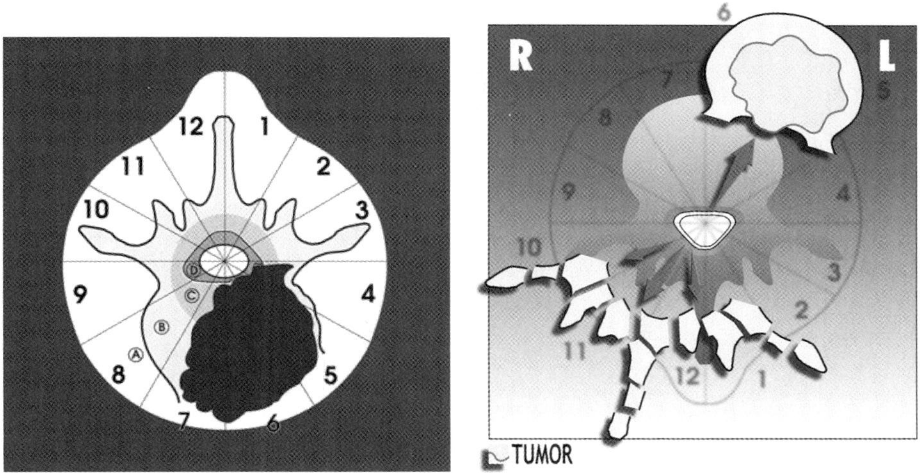

A B

FIGURE 12.1 **A:** Indication for *en bloc* resection of the vertebral body according to the WBB system (4). The transverse extension of the tumor is described with reference to 12 radiating zones (numbered 1 to 12 in clockwise order, starting from the left side) and to five concentric layers (A to E). **B:** When the tumor invades layer A, a double approach is suggested to allow direct visualization of the tumor.

resection of the vertebral body (sectors 4 to 8 or 5 to 9). The vertebral body can be resected by a posterior approach alone (10,13) in the thoracic spine, but the procedure will be oncologically appropriate only if the tumor is not expanding in layer A AU1 (Fig. 12.2A and B). In this case, this technique (10,13) exposes to violate the margin. The anterior step of the procedure will permit leaving a sheet of continuous healthy tissue over the tumor (5).

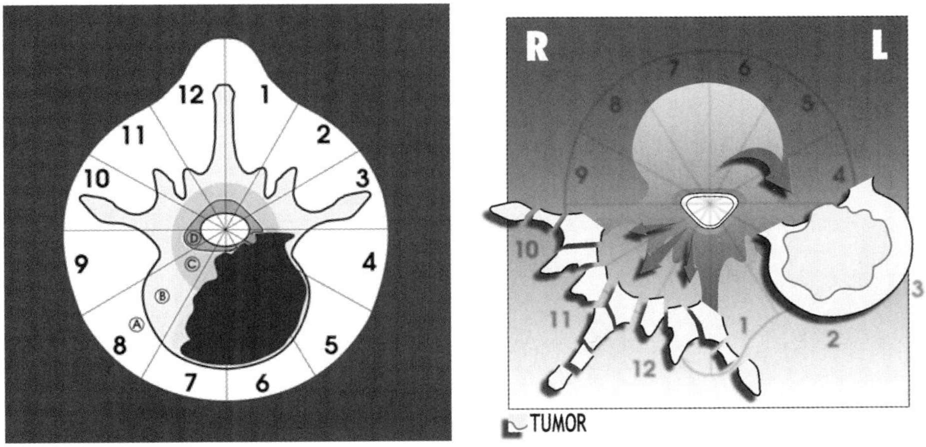

A B

FIGURE 12.2 **A, B:** If the tumor is contained in the vertebral body (no layer A invasion), a single posterior approach (20,28) is appropriate.

A 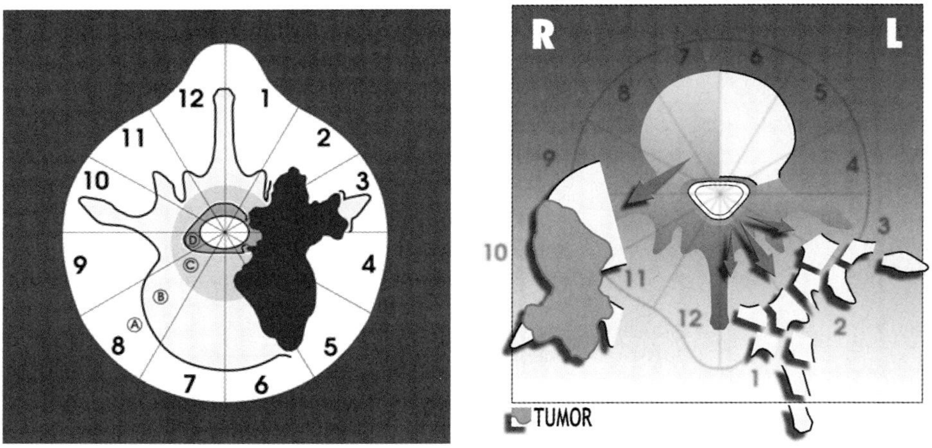 B

FIGURE 12.3 **A:** Indications for *en bloc* resection of eccentrically growing tumor (sagittal resection), according to the WBB staging system. (From Boriani S, Weinstein JN, Biagini R. Spine update: primary bone tumors of the spine: terminology and surgical staging. Spine 1997;22:1036–44, with permission.). **B:** Intralesional excision of the sectors 4 to 12 is required to visualize, protect, and separate the dura from the tumor involving sectors 7 to 11 to be resected *en bloc*. An anterior approach is frequently required to leave appropriate margins and to protect the anterior structures.

Sagittal resection is as well performed by a double approach: the target is to remove *en bloc* an eccentrically growing tumor (sectors 2 to 5/6 or 7/8 to 11) (Fig. 12.3A and B).

Posterior resection is performed by a simple posterior approach: the criterion for an appropriate margin is that sectors 4 and 9 must be free from tumor (Fig. 12.4A and B). The appropriateness of the procedures must be confirmed by the pathologist, who will

A 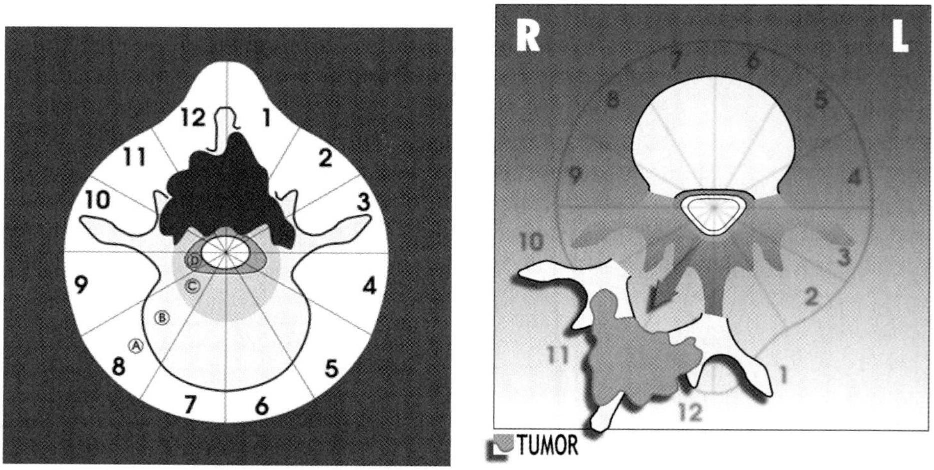 B

FIGURE 12.4 **A:** Indications for *en bloc* resection of a posteriorly located tumor (posterior resection) according to the WBB staging system (From Boriani S, Weinstein JN, Biagini R. Spine update: primary bone tumors of the spine: terminology and surgical staging. Spine 1997;22:1036–44, with permission.) To achieve appropriate margins, sectors 4 and 9 must be free from tumor growth. **B:** Posterior approach only is required.

dictate the margins achieved (wide, marginal, intralesional) for prognostic evaluation and for indications for adjuvant therapies.

The oncologic approach to bone tumor of the spine by *en bloc* resection was started in the 1970s by B. Stener (11) and R. Roy-Camille (10), who first described surgical techniques of *en bloc* resection in the thoracic and lumbar spine with an appropriate oncologic view. K. Tomita (13) later described a similar technique of vertebrectomy by posterior approach in the thoracic and lumbar spine. Recently, *en bloc* resection of the cervical vertebral body was described in a single case report (12), but it contaminated the epidural area, confirming the doubts about the oncologic value of *en bloc* resection in the cervical spine because of the frequent invasion of the epidural space at diagnosis and the anatomic restrictions to the required circumferential visualization of the vertebral components. The most interesting feature of Stener's work (11), not found in the article published later, is the concept that to achieve an appropriate *en bloc* excision, each tumor extension must be carefully evaluated, and the surgical resection must be "personalized." Our attitude has been to develop this philosophy further by setting up a surgical staging [so-called WBB system (3,4)] for planning the surgical procedure in each tumor (2–4,9,14), based on the oncologic staging (7), which is the guide to deciding the appropriate anatomic margin.

MATERIAL AND METHODS

Starting in October 1991, a prospective study was settled by applying to the spine the same criteria adopted for bone tumors of the limbs. The articulation staging versus margins proposed by Enneking (7) (Fig. 12.5) and the planning according to the WBB system (3,4) was performed in all cases.

All the specimens were submitted to the pathologist's analysis for histologic evaluation of margins.

One hundred twenty-five *en bloc* resections were performed till December 2003, and the outcomes were evaluated according to diagnosis, staging, previous surgery, and margins.

RESULTS

En bloc resections were performed in 27 benign stage 3 aggressive, in 41 low-grade (stage I), in 20 high-grade (stage II) malignant primary tumors, and also in 37 solitary metastases. Resection of the vertebral body was performed in 70 cases, sagittal in 17, posterior resections in 38.

Follow-up ranged from 24 to 180 months; 87 cases were followed up for longer than 24 months. No case was lost; all cases had clinical and radiographic follow-ups to date or until death.

The rate of local control after *en bloc* resection (continuously disease free) was 70.4% at 89 months average follow-up, ranging from 90.7% in intact cases to 54.8% in previously treated cases; 75% of the patients had no sign of disease at the final follow-up.

Full local control was achieved in nine *en bloc* resections performed in a series of 31 stage 3 GCTs at 6 to 172 months of follow-up. One patient died in the early postoperative course of pulmonary embolism. This figure was compared with the whole series of

Stage	Margin for ontrol
Benign 3	Wide (or Intralesional plus Adjuvants)
Malignant IA/B	Wide
Malignant IIA/B	(Radical) Wide plus Adjuvants

FIGURE 12.5 Articulation between staging and margins.

TABLE 12.1

TREATMENT	n.	Rec/Prog.	A.W.D.	N.E.D.	C.D.F.	DEAD
Intralesional exc.	6	2 (2 mos)	0	5 (60–251; av. 148 mos)	4 (111–251; av. 170 mos)	1 (19 mos)
Intralesional exc. + RT	15	8 (3–53; av. 17 mos)	0	13 (24–328; av. 136 mos)	6 (60–262; av. 121 mos)	2 (56, 76 mos)
En bloc exc	10	0	0	9 (28–172; av. 68 mos)	9 (28–172; av. 68 mos)	1 (0)
TOTAL	31	10	0	27	19	4

GCT of the spine treated by our team (Table 12.1): two of six recurred within 2 months, and one died 19 months later. Eight local recurrences followed 15 intralesional excisions combined with radiation: two patients died (one of radiation-induced osteosarcoma). Only six of 15 were continuously disease free at an average of 121 months of follow-up.

Fifty-one cases of chordoma were reviewed (Table 12.2), including 21 *en bloc* resections. Two local recurrences occurred of 12 resections with appropriate margins, five of nine with contamination of the tumor, even if given adjuvant radiation. Recurrences were clinically and radiographically evident at 8 to 93 months after the surgery (average, 48 months), and one patient died. Six patients are living with progressive disease; 14 are continuously disease free at 25 to 151 months after surgery. All the cases given radiation therapy, even if palliative surgery was associated, had recurrences, even very

TABLE 12.2

TREATMENT	n.	Rec/Prog.	A.W.D	N.E.D.	C.D.F.	DEAD
RT + Palliative	10	10 (1–140; av. 57 mos)	0	0	0	10 (1–155; av. 57 mos)
Intralesional exc.	4	4 (5–41; av. 18 mos)	2 (44 and 54 mos)	1 (47 mos)	0	1 (153 mos)
Intralesional exc. + RT	16	12 (5–87; av. 29 mos)	5 (24–153; av. 84)	2 (34 and 68 mos)	2 (34 and 68 mos)	9 (12–129; av. 58)
En bloc exc.	12	2 (56 and 93 mos)	2 (62 and 123 mos)	10 (25–113; av. 60 mos)	10 25–113; av. 60 mos)	0
En bloc exc. + RT	9	5 (8–52; av. 35 mos)	4 (44–123 av. 87 mos)	4 (55–151; av. 125 mos)	4 (55–151; av. 125 mos)	1 (102 mos)
TOTAL	51	33	13 (24%)	17 (31%)	16 (29%)	21 (38%)

TABLE 12.3

TREATMENT	n.	Rec/Prog.	A.W.D	N.E.D.	C.D.F.	DEAD
Intralesional exc.	10	5 (17–131; av. 74)	0	3 (41–243; av. 148)	0	7 (1–169; av. 33)
Intralesional exc. + RT	5	3 (5–64; av. 33)	0	1 (21 mos)	1 (21 mos)	4 (1–87; av. 48)
En bloc exc. Wide/Marginal Contam.	8	3 (6–55; av. 36)	1 (83 mos)	4 (30–165; av. 83)	4 (30–165; av. 83)	3 (5–65; av. 28)
En bloc exc. Wide/Marginal	12	0	0	11 (6–168; av. 108)	11 (6–168; av. 108)	1 (7 mos)
TOTAL	35	11	1	19	16	15

late, and all died an average of 57 months after diagnosis. Intralesional excisions too proved ineffective for local control. A combination of intralesional excision and radiation was performed in 16 cases, mostly in the cervical spine or for huge, unresectable tumors. Twelve recurred 5 to 87 months after surgery; nine patients died. Only two in this group are continuously disease free at 34 and 68 months of follow-up.

In a series of 35 stage IA/B chondrosarcoma, full local control was achieved in 12 *en bloc* resections with appropriate margins at 6 to 168 months of follow-up. One of these patients died of a late complication of the procedure. In eight cases with tumor contamination (intralesional margin), three local recurrences occurred: one of these patients is living at 83 months with local disease, and two died. Another patient died of lung metastases without local tumor. Only four of these eight are continuously disease free at an average 83 months. Eight of 15 had recurrences after intralesional excision (three of five given surgery and radiation). Eleven of 15 died of the disease (Table 12.3).

In osteosarcoma, the combination of appropriate margins and a full course of multiple-drug chemotherapy is critical (six cases, no local recurrences at 24 to 108 months), whereas inappropriate margins, incomplete chemotherapy, and chemotherapy alone were always followed by a local recurrence (Table 12.4). One cervical case treated in 1984 with intralesional extracapsular excision followed by radiation is continuously disease free, although she refused chemotherapy and represents an exception to the apparent rule.

COMPLICATIONS

The morbidity of these procedures is very high. Vertebrectomy and sagittal resections combine all the risks and complications of anterior surgery (8) with all the possible problems connected with a long and difficult posterior approach with possible careful dissection of the dura, sometimes strictly adherent to the tumor. The complications related to long-duration procedures must also be considered (6).

The risk of damaging large vessels is increased by the need to leave healthy tissues around the tumor. If previous surgery or radiation or both were performed, the risk would be higher, and scar dissection would expose to lesions the neighboring structures

TABLE 12.4

TREATMENT	n. of cases	Progression/ Local recurrence	Bone/ST mets	Lung Mets	NED	AWD	Dead
CHT only	1	1	0	1	0	0	1 (6 mos)
I.L. Intracapsular excision + CHT + RT	5	4 (1–38; av. 19 mos)	1 (40 mos)	1	1 (26 mos)	0	4 (2–68; av. 33 mos)
I.L.excision Extracapsular + RT	1	0	0	0	1 (234 mos)	0	0
En Bloc excision + Incomplete CHT	3	3 (5–20; av. 12 mos)	1 (20 mos)	2 (6 and 20 mos)	0	0	3 (4–37; av. 23 mos)
En Bloc excision + Complete CHT	6	0	1	2 (10–65 mos)	6 (23–108; av. 61 mos)	0	0
TOTAL	16	8	3	7	8	0	8

(ureter, cisterna magna, segmental vessels, nerve roots, and so on). The most severe late complications after vertebrectomy performed in patients who previously had an anterior approach and radiation was dissection of the aorta wall, which was lethal in one case. Among late complications, infection is particularly threatening because of the wide exposure and the reduced immunocompetence of these patients. Posterior resection is a shorter procedure; its possible complications are connected with dura dissection from the tumor and with possible damage of vessels and viscera by dissection of the tumoral mass from the posterior.

CONCLUSIONS

Knowledge of the biologic behavior of the different tumor types is mandatory to decide which is the most appropriate surgical margin for any tumor and therefore to decide the extent of surgical *en bloc* or intralesional excision. To popularize this concept, the Enneking staging system was set up (7). A surgical staging system is also required for planning the surgical procedure to achieve such margins (4).

The combination of Enneking staging (7) and WBB staging (4) should aim to

- avoid high-morbidity surgery when not necessary (for example, in stage 2 benign or in metastatic tumors);
- achieve the appropriate margin by correctly performed *en bloc* resections in selected cases; and
- increase the knowledge of these tumors by comparing uniform reports on outcomes of series homogeneously treated.

REFERENCES

1. Biagini R, Casadei R, Boriani S, et al. En bloc vertebrectomy and dural resection for chordoma: a case report. Spine Sep 2003;15:E368–372.
2. Boriani S, Biagini R, De Iure F, et al. En bloc resection of bone tumors of the thoracolumbar spine: a preliminary report on 29 patients. Spine 1996;21:1927–1930.
3. Boriani S, Weinstein JN. Differential diagnosis and surgical treatment of primary benign and malignant neoplasm. In: Frymoyer JW, ed. The Adult Spine: Principles and Practice, 2nd ed. Philadelphia: Lippincott-Raven, 1996:951–987.
4. Boriani S, Weinstein JN, Biagini R. Spine update: primary bone tumors of the spine: terminology and surgical staging. Spine 1997;22:1036–1044.
5. Boriani S. Subtotal and total vertebrectomy for tumours. In: Surgical Techniques in Orthopedics and Traumatology. Paris: Editions Scientifiques et Medicales Elsevier, 2000;A10:55–70.
6. Di Fiore M, Lari S, Boriani S, et al. Major vertebral surgery: intra- and postoperative anaesthesia-related problems. Chir Org Mov 1998;83:65–72.
7. Enneking WF. Muscoloskeletal Tumor Surgery. New York: Churchill Livingstone, 1983:69–122.
8. Faciszewski T, Winter RB, Lonstein JE, et al. The surgical and medical perioperative complications of anterior spinal fusion surgery in the thoracic and lumbar spine in adults: a review of 1223 procedures. Spine 1995;20:1592–1599.
9. Hart RA, Boriani S, Biagini R, et al. A system for surgical staging and management of spine tumors: a clinical outcome study of giant cell tumors of the spine. Spine 1997;22:1773–1783.
10. Roy-Camille R, Mazel Ch, Saillant G, et al. Treatment of malignant tumors of the spine with posterior instrumentation. In: Sundaresan N, Schmidek HH, Schiller AL, et al., eds. Tumors of the Spine: Diagnosis and Clinical Management. Philadelphia: Saunders, 1990:473–492.
11. Stener B. Complete removal of vertebrae for extirpation of tumors. Clin Orthop Rel Res 1989; 245:72–82.
12. Takuya Fujita, Norio Kawahara, Tadami Matsumoto, et al. Chordoma in the cervical spine managed with en bloc excision. Spine 1999;24: 1848.
13. Tomita K, Kawahara N, Baba H, et al. Total en bloc spondylectomy for solitary spinal metastases. Int Orthop (SICOT) 1994;18:291–298.
14. Weinstein JN. Differential diagnosis and surgical treatment of primary benign and malignant neoplasm. In: Frymoyer JW, ed. The Adult Spine: Principles and Practice. New York: Raven Press, 1991:830–850.

Management of Spinal Metastases

Charles S.B. Galasko

13

Diagnosis and treatment of spinal metastatic tumors is an increasing part of an orthopedic spinal surgeon's role, as the life expectancy of patients with treatable malignancy increases. The spine is the commonest site of skeletal metastases. Traditionally, metastatic tumors involving the spine have been treated palliatively with increasing opiate-based analgesics, but over the past 3 decades, a growing interest has been expressed in the surgical management of these patients, with an aim of stabilization of the spine and decompression of the spinal cord, when appropriate, to increase the patient's quality of life and reduce the analgesic requirements. In the vast majority of cases, spinal surgery is still palliative, as even total resection of the metastatic lesion will not affect the outcome, which is usually determined by other secondaries. Rarely an isolated spinal metastasis may be noted.

The three main aspects to the management of spinal metastases are as follows.

- Diagnosis
- Treatment
- Education

The diagnosis must include not only the presence of spinal metastases but also their site, including the amount of bone destruction; the degree of dissemination of the metastatic cancer; the presence or absence of complications, such as hypercalcemia, spinal instability, and spinal cord or cauda equina compression; the degree of soft tissue involvement; and the vascularity of the lesion. Magnetic resonance scanning is the optimal method of assessing the presence, site, amount of destruction, and soft tissue involvement, including neural compression. Skeletal scintigraphy is still probably the optimal method of assessing the overall skeletal dissemination, although whole-body MR scanning also can be satisfactory. The degree of involvement of other organs is necessary, as the final decision on treatment will partly depend on whether the patient's life expectancy justifies major surgery. All patients require full staging before surgery. Our own protocol includes magnetic resonance imaging (MRI) of the whole spine (to rule out other spinal lesions), skeletal scintigraphy, ultrasound of the abdomen, chest radiograph, and a full hematologic workup.

Provided that no contraindication to surgery exists, the decision as to whether the treatment should be surgical will depend on the presence of complications that require surgery: instability and/or spinal cord or cauda equina compression. If surgery is indicated, it must be supplemented by adjuvant therapy.

Some lesions can be very vascular, and if this is the case, preoperative embolization may be essential. This occurs particularly with metastases from renal carcinoma but can occur with other lesions. Depending on the primary tumor and the radiologic appearance of the metastasis, preoperative arteriography and, if necessary, embolization may be required (Guzman et al., 2005; Roscoe et al., 1989; Olerud et al., 1993; Sun and Lang, 1998; Gellad et al., 1990).

TREATMENT

The minority of patients with spinal metastases require surgery. In a study of 31 consecutive patients who had an underlying carcinoma and who initially had back pain (Galasko and Sylvester, 1978), we found that 11 patients had a benign lesion causing their back pain, seven had painful metastases that did not warrant surgical intervention, three had spinal instability with symptoms of sufficient severity to warrant surgical intervention, and ten had evidence of malignant spinal cord or cauda equina compression.

The majority of painful metastases can be treated with radiotherapy, usually combined with adjuvant treatment, such as chemotherapy or endocrine therapy, and frequently combined with bisphosphanates. Recent studies suggest that zoledronic acid, a third-generation bisphosphanate, may be the most useful in patients with skeletal metastases (Hortobagyi, 2005). These forms of treatment are reviewed in other chapters. Radiopharmaceuticals also have been used.

This chapter concentrates on the surgical management of spinal instability and/or malignant spinal cord or cauda equina compression. Surgery also may be occasionally indicated in patients with spinal metastases that have not responded to other forms of treatment and are still painful. Surgery also includes biopsy of a lesion for which the diagnosis is not known, but this aspect is not considered further in this chapter.

A variety of surgical techniques are available. As indicated earlier, preoperative embolization may be essential. The stabilization can be anterior, posterior, or combined anterior and posterior. More recently, minimal-access surgery (Huang et al., 2006) and endoscopically assisted decompression was undertaken (McLain, 1998). McLain concluded that endoscopic-assisted decompression can reduce morbidity and may aid surgery, improving the surgeon's vision, providing light and magnification as well as a more direct view.

Spondylectomy has been advocated for patients with a single metastasis and in whom the primary tumor has been successfully excised (Sakaura et al 2004, Tomita et al 1994, Abe et al 2001).

Vertebroplasty can be used for painful metastases that have not responded to other treatment or if the instability can be controlled by vertebroplasty without the necessity for instrumentation, as may be the case with a painful compression fracture secondary to spinal metastasis (Alvarez et al., 2003; Cotton et al., 1996; Weill et al., 1996; Gaitanis et al., 2005; Hadjipavlou et al., 2005; Yamada et al., 2004; Barragen–Campos et al., 2006; Vrionis et al., 2005; Dudeney et al., 2002; Burton et al., 2005). This involves the percutaneous injection of bone cement into lytic lesions in the vertebral body to provide support and prevent collapse of the vertebral body. Basically, it takes advantage of interventional radiologic techniques. It has been used in the treatment of osteolytic lesions, including myeloma and spinal metastases. Although a number of articles have been published on this procedure, few have clearly defined the outcome measures, and virtually none has provided a long-term follow-up in terms of the clinical indications, expected complications, and inherent risks in patients with skeletal metastases.

Approximately 80% of the forces to the spinal column are transmitted through the anterior column (Lowery and Harms, 1997). Metastases are more common in the vertebral body as opposed to the posterior elements, and this predisposes to kyphotic collapse, as the metastatic tissue is structurally less able to transmit these forces than is normal cancellous bone. Not all patients are suitable for anterior surgery because of the widespread nature of their metastases, and some patients, because of their poor medical fitness, may not be suitable for major surgery, even though it is indicated. Tokuhashi (1994, 2005, (Table 13.1) made an attempt at a scoring system to determine whether palliative stabilization or a more radical palliative resection should be undertaken. The system uses six parameters: the general condition of the patient; the number of extraspinal bone metastases; the number of metastases in the vertebral body; metastases to major internal organs (lungs, liver, kidneys and brain); the primary site

TABLE 13.1 Tokuhashi's Revised Evaluation System for the Prognosis of Metastatic Spine Tumors

Characteristic		Score
General condition (Karnofsky's performance status)		
Poor	(PS 10%–40%)	0
Moderate	(PS 50%–70%)	1
Good	(PS 80%–100%)	2
Number of extraspinal bone metastases foci		
3 or more		0
1–2		1
0		2
Number of metastases in the vertebral body		
3 or more		0
2		1
1		2
Metastases to the major internal organs		
Unremovable		0
Removable		1
No metastases		2
Primary site of the cancer		
Lung, osteosarcoma, stomach, bladder, esophagus, pancreas		0
Liver, gallbladder, unidentified		1
Others		2
Kidney, uterus		3
Rectum		4
Thyroid, breast, prostate, carcinoid tumor		5
Palsy		
Complete	(Frankel A, B)	0
Incomplete	(Frankel C, D)	1
None	(Frankel E)	2

Total score	0–8	Predicted prognosis, <6 mo	Conservative treatment
Total score	9–11	Predicted prognosis, 6 mo plus	Palliative surgery (Excisional surgery if single lesion and no metastases to major internal organs.)
Total score	12–15	Predicted prognosis, 12 mo plus	Excisional surgery

of the cancer; and the severity of spinal cord palsy. They concluded that the total score obtained for each patient could be correlated with the prognosis but that the prognosis could not be predicted from a single parameter. They advised an excisional operation in patients with a good prognosis and a palliative procedure in those with a poor prognosis. The latter was aimed only at securing support with no or only partial resection of the lesion. To assess the general condition of the patient they used the criteria established by Karnofsky (1967). The Tokuhashi score tends to segregate those who would benefit from conservative treatment and those who would benefit from surgery. It is a useful tool but has not been fully validated and is only a guide to selection. The Karnofsky score (Karnofsky, 1967) is a functional score that can be used to assess changes in outcome after major surgery for spinal metastases, as is the Eastern Cooperative Oncology Group (ECOG) performance status (Oken et al., 1982).

Tomita et al. (2001) based their surgical strategy on a prognostic scoring system that used the grade of malignancy, visceral metastases (no metastases, treatable, untreatable), and skeletal metastases (solitary or isolated, multiple). The surgical strategy was based on a prognostic score. They divided their patients into four groups depending on the prognostic score. Those with the best prognosis were treated with wide or marginal excision, the next group by marginal intralesionary excision, the third group by palliative surgery with stabilization, and those with the worst prognosis, with nonoperative supportive care. The mean survival in their first group was 38.2 months; in the second group, it was 21.5 months; and in those treated with palliative surgery and stabilization, 10.1 months. The mean survival time of patients treated with terminal care was 5.3 months. It is my view that if a patient is in excruciating pain, spinal stabilization is warranted, even if the survival is no more than 2 to 3 months.

Taneichi et al. (1997) attempted to assess whether impending vertebral collapse could be assessed and prophylactic stabilization carried out. They suggested that a significant risk of collapse of thoracic vertebrae exists with a 50% to 60% tumor involvement of the vertebral body with no destruction of other structures or 25% to 30% involvement of the vertebral body with costovertebral joint destruction, and in the thoracolumbar and lumbar spine, if 35% to 40% involvement of the vertebral body or 20% to 25% of the vertebral body with pedicle destruction was found.

Posterior stabilization is less invasive, and the postoperative management usually requires less monitoring and is less intensive. It is usually a smaller surgical insult and can be carried out on less medically fit patients. As has already been indicated, most of the metastatic deposits are anterior and, therefore, the posterior structures at the level of pathology are relatively strong, consisting of pedicles and laminae unaffected by the disease process. If stabilization is combined with a decompressive procedure, these relatively intact structures (spinous processes, interspinous ligaments, and laminae) require removal for the decompression to be undertaken. Thus, in a posterior decompression, the spine is destabilized further by sacrificing intact bony elements to decompress indirectly the neural elements.

Posterior decompression alone, without stabilization, is contraindicated because of the further destabilizing effect. If a posterior decompression is thought to be appropriate, it should **always** be combined with posterior instrumentation to restore stability. It is usually possible, when carrying out posterior stabilization, to use pedicle screws, sublaminar hooks, or sublaminar wires. However, implant failure will occur, either by implant breakage or implant pull-out unless either a sound bony fusion occurs or the patient dies of the malignancy. Posterior stabilization also is mechanically inferior as a deficient anterior column is not reconstructed. Therefore, force must be transferred to the posterior elements. At least two spinal segments must be stabilized on each side of the pathologic level, so in total, five levels or more require instrumentation when combined with a one-level posterior decompression. Posterior stabilization alone is inadequate for lesions at L-5 and usually L-4. Posterior surgery has a number of drawbacks compared with anterior surgery.

- The indirect decompression may be inferior, as the compression is anterior to neural elements.
- Posterior decompression destabilizes the spine further, making instrumentation necessary.
- A long construct is necessary to achieve stability, but without anterior column reconstruction, this is mechanically inferior.

Nevertheless, posterior stabilization alone rarely fails, if carried out properly and patient selection is correct.

Anterior decompression and stabilization has become the approach of choice when treating neurologic compression. This is because it allows direct decompression and stabilization, restoring anterior column function and allowing a better biomechanical reconstruction. Anterior stabilization requires normal bone quality cephalad and caudad to the level of vertebrectomy to obtain secure fixation. During the procedure, the posterior longitudinal ligament is visualized and well decompressed. An appropriate-sized cage can be inserted to restore vertebral height, therefore reducing the kyphosis and allowing restoration of anterior column support. Depending on the prognosis, the cage can be filled with cement or bone graft. The reconstruction is completed with the use of a screw-and-rod system such as the Kaneda- or Ventrafix-type device. Multiple-level vertebral metastases, even when they do not cause compression, interfere with secure fixation and are therefore a relative contraindication to anterior surgery. Severe osteoporosis is also a relative contraindication, as construction failure, by cage sinkage or screw pull-out, can occur. Anterior stabilization, with or without decompression, is relatively easy from T-6 to L-3. Stabilization of T-5 would require screws being inserted into T-4. This is contraindicated because of metalwork close to the great vessels. An L-4 vertebrectomy is surgically more demanding and often requires posterior stabilization with pedicle screws, as it is difficult to instrument L-5 because of the proximity of the great vessels. An L-5 vertebrectomy has unique problems. It may not be possible to insert an anterior screw into S-1 and, therefore, posterior stabilization is necessary. If an L-5 vertebrectomy is to be carried out, it is probably easiest through a transperitoneal approach, although a retroperitoneal approach also is possible.

Occasionally the neurologic compression is caused by circumferential tumor. If this is the case, anterior and posterior stabilization may give the best palliative approach, allowing debulking of tumor from both anterior and posterior approaches with rigid stabilization. It is my current preference, wherever possible, to perform anterior surgery alone. However, where significant posterior tumor requires decompression or osteoporosis, which would increase the risk of anterior construct failure, anterior surgery is supplemented by posterior stabilization. Posterior stabilization is used where multiple lesions must be stabilized.

SPINAL INSTABILITY

Back pain is a frequent symptom of disseminated carcinoma, and in 10%, is due to spinal instability (Galasko and Sylvester, 1978). Carcinoma of the breast is the commonest primary tumor associated with spinal instability, but any tumor can metastasize to the spine and can cause sufficient destruction to render the spine unstable. Spinal instability can cause excruciating pain, which is mechanical. In its severe form, the patient is comfortable only when lying absolutely still. Any movement, including log-rolling by two or three trained nurses, may be associated with agonizing pain, and the patient may not be able to sit, stand, or walk because of the pain, even with the use of a spinal orthosis. In its milder form, which is more usual, the patient may be relatively free from pain when not moving, but any movement of the back, for example, turning in bed, may be extremely painful. Plain radiographs show the amount of destruction. Two causes exist for spinal instability in metastatic cancer: bone destruction, due to the tumor and iatrogenic, due to posterior decompression (laminectomy) without concomitant stabilization. Plain radiographs show destruction of bone with vertebral collapse of a greater or lesser degree.

Stabilization is required for pain relief. The decision as to whether the spine should be stabilized from an anterior or posterior approach depends on the site and the extent of the lesions. Spinal metastases usually initially involve the vertebral body, and if the instability is limited to one or possibly two adjacent vertebrae, anterior resection of the lesion with anterior instrumentation is usually indicated. However, if the lesion is more extensive or more than one area requires stabilization, posterior stabilization may be indicated; occasionally, because of the site of the lesion, both anterior and posterior instrumentation might be indicated (see earlier). At the time of spinal stabilization, if any tumor lies in the spinal canal, irrespective of whether the patient has neurologic symptoms, the spinal cord or cauda equina (depending on the level of the lesion) should be decompressed.

In our first study (Galasko et al., 2000), we reported on 80 patients with spinal instability secondary to tumor-induced bone destruction. Of these, 70 were treated with posterior stabilization, five by anterior stabilization and five by combined anterior and posterior stabilization. Seventy-one (89%) had complete relief of pain, and four (5%) patients had partial relief. In five patients, treatment failed. One patient died of septicemia after a wound infection; in a second patient, a deep infection developed, requiring removal of the implant. In two patients, the implant failed. In the beginning of this study, we used Harrington rods, but the risk of this complication has diminished considerably with current instrumentation. Since modern instrumentation became available, we have not had a further case of loosening. The fifth patient initially had complete relief of pain, but paraplegia developed as a result of an extradural bleed. Despite removal of the clot, no recovery occurred. This patient had been taking anticoagulants for an intercurrent illness. Preoperative radiation therapy predisposed to wound infection and breakdown, and after this study, we have tried to persuade our radiotherapy colleagues that preoperative radiotherapy should not be given.

Ghogawala et al. (2001) reported that patients who had radiation before surgical decompression and stabilization had a threefold greater wound complication rate ($p < 0.05$) than did patients who had surgery followed by radiation.

Ideally, patients should receive postoperative irradiation, which should be given once the wound has healed. On some occasions, however, when the patient has received the maximal tolerable preoperative dose, further radiotherapy would put the cord at risk of developing transverse myelitis. The underlying tumor may require treatment with endocrine therapy or chemotherapy, and bisphosphonates may be indicated for other small skeletal metastases demonstrated in the preoperative investigations.

In our next 42 patients, 25 underwent anterior decompression and stabilization, 15 underwent posterior decompression and stabilization, and two underwent combined anterior and posterior stabilization with decompression. One patient with breast carcinoma underwent anterior decompression and stabilization, but the tumor did not respond to treatment, and 7 months later, she required posterior decompression and stabilization for neural compression.

In a more recent study (Galasko and Spilsbury, 2002), we evaluated 23 patients who were treated with anterior vertebrectomy, insertion of a Moss cage, and Kaneda fixation. None of the patients deteriorated neurologically. The pre-operative Karnofsky score (1967) was 57% (30% to 80%) and postoperatively was 85% (70% to 90%). This calculates to a change in Karnofsky score of 27%, which equates to most patients becoming independent, whereas previously they were dependant for most activities of daily living. A marked decrease in the consumption of opiates and analgesics was found after the operation.

In both studies, some of the patients had malignant cord compression. In this study, no patient deteriorated neurologically; 62% started at Frankel E, where they remained; 30% improved from Frankel D to Frankel E; and one patient improved from Frankel C to Frankel E.

O'Donoghue et al. (1997a) found that in patients with structurally significant bone destruction secondary to metastases from breast cancer, surgery and radiotherapy were associated with a speedier resolution of symptoms, a longer symptom-free survival, a lower incidence of symptom recurrence, and a longer survival overall than was radiotherapy alone. The symptom-free survival in patients with structurally significant bone destruction of their axial skeleton was 11 weeks in patients treated with radiotherapy alone compared with 39 weeks in patients treated with surgery and radiotherapy ($p < 0.5$). The overall survival was 9.4 months in patients treated with radiotherapy alone, compared with 22.3 months in those treated with surgery and radiotherapy ($p < 0.05$).

Onimus et al. (1996) reported the results of operative intervention in 100 patients with spinal metastases. Anterior stabilization was carried out in 58, posterior stabilization in 33, and combined anterior and posterior stabilization in nine. Preoperatively, 96 patients had vertebral pain, and 43 had radicular pain. Walking was impossible for 50 patients because of either neural compression or pain caused by spinal instability. Thirty-five (70%) of the 50 patients were able to walk after decompression and stabilization. Of the 38 patients with a preoperative neurologic deficit, 30 had a postoperative decrease of the deficit. Sixty-two patients completely stopped using analgesics after the operation. Overall, clinical improvement occurred in 80 of the 100 patients.

Weigel et al. (1999) retrospectively assessed 86 surgical interventions in 76 consecutive patients with symptomatic spinal metastases. Back pain or radicular pain or both was present in all patients before surgery, and in 76% of patients, it was severe. Sixty percent of patients obtained marked pain relief after surgery, and 29%, moderate improvement. In 11%, no change was found. No patients reported worsening of pain. The relief of pain was permanent, returning only in patients in whom local tumor recurrence of new metastatic spinal disease developed. The mean postoperative survival was 13.1 months, the highest survival rates being seen in patients with multiple myeloma and breast carcinoma, with very poor survival in patients with lung carcinoma (2.1 months) and melanoma (1.5 months). Survival in patients with these tumors was significantly shorter than the overall survival of the other 64 patients ($p < 0.0001$). In 45 instances, a neurologic deficit occurred. Improvements were observed in 58%.

They found that 19% of the operations were associated with complications. Hatrick et al. (2000) evaluated 42 patients who underwent surgery for metastatic disease of the spine. Postoperatively, pain improved in 38 (90%), the neurologic deficit in 20 of the 29 patients with a deficit (69%), and ambulatory ability in 25 (78%) of the 32 patients with very restricted mobility.

Jackson et al. (2000) reviewed 79 patients who underwent 107 spinal operations for metastatic renal cell carcinoma. Indications for surgery included disabling pain or neurologic dysfunction or both. Preoperative embolization was required in approximately one half of the patients. The median postoperative survival was 12.3 months. Significant pain reduction was achieved in 84 (89%) of the 94 cases with disabling pain. Neurologic improvement was seen in 36 (65%) of the 55 patients with neurologic dysfunction.

MALIGNANT COMPRESSION OF THE SPINAL CORD OR CAUDA EQUINA

Schaberg and Gainor (1985) reported that cord compression occurred in 20% of patients with vertebral metastases. Constance et al. (1983) thought it likely that in 5% to 10% of patients with spinal metastases, symptomatic neurologic manifestation of their metastases developed. Galasko and Sylvester (1978) indicated that such compression may occur in one third of patients with spinal metastases. Compression of the spinal cord or cauda equina may occur in association with spinal instability or in isolation. Pain is almost invariable and persisting, and increasing back pain may herald spinal cord compression. The pain is frequently localized to the site of the disease and is probably caused by stimulation of pain receptors in the longitudinal ligaments, dura, or periosteum as the tumor expands. Radicular pain is less common. Nevertheless, by the time treatment is started, up to 50% of patients will no longer be able to walk, and 10% to 30% will be paraplegic (Galasko, 1986; Fidler, 1987). Other symptoms include weakness, disturbance of gait, paresthesiae, urinary hesitancy or precipitance, and constipation or spurious diarrhea. The sequence of events is often pain, motor dysfunction, paresthesia, and sensory loss. The pain from malignant spinal cord compression is often deep, unremitting, worsening, and severe.

The choice of treatment of spinal cord compression, without deformity or instability, depends on the duration, severity, and speed of progression of the neurologic symptoms and the radiosensitivity of the tumor. Patients with minor neurologic symptoms that have been slow in onset tend to respond favorably to irradiation. Dense paraparesis and rapid neurologic deterioration are poor prognostic indicators, irrespective of treatment. Under these circumstances, the only chance of achieving a functional recovery lies in rapid decompression of the spinal cord. If the tumor is radiosensitive, irradiation may affect cord compression as rapidly as surgery. Radioresistant tumors are slow to respond and require urgent surgical decompression. Radiotherapy will not be as effective in symptomatic patients with progressive kyphotic spinal deformity or spinal instability. These patients require decompression and stabilization.

The results of treatment depend heavily on the neurologic status of the patient at the time of starting treatment, and it is important, therefore, to make the diagnosis urgently. Surgery is indicated in patients with recent onset of symptoms, particularly a developing paraplegia or urinary retention of less than 24 hours' duration; a block shown on the preoperative MRI localized to no more than two or three segments; and a life expectancy of at least 2 to 3 months. It is also indicated in patients whose compression is associated with spinal instability, as other treatments are not likely to resolve the pain caused by the spinal instability. Once paraplegia has been established for some days, or urinary retention has been present for more than 24 to 30 hours, surgery is often associated with some return of sensation or pain relief or both, but not with useful recovery of bladder or motor function.

Occasionally, anterior decompression and stabilization may be associated with major neurologic recovery in patients with long-standing neurologic disturbances in which the onset of the symptoms has been gradual. In general terms, patients with a gradual onset of neurologic disturbances do better than those in whom paraplegia and urine retention developed extremely rapidly. Decompression should never be carried out without simultaneous stabilization. Laminectomy alone is contraindicated. It leads to increased instability of the spine with increasing kyphosis, increasing pain, and increased neurologic deficit. Studies that compare laminectomy and radiotherapy with radiotherapy alone are flawed, in that they compare a destabilizing operation with radiotherapy. Decompression and stabilization may be either posterior or anterior (see earlier). The question arises as to whether treatment should also be combined with a short course of high-dose corticosteroids to minimize the edema. Until recently, this was standard practice, but the value of steroids is currently being questioned.

Jansson and Bauer (2006) evaluated 282 consecutive patients operated on for spinal metastases. Their main surgical indication was neurologic deficit. Metastases from cancer of the prostate accounted for 40%; breast, 15%; kidney, 8%; and lung, 7%. In 78%, the level of decompression was thoracic, and in 22%, it was lumbar. Thirteen percent had a single metastasis only. Preoperatively, 64% were nonwalkers (Frankel A–C), 30% could walk with aids (Frankel D), and 8% had normal motor function (Frankel E). Posterior decompression and stabilization was carried out in 212 patients; 47 underwent laminectomy alone; and 23 underwent anterior decompression and reconstruction. Complications were recorded in 20%, and systemic complications were often associated with early death. Twelve (55%) of 255 patients with motor deficits were worse postoperatively, whereas 179 (70%) improved at least one Frankel grade. Pathologic fracture was present in 55% of cases. None of the 65 patients with nonskeletal metastases survived 2 years. Laminectomy alone was reserved mostly for patients without pathologic fracture and particularly for those with epidural compression posteriorly from metastasis to the spinous process. Reoperation for recurrence of epidural compression at the previously operated-on level was carried out in 17 (6%) of the 282 patients. Fourteen of these operations occurred more than 1 year after the initial procedure.

Saito et al. (2006) reviewed 74 patients who underwent posterior spinal surgery combined with intraoperative radiotherapy for spinal paresis due to spinal metastases. Improvement of at least one level, according to Frankel's classification, was attained in 86%. Of the 58 patients unable to walk preoperatively, 45 (78%) patients regained walking ability postoperatively. The rate of local recurrence was 2.5%. Some patients also received preoperative or postoperative external radiotherapy.

Surgery also is indicated where the malignant neural compression is associated with retropulsed bone, producing neural compression, spinal deformity producing the neural compression, and failure of radiation. In our study (Galasko et al. 2000) of 80 patients who underwent surgery for spinal instability or neural compression or both, 34 patients had malignant cord or cauda equina compression associated with the neurologic deficit. Twenty-three (67.6%) obtained a major/complete recovery of bladder function and walking ability. In one patient who appeared to obtain a full recovery, recurrence of his neurological symptoms developed 8 months later.

In a more recent study, Patchell and colleagues (2005) carried out a randomized, multi-institutional, nonblinded trial comparing surgery and radiotherapy with radiotherapy alone, by using the same radiotherapy protocol in both arms of the study. They noted that metastatic epidural spinal cord compression occurred in 5% to 14% of cancer patients; more than 20,000 new cases being reported every year in the United States.

They also noted that the standard nonsurgical treatment for malignant neural compression was radiotherapy and corticosteroids, but that with such treatment, few nonambulatory patients ever walked again, and that the results of laminectomy and radiation did not seem to differ from results with radiation alone. As a result, referrals for surgical treatment were largely abandoned by many oncologists and radiotherapists, but as indicated earlier, laminectomy without stabilization destabilizes the spine and is contraindicated for metastatic disease. Subsequently, several uncontrolled surgical series (Siegel et al., 1982; Harrington, 1984; Sundaresan et al., 1984; Overby and Rothman, 1985; Siegel et al., 1985) and a meta-analysis (Klimo et al., 2005) showed that direct decompressive surgery with instrumentation is superior to radiation therapy.

In their study, Patchell et al. defined metastatic epidural spinal cord compression (MESCC) as a true displacement of the spinal cord (by an epidural mass) from its normal position in the spinal canal. Patients had to have had at least one neurologic sign or symptom and not to have been totally paraplegic for longer than 48 hours before entry into the study. The MESCC had to be restricted to a single area, which could include several contiguous spinal or vertebral segments. Patients with a mass that compressed only the cauda equina or spinal roots were excluded, as were those with multiple discrete compressive lesions, unless they had one area of compression and multiple noncompressive lesions. Patients with certain radiosensitive tumors (lymphomas, leukemia, multiple myeloma, and germ cell tumors) were excluded, as were patients with preexisting or concomitant neurologic problems not related directly to the MESCC, such as brain metastases. Patients with previous MESCC and those who had received previous spinal radiation such that they were unable to receive the study dose also were excluded. Patients had to have a general medical status good enough to be accepted surgical candidates and an expected survival of at least 3 months. All patients were given the same corticosteroid regimen starting with 100 mg dexamethasone immediately on diagnosis. Spinal stability was ascertained according to Cybulski's guidelines (1989). All patients received the same radiotherapy regimen, but the surgery was tailored for each patient depending on the level of the spine involved and the patient's circumstances.

The primary end point of the study was the ability to walk after treatment. The secondary end points were urinary continence, changes in Frankel functional scale scores (Frankel et al., 1969), American Spinal Injury Association (ASIA) motor scores, and the use of corticosteroids and opioid analgesics.

They had initially planned to include 100 patients in each treatment group, but because of proven superiority of surgical treatment, the data-safety and -monitoring committee deemed that the trial should be stopped early. When the trial was closed 101 patients had been entered: 51 patients in the radiotherapy group and 50 patients in the surgery-plus-radiotherapy group.

The posttreatment ambulatory rate in the surgery group was 84% (42 of 50) compared with 57% (29 of 51) in the radiation group ($p = 0.001$). Patients in the surgery group retained the ability to walk for significantly longer than did those in the radiation group (median, 122 days vs. 13 days; $p = 0.003$). Multivariate analysis showed surgery ($p = 0.0017$) and pretreatment Frankel score ($p = 0.0008$) to be associated with longer ambulatory times.

In the subgroup of patients who could walk at study entry, 94% (32 of 34) in the surgery group continued to walk after treatment compared with 74% (26 of 35) in the radiation group ($p = 0.024$). Patients in the surgical group were able to walk for a median of 153 days compared with 54 days in the radiation group ($p = 0.024$). Multivariate analysis showed surgery ($p = 0.0048$), Frankel score ($p = 0.016$), and primary breast tumor ($p = 0.029$) to be associated with longer ambulatory time.

Thirty-two patients (16 in each group) entered the study unable to walk; of these, 10 (62%) patients in the surgery group regained the ability to walk compared with only three (19%) patients in the radiotherapy group ($p = 0.012$). Nonambulatory patients treated with surgery walked for a median 59 days compared with a median of 0 days for patients in the radiotherapy group ($p = 0.04$).

Surgical treatment resulted in significant differences in maintenance of continence, muscle strength (ASIA scores), functional ability (Frankel scores), and increased survival time. The surgical group also had a substantial reduction in the use of corticosteroids and opioid analgesics. The 30-day mortality rate was 6% in the surgery group and 14% in the radiotherapy group ($p = 0.32$). Surgery did not result in increased hospitalization; the median hospital stay was 10 days in both groups. The 30-day morbidity was substantially worse in the radiation group.

The cause of damage to the spinal cord from compression is complex and multifactorial. Direct compression results in edema, venous congestion, and demyelination. If the compression is of short duration, the effects are reversible; remyelination and recovery of function is possible. However, with prolonged compression, secondary vascular injury occurs with infarction of the spinal cord (Patchell et al., 2005). After this type of injury, no meaningful recovery is possible. Surgical decompression is immediate, whereas radiotherapy takes several days to have an effect. Surgery was probably able to provide relief from compression before irreversible vascular injury occurred in a substantial number of patients in their study (which probably explains the better results obtained in the surgery group).

SPONDYLECTOMY

A number of authors reported on small series of total *en bloc* spondylectomy for solitary metastasis of the thoracolumbar spine. Tomita et al. (1994) reported that local recurrences were absent in all of the 20 patients at an average follow-up of 13 months after total *en bloc* spondylectomy, whereas Abe et al. (2001) reported that local recurrences developed in two of eight patients at an average follow-up of 32 months after surgery. Sakaura et al. (2004) noted that the indication for total *en bloc* spondylectomy was a solitary spinal metastasis localized to one level and that did not invade adjacent visceral organs; a controllable primary tumor; and no evidence of metastases in other organs, such as brain, lung, and liver. They evaluated 12 patients whose primary tumors included breast cancer in four, thyroid cancer in three, renal cell carcinoma in three, and lung cancer in one. In the 12th patient, the tumor was of unknown origin. In two of the four patients with paraspinal tumor extension, local recurrences developed at 26 months after surgery. Seven patients survived for an average of 61 months, whereas the remaining five died of disseminated metastases, with a mean survival of 23 months after surgery. They concluded that *en bloc* spondylectomy failed to prove curative resection of the tumor if a paraspinal extension was present.

PREVENTION OF BONE LYSIS

The main role of the orthopedic or spinal surgeon, in the palliation of pain for patients with skeletal metastases, is in the treatment of the complications of these lesions. These complications are usually caused by bone lysis, resulting in spinal instability or malignant neural compression or both. The aim of treatment, in the future, must be to prevent this progressive bone destruction. If it is not possible to destroy the cancer cells, the treatment of choice for skeletal metastases may be to inhibit the secondary bone resorption that subsequently occurs and that is responsible for much of the morbidity associated with skeletal metastases. The tumor-induced osteolysis is mediated by osteoclasts, the osteoclasts being stimulated by cytokines and growth factors secreted by the tumor (Galasko, 1976). Some of these factors may also affect the cell-adhesion molecules (Evans et al., 1992). Bisphosphonates inhibit osteoclast bone resorption. They are useful in the management of small lesions but have not yet been shown to be of benefit in large, lytic lesions. In the future, it is likely that other drugs will be developed to inhibit the osteoclastic response to tumors, such as those inhibiting the nuclear factor (NF)–κB (RANK) ligand.

Tumors grow only if they develop their own blood supply. This is dependent on local angiogenetic factors; another possibility for controlling tumor growth is by the use of antiangiogenic drugs such as anti–vascular endothelial growth factor (VEGF) therapy.

It is likely that in the future, the development and use of such agents will minimize tumor-induced bone osteolysis and the subsequent complications that develop and require orthopedic intervention.

FAILURE OF EDUCATION

Although orthopedic surgery can do much to improve the quality of life of patients with metastatic cancer, many suitable patients are not being referred. Galasko et al. (2000) analyzed the records of 1,412 women who were diagnosed with untreatable breast cancer in 31 hospitals. Of these, 963 had complete records that were used for the analysis.

The results are shown in Table 13.2. All patients in whom a pathologic fracture of the femur developed were referred for an orthopedic appointment. Only four of ten patients in whom a pathologic fracture of the humerus developed were referred for an orthopedic opinion. It is possible that surgery may not have been the optimal form of providing palliative care in all the other six patients, but it is likely that it would have been the optimal form of treatment in some of them. Of the six patients in whom neurologic compression developed, only two were referred for an orthopedic opinion More worrying is that only six (11.8%) of the 51 women in whom spinal instability developed were referred for an orthopedic opinion. An analysis of textbooks available in 2000 revealed that only two of nine oncologic textbooks and one of 12 textbooks on breast cancer mentioned spinal instability secondary to metastatic disease of the spine.

O'Donoghue et al. (1997a, 1997b) reported similar results. They evalued 269 consecutive patients with breast cancer who had been seen in internationally known breast units. They found that patients who had a pathologic fracture did better after operative

TABLE 13.2 Complications of Skeletal Metastases in 207 Patients with Mammary Cancer

Complication	Number	Number referred to orthopedic surgeon	Treated surgically
Pathologic femoral fracture	22	22 (100%)	19 (86.4%)
Pathologic humeral fracture	10	4 (40%)	2 (20%)
Neural compression	6	2 (33%)	1 (16.6%)
Spinal instability	51	6 (11.8%)	0 (0%)

From Galasko et al., 2000, with permission.

intervention with adjunctive therapy than did those who had nonoperative treatment alone. Forty-seven women had a total of 82 instances of structural bone destruction, 52 (63%) of which involved the spine and 11 of which were associated with cord compression. The average duration of symptom-free survival was 39 weeks in the group that was treated surgically for spinal structural bone destruction compared with 11 weeks in the group treated nonoperatively. The average duration of overall survival was 22 and 9 months, respectively ($p < 0.05$ for both comparisons). They concluded that clinical review by an orthopedic surgeon would have been appropriate in 89% of the instances but was sought in only 46% and that operative intervention was feasible in 65% but was carried out in only 31%.

The role of the orthopaedic and spinal surgeon must include education of oncologists, radiotherapists, breast surgeons, and others as to the indications and benefits of spinal surgery when appropriate.

SUMMARY

The development of spinal instability or spinal cord or cauda equina compression or both in patients with metastatic cancer is not necessarily a terminal event. These lesions are associated with severe pain and severe morbidity. The aims of treatment are to alleviate pain, restore mobility, prevent neurologic compression, and restore neurologic function.

Before the lesion is treated, the patient must be carefully evaluated to determine the degree of dissemination of the cancer and the general medical condition. Optimal treatment of many of these lesions requires major surgery, which should not be carried out if a patient is terminal. The aim of treatment is to palliate the symptoms and improve the patient's quality of life. Surgical treatment does not affect the life expectancy, except in the very rare instance in which a single isolated metastasis is amenable to *en bloc* spondylectomy. Irrespective of whether surgical reconstruction is possible, the patient should always be made comfortable, kept comfortable, and be allowed to die with dignity.

Contraindications to surgery include a terminally ill patient, a high risk of fixation failure due to the extent of bone destruction, or severe osteoporosis that militates against instrumentation. Spinal instability requires stabilization with decompression as necessary, supplemented by postoperative radiotherapy (if feasible), chemotherapy, or endocrine therapy and bisphosphanates if indicated. Malignant neural compression requires decompression combined with stabilization, postoperative radiotherapy, and adjuvant therapy.

In patients with metastatic cancer of the spine, spinal decompression must always be supplemented by spinal stabilization to prevent progressive collapse of the spine, resulting in kyphosis and stretching of the spinal cord.

Although orthopedic surgery has much to offer in the palliation of the pain of patients with spinal complications from skeletal metastases, the minority of patients with these spinal disorders have been referred for treatment. Better education of oncologists, radiotherapists, cancer surgeons, and others is required.

The role of the orthopaedic and spinal surgeon must include the education of other medical specialists as to the potential benefits of spinal surgery.

It is hoped that improved understanding of the underlying pathophysiologic changes that occur when tumor invades bone may lead to effective osteoclast-inhibiting drugs and other agents that may obviate the development of large lytic metastases in the future.

REFERENCES:

Alvarez L, Pereze-Higueras A, Quinones D, et al. (2003) Vertebroplasty in the treatment of vertebral tumours: procedural outcomes and quality of life. Eur Spine J 12:356–360.

Barragen-Campos HM, Vallee J-N, Lo D, et al. (2006) Percutaneous vertebroplasty for spinal metastases: complications. Radiology 238:354–362.

Burton AW, Reddy SK, Shah HN et al. (2005) Percutaneous vertebroplasty: a technique to treat refractory spinal pain in the setting of advanced metastatic cancer: a case series. J Pain Symptom Manage 30:87–95.

Constans JP, de Divitiis E, Donzelli R, et al. (1983) Spinal metastases with neurological manifestations: review of 600 cases. J Neurosurg 59:111–118.

Cotton A, Dewatre F, Cortet B, et al. (1966) Percutaneous vertebroplasty for osteolytic metastases and myeloma: effects of the percentage of lesion filling and the leakage of methyl methacrylate at clinical follow-up. Radiology 200:525–530.

Cybulski GR, (1989) Methods of surgical stabilization for metastatic disease of the spine. Neurosurgery 25:240–252.

Dudeney S, Lieberman IH, Reinhardt M-K, et al. (2002) Kyphoplasty in the treatment of osteolytic vertebral compression fractures as a result of multiple myeloma. J Clin Oncol 20:2382–2387.

Evans CE, Ward C, Rathour L, et al. (1992) Myeloma affects both the growth and function of human osteoblast-like cells. Clin Exp Metastases 10:33–38.

Frankel HI, Hancock DO, Hyslop G, et al. (1969) The value of postural reduction in the initial management of closed injuries to the spine with paraplegia and tetraplegia. Paraplegia 7:179–192.

Fidler MW. (1987) Pathological fractures of the spine including those causing anterior spinal cord compression: surgical management. In: Galasko CSB, Noble J (eds). Recent developments in orthopaedic surgery; Festschrift to Sir Harry Platt. Manchester, Manchester University Press, pp 94–103.

Gaitanis IN, Hadjipavlou AG, Katonis PG, et al. (2005) Balloon kyphoplasty for the treatment of pathological vertebral compression fractures. Eur Spine J 14:250–260.

Galasko CSB. (1976) Mechanisms of bone destruction in the development of skeletal metastasis. Nature 263:507–508.

Galasko CSB. (1986) Skeletal Metastasis. London: Butterworths.

Galasko CSB, Norris HE, Crank S. (2000) Spinal instability secondary to metastatic cancer: current concepts review. J Bone Joint Surg 82-A:570–576.

Galasko CSB, Spilsbury JB. (2002) Treatment of secondary spinal tumours. In: Bone Metastases. Medical, Surgical and Radiological Treatment. (Ed. DG Poitout), London, Springer, pp. 115–128.

Galasko CSB, Sylvester BS. (1978) Back pain in patients treated for malignant tumours. Clin Oncol 4:273–283.

Gellad FE, Sadato N, Numaguchi Y, Levine AM (1990) Vascular metastatic lesions of the spine; preoperative embolization. Radiology 176:683–686.

Ghogawala Z, Mansfield FL, Borges LF. (2001) Spinal radiation before surgical decompression adversely affects outcomes of surgery for symptomatic metastatic spinal cord compression. Spine 26:818–824.

Guzman R, Dubach-Schwizer S, Heini P, et al. (2005) Preoperative transarterial embolization of vertebral metastases. Eur Spine J 14:263–268.

Hadjipavlou AG, Tzermiadianos MN, Katonis PG, Szpalski M (2005) Percutaneous vertebroplasty and balloon kyphoplasty for the treatment of osteoporitic vertebral compression fractures and osteolytic tumours: review article. J Bone Joint Surg 87B:1595–1604.

Harrington KD. (1984) Anterior cord decompression and spinal stabilization for patients with metastatic lesions of the spine. J Neurosurg 61:107–117.

Hatrick NC, Lucas JD, Timothy AR, Smith MA. (2000) The surgical treatment of metastatic disease of the spine. Radiother Oncol 56:335–339.

Hortobagyi GN (2005) Moving into the future: treatment of bone metastases and beyond. Cancer Treat Rev 31:S9–S18.

Huang T-J, Hsu RW-W, Li Y-Y, Cheng C-C (2006) Minimal access spinal surgery (MASS) in treating thoracic spine metastases. Spine 31:1860–1863.

Jackson RJ, Gokaslan ZL, Loh S-CA (2000) Metastatic renal cell carcinoma of the spine: surgical treatment and results. J Neurosurg (Spine 1) 94:18–24.

Jansson K-A, Bauer HCF (2006) Survival, complications and outcomes in 282 patients operated for neurological deficit due to thoracic or lumbar spinal metastasis. Eur Spine J 15:196–202.

Karnofsky DA (1967) Clinical evaluation of anticancer drugs: cancer chemotherapy. GANN Monogr 2:223–231.

Klimo P, Thompson CJ, Kestle JRW, Schimdt MH (2005) A meta-analysis of surgery versus conventional radiotherapy for the treatment of metastatic spinal epidural disease. Neuro-oncol 7:64–76.

Lowery GL, Harms J (1997) Principles of load sharing. In: Bridwell KH, De Wald RL (eds). Text Book of Spinal Surgery, 2nd ed. Lippincott-Raven, Philadelphia.

McLain RF. (1998) Endoscopically assisted compression of metastatic thoracic neoplasms. Spine 23:1130–1135.

O'Donoghue DS, Howell A, Walls J (1997a) Orthopaedic management of structurally significant bone destruction in breast cancer bone metastases. J Bone Joint Surg 79B (suppl i):98.

O'Donoghue DS, Howell A, Walls J (1997b) Implications of fracture in breast cancer bone metastases. J Bone Joint Surg 79B(suppl. i):97.

Oken MM, Creech RH, Tormey DC, et al. (1982) Toxicity and response criteria of the Eastern Cooperative Oncology Group. Am J Clin Oncol 5:649–655.

Olerud C et al. (1993) Embolization of spinal metastases reduces perioperative blood loss: twenty-one patients operated on for renal carcinoma. Acta Orthop Scandi 64:9–12.

Onimus M, Papin P, Gangloff S (1996) Results of surgical treatment of spinal thoracic and lumbar metastases. Eur Spine J 5:407–411.

Overby MC, Rothman AS (1985) Anteriolateral decompression for metastatic epidural spinal cord tumours. J Neurosurg 62:344–348.

Patchell RA, Tibbs PA, Regine WF, et al. (2005) Direct decompressive surgical resection in the treatment of spinal cord compression caused by metastatic cancer: a randomised trial. Lancet 366:643–648.

Roscoe MW et al. (1989) Preoperative embolization in the treatment of osseous metastases from renal cell carcinoma. Clin Orthop Relat Res 238:302–307.

Saito T, Kondo T, Hozumi T et al. (2006) Results of posterior surgery with intraoperative radiotherapy for spinal metastases. Eur Spine J 15:216–222.

Sakaura H, Hosono N, Mukai Y, et al. (2004) Outcome of en bloc spondylectomy for solitary metastasis of thoracolumbar spine. J Spinal Disorder Tech 17:297–300.

Schaberg J, Gainor BJ (1985) A profile of metastatic carcinoma of the spine. Spine 10:19–20.

Siegal T, Siegal T, Robin G, et al. (1982) Anterior decompression of the spine for metastatic epidural cord compression: a promising avenue of therapy. Ann Neurol 11:28–34.

Siegal T, Siegal T (1985) Vertebral body resection for epidural compression by malignant tumours. J Bone Joint Surg. 67A:375–382.

Sun S, Lang EV. (1998) Bone metastasis from renal cell carcinoma: preoperative embolization. J Vasc Intervent Radiol 9:263–269.

Sundaresan N, Galicich JH, Bains MS, et al. (1984) Vertebral body resection in the treatment of cancer involving the spine. Cancer 53:1393–1396.

Taneichi H, et al. (1997) Risk factors and probability of vertebral body collapse in metastases of the thoracic and lumbar spine. Spine 22:239–245.

Tokuhashi Y (1990) Scoring system for the preoperative evaluation of metastatic spine tumour prognosis. Spine 15:1110–1113.

Tokuhashi Y, Matsuzaki H, Oda H et al. (2005) A revised scoring system for preoperative evaluation of metastatic spine tumour prognosis. Spine 30:2186–2191.

Tomita K, Kawahara N, Baba H, et al. (1994) Total en bloc spondylectomy for solitary spinal metastases. Int Orthop 18:291–298.

Tomita K, Kawahara N, Kobayashi T, et al. (2001) Surgical strategy for spinal metastasis. Spine 26:298–306.

Vrionis FD, Hamm A, Stanton N, et al (2005) Kyphoplasty for tumour-associated spinal fractures. Tech Region Anaesthesia Pain Manage 9:35–89.

Weill A, Chiras J, Simon JM, et al. (1996) Spinal metastases: indications for and results of percutaneous injection of acrylic surgical cement. Radiology 199:241–247.

Weigel B, Maghsudi M, Neuman C, et al. (1999) Surgical management of symptomatic spinal metastases: postoperative outcome and quality of life. Spine 24:2240–2246.

Yamada K, Matsumoto Y, Kita M, et al. (2004) Long-term pain relief effects in four patients undergoing percutaneous vertebroplasty for metastatic vertebral tumour. J Anesth 18: 292–295.

Intraoperative ISO-C Navigation in Treatment of Difficult Spine Fractures and Spine Tumors

14

S. Rajasekaran

Spinal instrumentation has become an integral part of modern spinal surgery as it allows us to achieve the goals of spinal decompression, stabilization in the presence of instability, correction of deformities, or excision of tumors very successfully. However, spinal instrumentation is not without risk, and ample evidence indicates that it has a high potential for dangerous complications (1–4). Pedicle screw fixation, with its numerous advantages over other methods of fixation, has become the most commonly used form of spinal fixation, but it requires a significant learning curve and has the potential for neural and vascular complications, especially in the thoracic (1,2,5) and cervical spine (3,4).The pedicles of the thoracic spine are smaller, and more chance of neural damage exists because of a decreased canal-to-cord ratio in this region (1,2). Intracanal placements of the screws are more dangerous in the thoracic region because of cord injury than in the lumbar region, where only nerve roots are found. Similarly, the peculiar anatomy of the pedicles in the cervical spine, its wide anatomic variation within the population, and its proximity to both the vertebral artery and the cervical cord are serious deterrents for the spinal surgeon to use this method of fixation in this region (3)

The technique of pedicle screw insertion is usually "blind," because the pedicles are not visible directly, and the success of the procedure depends to a large extent on the anatomic landmarks and the experience of the surgeon. As a result, misplacement of the screws has been reported in 10% to 40%, especially when computed tomography (CT) scans are used to assess the postoperative position of the screws (6). The procedure becomes additionally challenging when the anatomy of the spine is altered, as in the presence of deformity such as scoliosis and kyphosis, or if an instability with altered intervertebral segmental displacement exists, such as seen in severe spondylolisthesis, posttraumatic displacements, or inflammatory disorders of the cervical spine (3,5,7,8).

Although freehand technique is commonly used, most surgeons opt for intraoperative fluoroscopic guidance in the presence of altered anatomy. These require the aid of an expert radiographer, as the fluoroscope tube must be tilted and rotated frequently to identify the end-on view of the respective pedicles. In the presence of severe deformities, exact identification of the pedicles is sometimes impossible. Multiple fluoroscopic exposures may be required, and the surgeon who is in the operating field has the risk of increased radiation exposure (9,10).

The need for improved accuracy and consistency in the placement of pedicle screws has led surgeons to probe into the application of computer-navigated spine surgery (11). Numerous reports prove the superiority and usefulness of navigation procedures in achieving a higher rate of accuracy in spinal instrumentation (8,11–14). The initial software for the navigation was CT-based; the data acquisition was secured by preoperative CT scans. The increased setup and surgical time due to the need for intraoperative registration at every single level and registration-related errors were a major drawback to the CT-based navigation systems, which rely on acquired data before surgery. The change in the intersegmental vertebral anatomic relations in unstable situations also has been reported with navigation systems using preoperative CT scans. It would be ideal to have intraoperative data acquisition, in which these disadvantages would be overcome. Intraoperative CT/magnetic resonance imaging (MRI)-based navigation systems are now more accurate but not widely applicable because of the unacceptably high cost (9,10). They also occupy much space in the operating theater and the specific compatible operating tables, anesthetic apparatus, and instruments increase the cost. The radiation exposure to the operating surgeon and the increased chances of infection are other added disadvantages.

Iso-C 3D navigation, which helps to acquire the data intraoperatively after the patient is positioned and surgical exposure is completed, overcomes these discussed disadvantages (9,12). The acquired data from the Iso-C 3D is directly transferred to the navigation machine by an interface, and this helps to obtain accurate real-time images, avoiding registration-related errors. Many reports detail the use and accuracy of Iso-C–based navigation in the spine literature (7,12–15).

ISO-C 3D C-ARM–BASED NAVIGATION

The procedure requires a modified C-arm CT system and navigation equipment. In our institution, a Siremobil Iso-C 3D C-arm (Siemens, Erlangen, Germany) and Vector Vision open platform navigation system (BrainLAB, Munich, Germany) is used. The other important requirement is an all-carbon operating table top with no metal that will interfere during the data acquisition. The patient is positioned as per the requirements of the surgical procedure. Preoperatively, the height of the table and the C-arm is adjusted so that the region of interest of the spine in which the instrumentation is going to be performed is in the center of the fluoroscope in both the anteroposterior (AP) and lateral views. After draping and completion of the exposure, a minimally invasive reference array (MIRA) is fixed firmly to the spine, either by using a 4-mm Schanz screw into the pedicle or by clipping it to the spinous process. During the process of acquisition, the camera on the navigation system is so positioned that it visualizes both the MIRAs on the marker range of the C-arm and the MIRA attached to the spine. The Iso-C then performs the three-dimensional image acquisitions as the motorized C-arm moves continuously with 190-degree orbital movement. During the rotation, 50 to 100 fluoroscopic images are taken, depending on the need for a low- or high-resolution image. After data acquisition, software in the ISO-C produces 3D and reformatted images, which are transferred directly to the Vector Vision by an interface. With each acquisition, the anatomy of a 12-cm cube is obtained and transferred to the navigation software. Good-quality sagittal, axial, and coronal reformatted images are produced on a virtual basis whenever the marker tool is brought into the field of data acquisition. The accuracy of the images produced is checked by using a navigator tool. The C-arm is then moved away from the operating field, with no need for any further fluoroscopic exposures during the entire procedure.

With the use of a tool and its trajectory shown on the screen, the starting point and the direction of the pedicle screw can be easily ascertained. The trajectory also has length-calibration markings that help in determination of the appropriate length. The software has provisions for "planning an ideal screw" and verifying the accurate positioning of the inserted screw by superimposition of the images (Fig. 14.1)

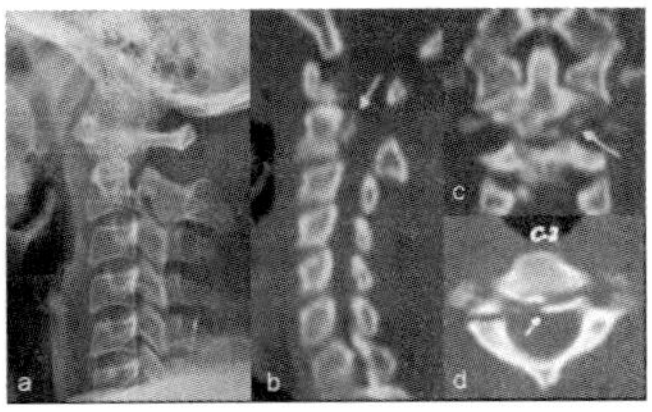

FIGURE 14.1 **A:** Lateral radiograph of an Effendi type II hangman's fracture with displacement and 20-degree angulation of the fractured fragments. **B:** Sagittal CT scan showing fracture through the pedicles and loose fragments in this canal. **C:** Coronal section CT scan with comminution of right pedicle. **D:** Axial CT showing the exact fracture configuration.

NAVIGATION IN SPINE FRACTURES

Although the role of navigation may appear superfluous to a well-trained surgeon in the treatment of routine thoracolumbar and lumbar injuries, it is helpful to place the screws accurately in upper thoracic, cervicothoracic, and cervical injuries. Fractures in the presence of ankylosing spondylitis, in which the anatomic landmarks are completely obscured, and in unstable cervical spine fractures with altered anatomy posing additional risk of injury to vertebral artery and spinal cord are the other areas for which spinal navigation is particularly helpful.

ILLUSTRATIVE CASES

Case 1

A 28-year-old male manual laborer had severe pain in the neck after a fall from a height of 6 feet. He was noted to have severe paraspinal muscle spasm with restriction of all neck movements. He was neurologically intact, and radiographs revealed bilateral pedicle fracture of axis with subluxation of C-2 over C-3. The fracture was classified as Effendi type II hangman's fracture with 20-degree angulation (Fig. 14.1a).

CT revealed a fracture line passing through the body at the base of the pedicle on the right side and through the pedicle on the left side. The fracture line on both sides involved the vertebral artery foramen and was associated with comminution (Fig. 14.1b–d). MRIs revealed cord edema at the C-2 to C-3 level. In view of the comminuted type II fracture with 20-degree angulation, surgical stabilization was chosen.

The fracture had reduced well after patient positioning with the neck in minimal extension. The patient was positioned prone on a carbon-fiber radiolucent operating tabletop (Hobo, Beijing, China), and a standard posterior exposure of C-2 to C-5 was performed. The MIRA was attached to the base of the C-5 spinous process, and the cervical spine was screened with the Iso-C 3D C-arm, and the acquired images were transferred to the computer navigation. Accurate axial and sagittal images of C-1 to C-4 were procured. The accuracy of the images was verified by using a tool navigator. In view of the excellent visualization of the fracture pattern, direct lag-screw osteosynthesis of the bipedicular fracture of the axis vertebra was planned to preserve the motion segments.

The tool navigator was used along with 3D fluoroscopic real-time images to determine the entry point and trajectory of the pedicle (Figs. 14.2a and b; Fig. 14.3a and b). The point of entry selected was marked and prepared by using a high-speed diamond burr. A 2.5-mm drill was then calibrated to the navigation system so that the real-time navigation images could be obtained during the drilling of the bones. The drilling was performed in stages, taking care to verify and double check the accuracy of the trajectory frequently by using the tool and also a pedicle probe. It was found that very accu-

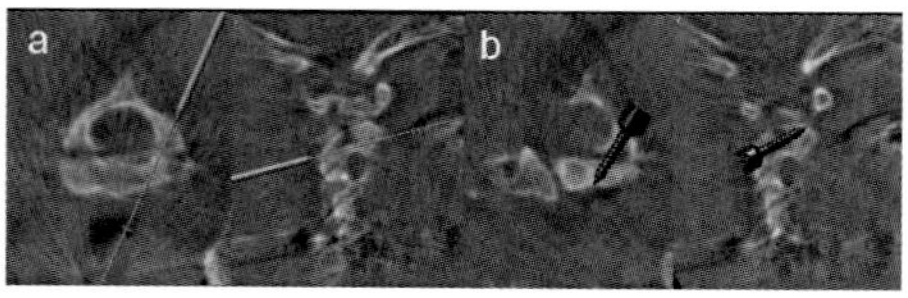

FIGURE 14.2 Intraoperative images from the navigation system. **A:** Trajectory to guide the direction and depth of drilling. **B:** Planning of the screw into the fractured left pedicle.

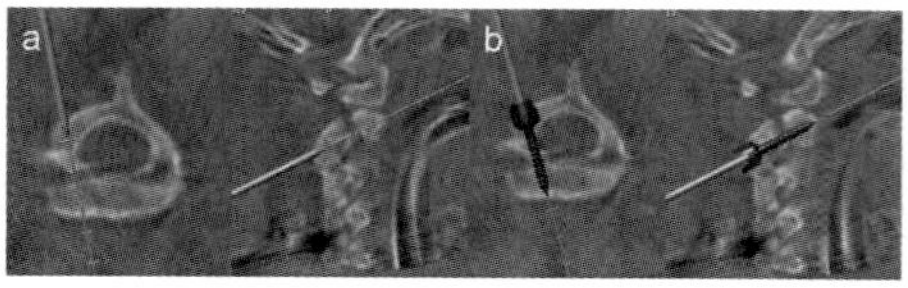

FIGURE 14.3 Images from the navigation system during surgery. **A:** Trajectory of drilling. **B:** Planning of the screw insertion into fractured right pedicle.

rate navigation is indeed possible for both fractured pedicles of the C-2 vertebra. The bicortical purchase of the pedicle screws was planned for during the surgery.

Screw sizes of 30 × 3.5 mm on the right side and 32 × 3.5 mm on the left side were chosen. Each of the chosen screws was then calibrated and verified with a navigator and threaded along the pretapped path with the guidance of the autopilot images. The real-time funnel-shaped spinal autopilot view was found to be very useful in accurate placement and verification of the screw during the entire process of screw insertion.

The accuracy of placement of this screw was again verified by acquiring coronal and sagittal images by using the Siremobil Iso-C 3D C-arm. Radiographs and CT scan of the cervical spine, done postoperatively to reassess the accuracy and length of the position of the screws, confirmed that both screws had been placed as per plan, with no breach of the cortex on either the side of the spinal canal or the vertebral artery canal (Fig. 14.4). Bicortical purchase on both sides allowed very stable fixation.

Case 2

A 43-year-old man with a history of ankylosing spondylitis and stiff spine had a whiplash injury 6 months earlier. Radiographs taken immediately did not reveal any skeletal injury, and the patient was treated with a soft collar of 4 weeks' duration. Some remission of pain occurred initially, but this was followed by increasing pain and progressive flexion deformity from the upper cervical region, once the patient started to mobilize (Fig. 14.5a and b). Repeated radiographs showed increasing deformity at the C-2 to C-3 level with a completely fused spine of both the anterior and posterior columns (Fig. 14.5c). An MRI showed the presence of pseudo arthrosis; this made it possible to correct the deformity with a halo sufficiently for the patient to have good vision. It was then planned to stabilize the spine posteriorly. After exposure, the entire posterior elements were found to be a single mass of bone with complete loss of anatomic details, making instrumentation difficult and risky (Fig. 14.6a).

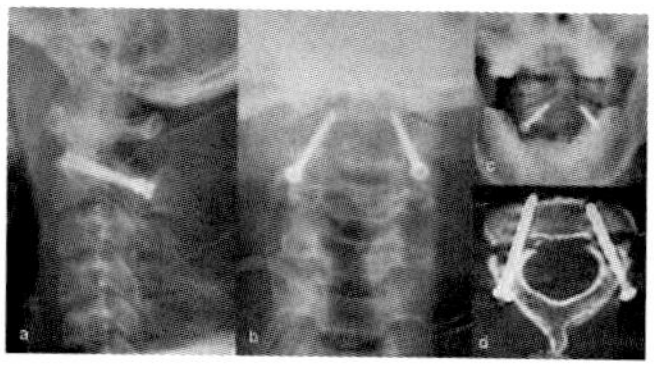

FIGURE 14.4 Postoperative imaging study depicting the accurate placement of the bicortical Judet screws into the fractured pedicles of the C-2 vertebra.

Spinal navigation was performed by anchoring the MIRA to the spinous process of the fifth cervical vertebra and acquiring a 3D image of the entire cervical spine. Excellent sagittal, coronal, and axial images were obtained (Fig. 14.6b and c), which made it possible to place both pedicle and lateral mass screws with excellent accuracy. The spine was stably fixed (Fig. 14.7). At 3-year follow-up, the patient has good fusion with excellent function.

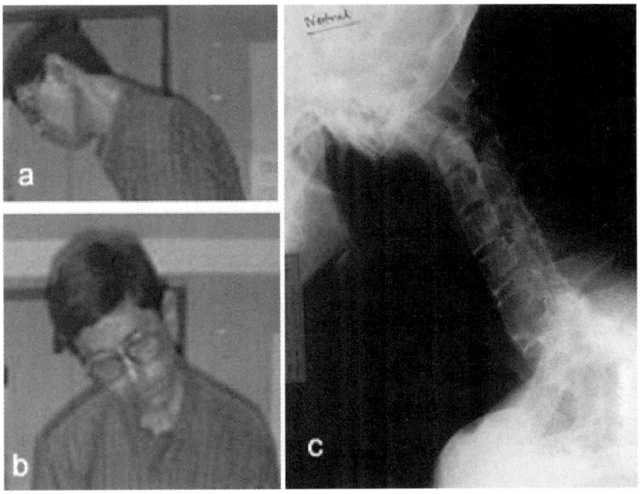

FIGURE 14.5 **A,B:** A 43-year-old man with ankylosing spondylitis and progressive deformity of the neck after whiplash injury. **C:** Radiograph shows pseudoarthrosis with angular and rotational deformity at the C-2 to C-3 level.

SPINAL TUMORS

The goal of curative treatment of a spinal tumor is its complete resection. The management of spinal tumors has always been challenging, owing to the complex anatomy in vicinity of critical neurovascular structures (16,17). Approach-related problems can further complicate the issue, as in some cases, both anterior and posterior elements are involved. The successful outcomes in spinal tumor surgery depend on accurate intraoperative localization of the extent of the tumor, complete excision with adequate margins, and secure stabilization with instrumentation if necessary (18,19).

Spinal navigation, by virtue of its ability to provide intraoperative 3D images, helps us to achieve these aims. Benign vertebral tumors are usually located in the pars, pedicle, and lamina (17). Their resection often leads to instability, requiring instrumentation, which can be avoided in most of the cases with use of navigation, as it allows resection with minimal collateral damage. Additionally, minimally invasive approaches are possible with the use of navigation, which is associated with lesser postoperative morbidity, early mobilization, and complete functional restoration. When the spine is destabilized

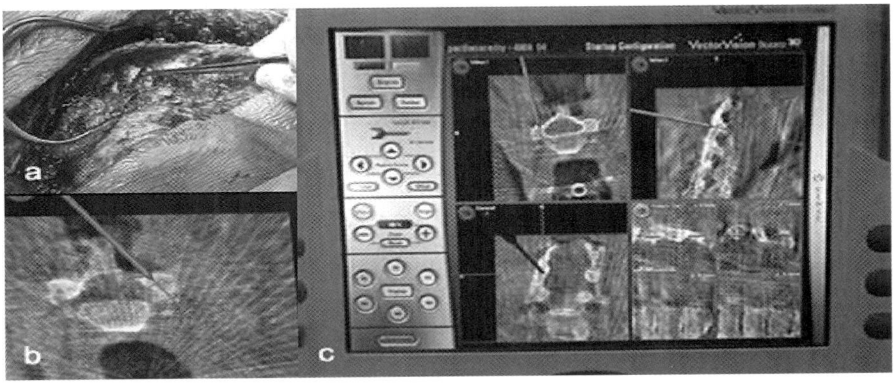

FIGURE 14.6 **A:** Intraoperative photograph after surgical exposure with completely fused spine and absence of anatomic landmarks. **B:** Intraoperative navigation-assisted identification of starting point and trajectory of lateral mass screw. **C:** Computer navigation allowed excellent reconstruction images of the axial, sagittal, and coronal sections of the spine with localization of the starting point and trajectory of the pedicle screw by using the tool.

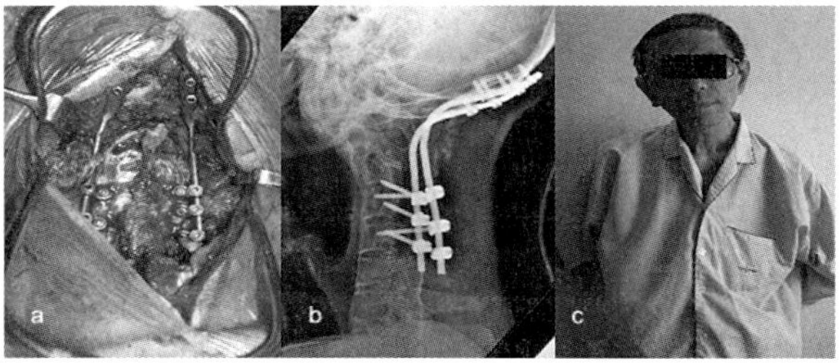

FIGURE 14.7 **A:** Intraoperative photograph after occipitocervical stabilization. **B:** Good correction was achieved, and the spine could be stabilized with occipitocervical fusion by using both lateral mass and pedicle screws inserted with image guidance **(C)**. The patient achieved good cosmetic and functional correction.

with tumoral destruction itself or because of access for its resection, then navigation helps in safe instrumentation, especially in surgically difficult locations like the upper cervical and cervicothoracic regions. Navigation has a role to play even in ablative surgery of metastatic tumors by locating adjacent vital neurovascular structures, ensuring decompression, and allowing safe instrumentation (20).

The surgical approach depends on the location of tumor and, in posteriorly located tumors, just unilateral subperiosteal elevation of paraspinal muscles to access the tumor will suffice. After exposure, the MIRA can be attached one or two levels adjacent to the tumor. A greater possibility of registration error exists while using preoperative CT-based navigation in cases of spinal tumors with distorted anatomic landmarks and exaggerated interpositional changes owing to tumoral destabilization of the segment. This limitation is overcome by Iso-C–based navigation by its intraoperative automated registration, thus enhancing the accuracy of the procedure. The Iso-C–based navigation is used to localize and outline precisely the margins of the tumor. Instruments required to remove the tumor, such as burr, drill, and osteotome, can be calibrated, which allows real-time multiplanar stereotactic localization of the instruments during surgery. Localization of the tip of the instrument will help to determine the adequacy of the tumor in all planes and also the extent of the margin of excision. Intraoperatively, spinal canal and vertebral foramen can be outlined precisely, avoiding inadvertent neurovascular injury during tumor resection. The biggest advantage is that after the surgical procedure; a repeated scan can be performed intraoperatively, which ensures the adequacy of resection, completeness of decompression, and secure placement of the implant in instrumented cases, before closure is done. This may obviate the need for a postoperative CT scan, thus avoiding additional radiation and expenditure. In our experience, Iso-C–based navigation is a useful adjunct in treatment of spine tumor, especially benign vertebral tumors.

Illustrative Case

A 27-year-old man reports progressive and severe pain in the neck with radiation to the right arm of 4 weeks' duration. The pain was particularly more severe in the night, disturbing his sleep, and was aggravated with activities that involved forward bending of his neck. No sensory motor deficit was found. Radiologic investigation, including a CT scan, showed a well-defined sclerotic lesion (10×11 mm) in the right pedicle of C-5, extending into adjacent lamina, abutting the vertebral artery foramen anteriorly and involving the margins of the spinal canal (Fig. 14.8a and b). The diagnosis was osteoid osteoma. Posterior unilateral exposure was done, and the MIRA was anchored rigidly to the C-6 spinous process, followed by image acquisition by the Iso-C arm. These images were automatically transferred to the navigation platform. After verification of registration, the navigator tool was used to localize the tumor and outline its margins, along with the neighboring spinal canal and vertebral artery foramen (Fig. 14.8c). The nidus was precisely deroofed by using a calibrated burr. It was removed with a curette and diamond burr, without transgressing either the vertebral artery foramen or the spinal canal. An intraoperative postprocedural scan (Fig. 14.8d) and postoperative CT scan (Fig. 14.8e) both revealed complete resection retaining the integrity of the adjacent healthy bone. The patient was mobilized on the next day, and no clinicoradiologic evidence of recurrence or instability was noted at the last follow-up.

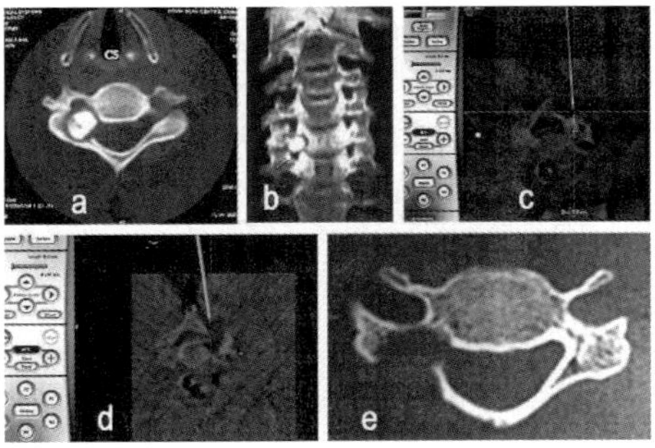

FIGURE 14.8 **A, B:** Nidus of osteoid osteoma located in right pedicle of C-5 vertebra abutting the vertebral artery and spinal canal. **C:** Intraoperative localization of nidus by using Iso-C 3D–based navigation clearly outlining the tumor margin and its relation with the vertebral artery foramen. **D:** Intraoperative postresection scan showing a small remnant of the tumor that requires removal. **E:** Postoperative CT scan shows complete removal of the tumor. No resultant instability required instrumentation.

LIMITATIONS OF ISO-C 3D

Navigation requires specialized equipment like the ISO-C 3D C-arm and also an all-carbon operating table top. The routinely used spinal radiolucent tables will not be sufficient, as they usually have metal strips on the sides. These will interfere with image acquisition when the ISO-C C-arm rotates around an arc of 190 degrees. The presence of metals in the field of image acquisition also distorts the images and can lead to a poor-quality image insufficient for accurate navigation. Another important requirement for ISO-C 3D navigation is that the anatomic region of interest should be in the center of the field both in the AP and lateral views before data acquisition. This is not possible in very obese patients and in patients who have a very severe deformity such as a kyphoscoliosis greater than 90 degrees. Obesity also can reduce the quality of image sufficiently to reduce the confidence of the surgeon to navigate.

REFERENCES

1. Brown CA, Lenke LG, Bridwell KH, et al. Complications of pediatric thoracolumbar and lumbar pedicle screws. Spine 1998;23:1566–1571.
2. Gertzbein SD, Robbins SE. Accuracy of pedicular screw placement in vivo. Spine 1990;15:11–14.
3. Abumi K, Shono Y, Ito M, et al. Complications of pedicle screw fixation in reconstructive surgery of the cervical spine. Spine 2000;25:962–969.
4. Abumi K, Kaneda K, Shono Y, et al. One-stage posterior decompression and reconstruction of the cervical spine by using pedicle screw fixation systems. J Neurosurg 1999;90:19–26.
5. Ebraheim NA, Jabaly G, Xu R, et al. Anatomic relations of the thoracic pedicle to the adjacent neural structures. Spine 1997;22:1553–1557.
6. Castro WH, Halm H, Jerosch J, et al. Accuracy of pedicle screw placement in lumbar vertebrae. Spine 1996;21:1320–1324.
7. Rajasekaran S, Vidyadhara S, Shetty AP. Intraoperative Iso-C 3D navigation for pedicle screw instrumentation of hangman's fracture: a case report. J Orthop Surg 2007;15:73–77.
8. Takahashi J, Shono Y, Nakamura I, et al. Computer-assisted screw insertion for cervical disorders in rheumatoid arthritis. Eur Spine J 2007;16: 485–494.
9. Gebhard F, Weidner A, Liener UC, et al. Navigation at the spine. Injury 2004;35(suppl 1): SA35–45.
10. Holly LT, Foley KT. Intraoperative spinal navigation. Spine 2003;28(suppl):54–61.
11. Laine T, Lund T, Ylikoski M, et al. Accuracy of pedicle screw insertion with and without computer assistance: a randomised controlled clinical study in 100 consecutive patients. Eur Spine J 2000;9:235–241.

12. Hott JS, Papadopoulos SM, Theodore N, et al. Intraoperative Iso-C C-arm navigation in cervical spinal surgery: review of the first 52 cases. Spine 2004;29:2856–2860.
13. Hott JS, Deshmukh VR, Klopfenstein JD, et al. Intraoperative Iso-C C-arm navigation in craniospinal surgery: the first 60 cases. Neurosurgery 2004;545:1131–6; discussion 1136–1137.
14. Rajasekaran S, Vidyadhara S, Ramesh P, et al. Randomized clinical study to compare the accuracy of navigated and non-navigated thoracic pedicle screws in deformity correction surgeries. Spine 2007;32:E56–64.
15. Acosta FL Jr, Thompson TL, Campbell S, et al. Use of intraoperative isocentric C-arm 3D fluoroscopy for sextant percutaneous pedicle screw placement: case report and review of the literature. Spine J 2005;5:339–343.
16. Raskas DS, Graziano GP, Herzenberg JE, et al. Osteoid osteoma and osteoblastoma of the spine. J Spinal Disord 1992;5:204–211.
17. Zileli M, Kilinçer C, Ersahin Y, et al. Primary tumors of the cervical spine: a retrospective review of 35 surgically managed cases. Spine J 2007;7:165–173.
18. Boriani S, Weinstein JN, Biagini R. Primary bone tumors of the spine: terminology and surgical staging. Spine 1997;22:1036–1044.
19. Fisher CG, Keynan O, Boyd MC, et al. The surgical management of primary tumors of the spine: initial results of an ongoing prospective cohort study. Spine 2005;15;30:1899–1908.
20. Arand M, Hartwig E, Kinzl L, et al. Spinal navigation in tumor surgery of the thoracic spine: first clinical results. Clin Orthop Relat Res 2002; 399:211–218.

Metastatic Epidural Spinal Cord Compression

Roy A. Patchell

15

INTRODUCTION

Metastatic epidural spinal cord compression (MESCC) occurs when cancer metastasizes to the spine and then secondarily compresses the spinal cord. It is a relatively common complication of cancer and develops in approximately 5% to 10% of all cancer patients (1,2). If left untreated, virtually 100% of these patients become paraplegic; therefore it is considered a true medical emergency, and immediate intervention is required. Even with aggressive therapy, results can often be unsatisfactory. Although most patients with MESCC have limited survival, up to one third will survive beyond 1 year (3). Thus it is essential to consider aggressive therapy to preserve or improve the quality of life and to prevent paraplegia.

PATHOPHYSIOLOGY

MESCC occurs in one of three ways: (a) continued growth and expansion of vertebral bone metastasis into the epidural space; (b) destruction of vertebral cortical bone, causing vertebral body collapse with displacement of bony fragments into the epidural space; or (c) neural foramina extension into the epidural space by a paraspinal mass. The cause of damage to the spinal cord from compression is complex and multifactorial, although two mechanisms predominate (1,2). Direct compression results in edema, venous congestion, and demyelination. If the compression is of short duration, the effects are reversible; remyelination and recovery of function is possible. However, with prolonged compression, a secondary vascular injury occurs with infarction of the spinal cord. After this type of injury, no meaningful recovery is possible (4).

Clinical Presentation

The vast majority of patients have a preexisting cancer diagnosis. Even without one, MESCC should be suspected in anyone who initially seen with progressively worsening back pain, incontinence, or paraplegia, especially in the high-risk population such as long-time smokers or women with a strong family history of breast cancer. In a review by Fuller et al. (5) of more than 1,000 patients with MESCC reported in the literature, the most common tumor type is breast cancer (29%), followed by lung cancer (17%) and prostate cancer (14%), which reflects the high natural incidence of these tumors. New-onset back pain in cancer patients must be taken very seriously, and a proper workup must be performed.

The osseous vertebral column is affected in 85% of cases, paravertebral sites in 10% to 15%, and rare cases exist of isolated epidural or intramedullary metastasis (6). Back pain is the most common presenting symptom (88% to 96%), followed by weakness (76% to 86%), sensory deficits (51% to 80%), and autonomic dysfunction (40% to 64%) (7–10). The most common level of the MESCC involvement is in the thoracic spine (59% to 78%), followed by lumbar (16% to 33%) and cervical spine (4% to 15%), whereas multiple levels are involved in up to half of the patients (5,7,11).

Diagnosis

Magnetic resonance imaging (MRI) is the standard modality for imaging of the central nervous system in cancer patients. It has a very high sensitivity (93%), specificity (97%), and accuracy (95%) in diagnosing MESCC (12). Because patients can have synchronous, multifocal MESCC, an MRI of the entire spine with and without contrast should be promptly performed in anyone suspected of having MESCC (13). High-resolution computed tomography (CT) scan or CT myelogram of the spine should be performed for those with contraindications to MRI.

Prognosis

Prognostic factors predicting survival are generally similar to those of patients with brain metastasis. In terms of predicting ambulatory outcome, one of the most important factors is the rapidity of symptom onset. Other important prognostic factors include radiosensitive histology (e.g., multiple myeloma, germ-cell tumors, lymphomas, and small cell carcinoma) and pretherapy ambulatory function. In a prospective study of 98 patients with MESCC reported by Rades et al. (14), the single strongest predictor for ambulatory status after therapy on multivariate ($p < 0.001$) analysis was time to development of motor deficits before radiation from the start of any symptoms. This cohort was separated into three groups according to the time to motor deficits before radiation therapy: 1 to 7 days (group I), 8 to 14 days (group II), and more than 14 days (group III). The ambulatory rates for groups I, II, and III were 35%, 55%, and 86% ($p < 0.001$), respectively. The symptom-improvement rates for groups I, II, and III were 10%, 29%, and 86% ($p = 0.026$), respectively. The other factor significant on the multivariate analysis for posttherapy ambulatory status was favorable histology ($p = 0\ 005$), and a trend was found regarding pretherapy ambulatory status ($p = 0.076$). Only 10% of the patients in group I had symptom improvement. Acute, rapid deterioration is predictive of irreversible spinal cord infarction; therefore recognition, prompt diagnosis, and treatment of MESCC are crucial.

THERAPY

Corticosteroids

Although multiple retrospective studies have demonstrated its clinical efficacy, Sorensen et al. (15) reported the only randomized controlled study on the utility of high-dose corticosteroids before definitive radiotherapy in MESCC from solid tumors. The treatment arm consisted of 96 mg of intravenous (i.v.) bolus of dexamethasone followed by 96 mg oral (p.o.) per day for 3 days and a 10-day taper, versus no corticosteroids before radiotherapy. This study demonstrated 3-month and 6-month ambulatory rates of 81% versus 63% and 59% versus 33% ($p < 0.05$), respectively, in favor of dexamethasone.

Corticosteroids must be started as soon as possible in anyone suspected of having MESCC even before radiographic diagnosis, because this can be rapidly discontinued with a negative diagnosis. Corticosteroids effectively decrease cord edema, and they serve as an effective bridge to definitive treatment.

Although a small randomized trial argued for a lower dexamethasone dose (4 mg per day) in patients with brain metastasis (16), the optimal maintenance dose of corticosteroids in patients with MESCC is unknown. With regard to i.v. loading dose for MESCC, Vecht et al. (17) reported the only randomized study comparing i.v. dexamethasone loading dose of 10 mg versus 100 mg, followed in both arms by the same p.o. regimen of 16 mg per day. Both arms demonstrated significant reductions in pain from baseline ($p < 0.001$); however, no difference was noted between the two arms with respect to pain reduction, ambulation, or bladder function.

Very high doses of corticosteroids are associated with significant side effects, mainly gastrointestinal (GI). The Sorensen phase III study reported an 11% frequency of serious side effects for patients in the treatment arm, whereas Heimdal et al. (15,18) reported a 14.3% frequency of serious GI side effects (one fatal ulcer, one rectal bleeding, and two bowel perforations) in 28 consecutive patients treated with 96 mg of i.v. dexamethasone per day. When the dexamethasone dose was decreased to 16 mg per day for the next 38 consecutive patients, no instances of serious side effects occurred in either group, with no difference in ambulatory rates between the groups.

Based on these data, a loading of 10 mg of i.v. dexamethasone and followed by a maintenance dose of 4 to 6 mg (i.v. or p.o.) every 6 to 8 hours should be sufficient for most patients. Furthermore, patients should be started on a proton-pump inhibitor for GI prophylaxis (19).

Radiotherapy

Palliative radiotherapy has long been the standard of care in the treatment of patients with MESCC. Although multiple fractionation schedules have been reported in the literature, a total of 30 Gy in 10 fractions is the one most frequently used (20). In one of the largest studies to date, Rades and colleagues (21) reported a retrospective series of 1,304 patients with MESCC. The patients were separated into five schedules: 8 Gy $\times$ 1 in 1 day ($n = 261$; group I), 4 Gy $\times$ 5 in 1 week ($n = 279$; group II), 3 Gy $\times$ 10 in 2 weeks ($n = 274$; group III), 2.5 Gy $\times$ 15 in 3 weeks ($n = 233$; group IV), and 2 Gy $\times$ 20 in 4 weeks ($n = 257$; group V). All of the groups had similar post-treatment ambulatory rates (63% to 74%) and motor-function improvements (26% to 31%). However, in-field recurrence rates were much lower for the protracted schedules. The 2-year in-field recurrence rates for groups I, II, III, IV, and V were 24%, 26%, 14%, 9%, and 7% ($p < 0.001$). They recommend that a single fraction of 8 Gy should be used in MESCC patients with limited survival expectations, and that 30 Gy in 10 fractions should be used for all other patients.

Maranzano and colleagues (22) reported the only randomized trial assessing radiation schedules for patients with MESCC. They compared two hypofractionation schemes, a short course (8 Gy $\times$ 1 followed by a 6-day break, then 8 Gy $\times$ 1; 16 Gy total in 1 week) versus a split course (5 Gy $\times$ 3 followed by a 4-day break, then 3 Gy $\times$ 5; 30 Gy total in 2 weeks). The study concluded that the treatment with short versus split courses of RT resulted in similar back-pain relief (56% vs. 59%), ambulatory maintenance (68% vs. 71%), and good bladder function (90% vs. 89%) rates. Therefore they recommend that an 8 Gy $\times$ 2 schedule be used for patients with MESCC.

However, design problems in the study by Maranzano et al. (22) call into question the validity of the conclusions (23). Although the response rates may seem impressive, when one limits the definition of response to regaining motor function and sphincter control, the rates of success decrease to 29% and 14%, respectively. Confounding variables included having patients with favorable histology, excellent performance status, and the use of nonstandard, large fraction sizes in both arms. It is entirely conceivable that the 5% who progressed to paraplegia without in-field recurrence may have had late radiation-induced toxicity, even if not scored as late toxicity by the authors. Therefore, it is difficult to interpret this study.

For patients with MESCC from solid tumors, 30 Gy in 10 fractions is considered the standard of care in the United States. Short schedules (e.g., 8 Gy × 1 or 4 Gy × 5) should be avoided in newly diagnosed, chemotherapy-naïve patients because the clinical course can be quite variable and unpredictable and should be reserved only for those with clear evidence of progressive, chemotherapy-refractory disease. Up-front chemotherapy (with a planned consolidative radiation) may be considered in selected, newly diagnosed patients with excellent neurologic status and very chemosensitive tumors (e.g., multiple myeloma, germ-cell tumors, lymphoma, or small-cell lung carcinoma).

If the patient is found to have unresectable/inoperable tumor and otherwise has a good performance status and controlled primary disease, then consideration should be made to escalate the dose beyond 30 Gy because this will not be sufficient to achieve long-term control of gross tumor. Special techniques, such as image-guided intensity modulated radiation therapy (IMRT) or stereotactic body radiation therapy (SBRT), should be considered. However, the routine use of IMRT or SBRT can not be recommended at this time because the technology is expensive, and it has yet to show definite benefit over conventional delivery of radiation in a patient population that has a median survival of 6 months or less.

Surgery

Radiation alone has been the standard treatment for MESCC, although results with radiation alone are disappointing. Fewer than 50% of patients so treated ever walk again, and few patients who begin treatment paraplegic ever regain the ability to walk (1,24–26). Several reasons exist for the relatively poor results: (a) some tumors (e.g., renal cell, sarcoma, and melanoma) are not radiosensitive; (b) even in radiosensitive tumors, it may take several days to deliver a radiation dose large enough to cause a response, during which time the spinal cord damage may continue; and (c) the most commonly used radiation dose and schedule (30 Gy in 10 fractions) is insufficient to provide long-term local control of gross tumor (except for radiosensitive tumors), so tumor may regrow to cause a recurrence of MESCC, even after an initial clinical response.

In the past, laminectomy and postoperative radiotherapy were frequently combined. However, retrospective studies suggested that radiotherapy alone was as effective as laminectomy plus postoperative radiotherapy in the treatment of MESCC (7,27). Nevertheless, combined treatment remained a standard treatment until 1980, when a small randomized trial suggested that radiotherapy alone was as effective as laminectomy plus radiotherapy in the treatment of MESCC. Young et al. (28) randomized 29 patients with MESCC to decompressive laminectomy followed by radiation versus radiation alone. Although this trial showed no benefit to surgery in terms of pain relief, ambulation, or sphincter function, it is impossible to draw any firm conclusion because of the small sample size. All of these studies used laminectomy in conjunction with radiotherapy; however, most of the lesions in MESCC involve the anterior portion of the vertebral body (1). Therefore a laminectomy does not effectively relieve the compression and may actually worsen the stability of the spine.

Recently, many have advocated the use of direct decompressive and maximal-debulking surgery with intraoperative stabilization of the spine (in appropriate cases) followed by postoperative radiation therapy. Because more than 85% of spinal metastases arise anterior to the spinal cord, direct attempts at anterior surgical decompression seem logical. In the less-common cases when the compressing tumor is located predominantly lateral or posterior to the spinal cord, direct surgical decompression involving removal of the tumor (using lateral or posterior approaches) is also possible and is a logical approach to treatment. The advantages of direct decompressive surgery include removal of the tumor with a resultant decrease in tumor burden that allows more effective postoperative radiotherapy; immediate relief of the cord compression; and immediate stabilization of the spinal column, which can be achieved by the same operation.

In preliminary uncontrolled studies using direct surgical decompression, results have been promising, with ambulatory rates greater than 75% (29). In several series, even about 50% of patients who could not walk at the time of treatment regained the ability to ambulate. These generally encouraging results were obtained in small series that contained only surgically treated patients. No control groups were used, and the patients were almost always selected from among those patients with the best overall prognoses. A controlled, randomized trial comparing direct decompressive surgery plus postoperative radiation therapy with radiation therapy alone was needed to determine the true value (if any) of the new treatment.

Patchell et al. (30) reported the first phase III randomized trial testing the efficacy of direct decompressive surgery in patients with MESCC. Table 15.1 summarizes the key findings of this trial. The study population consisted of patients with known cancer in whom symptoms of MESCC developed. These patients had MRI scans to confirm the presence of a true spinal cord compression. Patients were started on dexamethasone, 100 mg initially, followed by 24 mg every 6 hours until they began treatment. After that, steroids were decreased but continued until the completion of radiation therapy. After stratification for primary tumor type, ambulatory status, and presence or absence of spinal stability, patients were randomly assigned to one of two treatment groups. Patients randomized to the radiation-alone arm began radiation within 24 hours after study entry and received 30 Gy in 10 fractions. Patients randomized to the surgery-plus-radiation group were operated on within 24 hours after study entry and received radiation within 2 weeks after surgery. The intent of surgery in all cases was to remove as much tumor as possible and to provide immediate decompression and intraoperative spinal stabilization (when needed). The major end point of the study was the ability to walk after treatment. This was measured in two ways. The immediate success of treatment was determined by comparing the proportion of patients in each group who were able to walk after treatment. The long-term success of treatment was measured by comparing the length of time patients maintained the ability to walk. Secondary end points were posttreatment continence rates and length of time patients maintained muscle strength and functional status. Survival also was a secondary end point.

TABLE 15.1 Key Findings of the University of Kentucky Phase III Study of Patients with Metastatic Spinal Cord Compression

	Surgery + Radiation	Radiation Alone	
	Median (n = 50)	**Median (n = 51)**	***p* Value**
Primary end point			
Ability to walk			
Rate	84% (42/50)	57% (29/51)	0.001
Time	122 days	13 days	0.003
In patients ambulatory at study entry ability to walk (maintaining)			
Rate	94% (32/34)	74% (26/34)	0.024
Time	153 days	54 days	0.024
In patients nonambulatory at study entry ability to walk (regaining)			
Rate	62% (10/16)	19% (3/16)	0.012
Time	59 days	0 days	0.04
Secondary end points			
Maintenance of ASIA score[a]	566 days	72 days	0.001
Maintenance of Frankel score[a]	566 days	72 days	0.0006
Maintenance of continence	156 days	17 days	0.016
Overall survival	126 days	100 days	0.033
Other end points			
Mean daily morphine[b]	0.4 mg	4.8 mg	0.002
Mean daily dexamethasone[b]	1.6 mg	4.2 mg	0.0093

ASIA, American Spinal Injury Association.

[a]Measures of spinal function after injury.

[b]Converted into equivalent doses.

From Patchell RA, Tibbs PA, Regine WF, et al. Direct decompressive surgical resection in the treatment of spinal cord compression caused by metastatic cancer: a randomised trial. Lancet 2005;366:643–648, with permission.

The original study design called for a sample size of 200 patients. However, after an interim analysis, the study was stopped because the criterion of a predetermined early stopping rule was met. One hundred and one patients were entered into the study. The percentage of patients able to walk after treatment was significantly (p = 0.001) higher in surgical patients (84%) than in the radiotherapy-alone patients (57%). Patients treated with surgery also retained the ability to walk significantly longer than did those with radiotherapy alone (median, 122 days vs. 13 days; p = 0.003). Thirty-two patients (16 in each treatment group) entered the study unable to walk; patients in the surgery group regained the ability to walk in a significantly greater proportion than did patients in the radiation-alone group (62% vs. 19%; p = 0.01). The need for corticosteroids and opioid analgesics was significantly lower in the surgical group, and muscle strength and functional status were also maintained for significantly longer in patients treated with surgery. Survival times were also significantly longer in the surgery group (median, 126 days vs. 100 days; p = 0.033).

This phase III trial demonstrated that patients with MESCC treated with direct decompressive surgery plus postoperative radiotherapy *retain* the ability to walk longer and *regain* it more often than patients treated with radiotherapy alone. Surgery permits most patients to remain ambulatory for the remainder of their lives, whereas patients treated with radiation alone spend a large portion of their remaining time as paraplegic.

CONCLUSIONS

If the tumors are operable, patients with MESCC should undergo maximal tumor resection and stabilization, followed by postoperative radiotherapy. Even for radiosensitive tumors, surgery can often stabilize the spine. For patients with inoperable tumors, definitive radiotherapy still remains the standard of care. Although most patients with MESCC have short survivals, only through prompt multidisciplinary teamwork can the risks of paraplegia be minimized.

REFERENCES

1. Byrne TN. Spinal cord compression from epidural metastases. N Engl J Med 1992;327: 614–619.
2. Posner JB. Spinal metastases. In: Neurologic complications of cancer. Philadelphia: FA Davis, 1995:111–142.
3. Maranzano E, Latini P, Checcaglini F, et al. Radiation therapy in metastatic spinal cord compression: a prospective analysis of 105 consecutive patients. Cancer 1991;67:1311–1317.
4. Kato A, Ushio Y, Hayakawa T, et al. Circulatory disturbance of the spinal cord with epidural neoplasm in rats. J Neurosurg 1985;63:260–265.
5. Fuller BG, Heiss JD, Oldfield EH. Spinal cord compression. In: DeVita VT, Hellman S, Rosenberg SA, eds. Cancer: principles and practice of oncology. Philadelphia: Lippincott Williams & Wilkins, 2001:2617–2633.
6. Gerszten PC, Welch WC. Current surgical management of metastatic spinal disease. Oncology 2000;14:1013–1026.
7. Gilbert RW, Kim JH, Posner JB. Epidural spinal cord compression from metastatic tumor: diagnosis and treatment. Ann Neurol 1978;3: 40–51.
8. Heldmann U, Myschetzky PS, Thomsen HS. Frequency of unexpected multifocal metastasis in patients with acute spinal cord compression: evaluation by low-field MR imaging in cancer patients. Acta Radiol 1997;38:372–375.
9. Martenson JA, Evans RG, Lie MR, et al. Treatment outcome and complications in patients treated for malignant epidural spinal cord compression (SCC). J Neurooncol 1985;3:77–84.
10. Torma T. Malignant tumors of the spine and spinal epidural space: a study based on 250 histologically verified cases. Acta Chir Scand 1957; 225:1–176.
11. Schiff D, O'Neill BP, Wang CH, et al. Neuroimaging and treatment implications of patients with multiple epidural spinal metastases. Cancer 1998;83:1593–1601.
12. Li KC, Poon PY. Sensitivity and specificity of MRI in detecting malignant spinal cord compression and in distinguishing malignant from benign compression fractures of vertebrae. Magn Reson Imaging 1988;6:547–556.
13. Loughrey GJ, Collins CD, Todd SM, et al. Magnetic resonance imaging in the management of suspected spinal canal disease in patients with known malignancy. Clin Radiol 2000;55: 849–855.
14. Rades D, Heidenreich F, Karstens JH. Final results of a prospective study of the prognostic value of the time to develop motor deficits before irradiation in metastatic spinal cord compression. Int J Radiat Oncol Biol Phys 2002;53:975–979.
15. Sorensen S, Helweg-Larsen S, Mouridsen H, et al. Effect of high-dose dexamethasone in carcinomatous metastatic spinal cord compression

treated with radiotherapy: a randomised trial. Eur J Cancer 1994;30A:22–27.

16. Vecht CJ, Hovestadt A, Verbiest HB, et al. Dose-effect relationship of dexamethasone on Karnofsky performance in metastatic brain tumors: a randomized study of doses of 4, 8, and 16 mg per day. Neurology 1994;44:675–680.
17. Vecht CJ, Hovestadt A, Verbiest HB, et al. Dose-effect relationship of dexamethasone on Karnofsky performance in metastatic brain tumors: a randomized study of doses of 4, 8, and 16 mg per day. Neurology 1994;44:675–680.
18. Heimdal K, Hirschberg H, Slettebo H, et al. High incidence of serious side effects of high-dose dexamethasone treatment in patients with epidural spinal cord compression. J Neurooncol 1992;12: 141–144.
19. Lai KC, Lam SK, Chu KM, et al. Lansoprazole for the prevention of recurrences of ulcer complications from long-term low-dose aspirin use. N Engl J Med 2002;346:2033–2038.
20. Loblaw DA, Laperriere NJ. Emergency treatment of malignant extradural spinal cord compression: an evidence-based guideline. J Clin Oncol 1998; 16:1613–1624.
21. Rades D, Stalpers LJ, Veninga T, et al. Evaluation of five radiation schedules and prognostic factors for metastatic spinal cord compression. J Clin Oncol 2005;23:3366–3375.
22. Maranzano E, Bellavita R, Rossi R, et al. Short-course versus split-course radiotherapy in metastatic spinal cord compression: results of a phase III, randomized, multicenter trial. J Clin Oncol 2005;23:3358–3365. Epub 2005, Feb 28.
23. Kwok Y, Regine WF, Patchell RA. Radiation therapy alone for spinal cord compression: time to improve upon a relatively ineffective status quo. J Clin Oncol 2005;20:3308–3310. Epub 2005, Feb 28.
24. Faul CM, Flickinger JC. The use of radiation in the management of spinal metastases. J Neurooncol 1995;23:149–161.
25. Loblaw DA, Perry J, Chambers A, et al. Systematic review of the diagnosis and management of malignant extradural spinal cord compression. J Clin Oncol 2005;23:2028–2037.
26. Rades D, Blach M, Bremer M, et al. Prognostic significance of the time of developing motor deficits before radiation therapy in metastatic spinal cord compression. Int J Radiat Oncol Phys 2000;48:1403–1408.
27. Greenberg HS, Kim JH, Posner JB. Epidural spinal cord compression from metastatic tumor: results with a new treatment protocol. Ann Neurol 1980;8:361–366.
28. Young RF, Post EM, King GA. Treatment of spinal epidural metastases: randomized prospective comparison of laminectomy and radiotherapy. J Neurosurg 1980;53:741–78.
29. Klimo P, Thompson CJ, Kestle JRW, et al. A meta-analysis of surgery versus conventional radiotherapy for the treatment of metastatic spinal epidural disease. Neuro-Oncology 2005;7:64–76.
30. Patchell RA, Tibbs PA, Regine WF, et al. Direct decompressive surgical resection in the treatment of spinal cord compression caused by metastatic cancer: a randomised trial. Lancet 2005;366: 643–648.

Vertebral Augmentation and Radiosurgery in the Treatment of Osteolytic Vertebral Fractures

16

Krzysztof Siemionow and Isador H. Lieberman

INTRODUCTION

Osteolytic lesions of the spine are a growing problem, affecting as many as 70% of patients with metastatic disease or multiple myeloma (1,2). Although symptomatic spinal cord involvement has been estimated to occur in 18,000 patients per year (3), approximately one third of vertebral lesions are asymptomatic and discovered incidentally (4). Tumor-induced osteolysis may lead to pain, dysfunction, and ultimately vertebral collapse; unfortunately, pathologic fractures resulting from vertebral destruction may be the first presentation of a spinal tumor.

Recent advancements in the diagnosis and treatment of many types of cancers have prolonged and improved the quality of life for cancer patients. Unfortunately, the oncologic treatment itself also contributes to the already present osteolytic bone loss. With increased survival and ongoing bone loss, osteolytic lesions are becoming much more a functional and clinical problem for these patients. If left untreated, vertebral body compression fractures occur with progressive kyphosis over multiple levels, cord compromise, and intractable pain. In this scenario, comorbid conditions and poor bone quality contribute to the difficulties of surgical intervention in this patient group. To alleviate these issues, percutaneous minimally invasive vertebral-augmentation techniques have recently evolved and show promising results for this debilitated group of patients. In tandem to the development of these less invasive surgical techniques, contemporary image-guided focused-beam radiotherapy techniques have also been developed, which minimize the collateral tissue effects of ionizing radiation. In combination, vertebral augmentation and spinal radiosurgery can control the tumor and maintain spinal stability. Combining the two approaches offers the patient rapid pain relief and restores normal spinal biomechanics while sparing the patient significant surgical morbidity.

BIOMECHANICS

Tumors secrete a wide variety of inflammatory mediators and cytokines, which are known to stimulate osteolytic bone resorption by modulating osteoclast formation and function. The compressive strength of trabecular bone is proportional to the square of its density (5). Osteolytic bone resorption leads to a reduction in bone density, which decreases the ability of the vertebral body to withstand physiologic loads. This in turn leads to vertebral fracture, collapse, and eventually deformity progression.

The objective of a vertebral augmentation is to restore the strength and stiffness to the weakened vertebral body. In addition, the kyphoplasty technique attempts to reduce the existing deformity and provide structural support by enhancing the modulus of the vertebral body centrum. By preserving a trabecular mantle surrounding the cement bolus, vertebral stiffness and strength will not be significantly altered, thereby protecting the surrounding osteoporotic vertebrae from subsequent fractures. Kayanja et al. (6) biomechanically tested multilevel segments to determine whether the number and pattern of vertebral levels augmented with polymethylmethacrylate (PMMA) influenced strength and stiffness. The strength and stiffness of both the multilevel segments and individual vertebrae were dependent on BMD, and not the number of levels of prophylactic PMMA augmentation (6).

VERTEBRAL AUGMENTATION

In 1984, "percutaneous vertebroplasty" was conceived in France to reduce vertebral pain as a result of a hemangioma (7). A cervical vertebra was injected with acrylic cement during open surgery to strengthen the vertebral body. An analgesic effect was noted, and indications for the technique in neoplastic disease and osteoporosis expanded to include both primary and secondary pathology.

The "kyphoplasty" technique as first performed in 1998, is a "least invasive method" of restoring the vertebral body to its native height followed by the cement augmentation (8). It involves the percutaneous introduction of inflatable bone tamps into the vertebral body under fluoroscopic guidance. Once inflated, the bone tamps restore the vertebral body toward its original height, while creating a cavity that can be filled with bone cement.

The traditional indications for vertebral augmentation are progressive collapse and intractable pain. Either a transpedicular or extrapedicular approach is used to reach the vertebral body. Contraindications to vertebral augmentation are systemic pathology, such as sepsis, prolonged bleeding times, or cardiopulmonary pathology, which would preclude the safe completion of the procedure. Other contraindications include patients with neurologic signs or symptoms, nonosteolytic infiltrative spinal metastases, vertebral height collapse of more than 60%, burst fractures, or vertebral bodies with deficient posterior cortices (9,10). Control of local disease and potential dissemination of disease are concerns and potential limitations of these vertebral augmentation techniques.

The results of both vertebroplasty and kyphoplasty reveal that they are safe and effective for pain relief when performed for the correct indications. Currently both vertebroplasty and kyphoplasty are used in the treatment of osteolytic vertebral fractures, and these methods should not be considered mutually exclusive. They are tools in the treatment spectrum of osteoporotic and osteolytic vertebral compression fractures to be used under the correct circumstances for each.

CLINICAL EXPERIENCE IN METASTASES AND MULTIPLE MYELOMA

In our ongoing study of kyphoplasty for the treatment of compression fractures resulting from spinal metastases, we showed favorable preliminary results (11). We evaluated the safety and efficacy of kyphoplasty in the first 21 patients over a 3-year period for the treatment of spinal metastases. The mean age of the patients was 60.8 years (range, 40 to 88 years). The indication for the kyphoplasty procedure was painful osteolytic vertebral body compression fracture. Symptomatic levels were identified with plain radiographs and magnetic resonance imaging. The primary sources of the metastases included breast cancer (nine patients), lymphoma (four patients), lung cancer (three patients), and unknown primary location (five patients).

Postoperative evaluation showed that the procedure was well tolerated, with improvement in pain that resulted in early mobilization in all 21 patients. Preoperative and postoperative SF-36 data were available for 14 of the 21 patients, with a mean follow-up of 50 weeks (range, 3 to 206 weeks). Significant improvement (preoperative vs. postoperative scores, respectively) was noted in the following areas: physical function, 20.9 to 33.5 ($p = 0.036$); vitality, 31.2 to 42.9 ($p = 0.012$); and social function, 37.5 to 66.1 ($p = 0.011$). No significant changes occurred in mental health (60.0 to 62.0), role-emotional (55.5 to 51.3), general health (52.1 to 46.0), bodily pain (31.6 to 39.0), and pain, as measured by the visual analogue scale (6.5 to 3.9). All 21 patients tolerated the procedure well, and no substantial systemic complications occurred. The fact that we found statistically significant improvement in only three of the SF-36 subscores may be due to the relatively small number of patients currently available. A trend was noted toward decreased pain after kyphoplasty. It is important to note that our primary indication for the treatment of these patients was palliation and to avoid open conventional surgical procedures that could have had a negative impact on the general quality of life of these patients with multiple medical comorbidities and limited life expectancies. The fact that we were able to show a decrease in visual-analogue scale pain scores from 6.5 to 3.9, although not statistically significant, suggests that a trend toward pain control existed.

Dudeney et al. (12) reported satisfactory results after kyphoplasty as treatment for osteolytic vertebral compression fractures secondary to multiple myeloma. In an ongoing evaluation of this patient group, we treated and evaluated 80 patients with multiple myeloma and associated vertebral body compression fractures (13). The mean age of our patients at the time of the procedure was 60.6 years (range, 35 to 85 years). Preoperative and postoperative SF-36 scores were available for 61 of 80 patients, with a mean follow-up of 15.6 months (range, 2 to 59 months). No major complications related to the technique have been observed. Significant ($p < 0.05$) improvement in SF-36 scores (preoperative vs. postoperative, respectively) were observed for the following areas: bodily pain, 23.0 to 44.4 ($p < 0.001$); physical function, 25.5 to 36.6 ($p = 0.034$); vitality, 30.3 to 38.1 ($p = 0.039$); and social functioning, 35.4 to 67.5 ($p < 0.001$). Mental health scores showed an improvement of 60.3 to 66.2 ($p < 0.001$), whereas role-emotion and general health were essentially unchanged ($p = 0.086$ and $p = 0.054$, respectively).

Fourney et al. (14), Weill et al. (15), and Cotton et al. (16) also reported their results with vertebral augmentation in metastases and myeloma. Fourney et al. reported on a group of 56 patients (21 myeloma, 35 other metastases) with a mean follow-up of 4.5 months. In this group were 65 vertebroplasties and 32 kyphoplasties. They reported 84% marked or complete pain relief, and only 9% of the patients experienced no relief of their pain. Weill et al. reported a retrospective series of 37 patients who underwent 52 vertebroplasty procedures for spinal metastases. Twenty-four of 33 treatment sessions (73%) performed for pain relief resulted in clear improvement (15). Cotton et al. (16) also reported prospectively acquired data obtained in 37 patients who underwent 40 vertebroplasty procedures for osteolytic metastases (29 patients) and myeloma (eight patients). Partial or complete pain relief was observed after 36 (97%) of 37 procedures.

These outlined results suggest that vertebral augmentation is efficacious in the treatment of vertebral body compression fractures secondary to metastases and multiple myeloma.

RADIOSURGERY

The role of radiotherapy in the treatment of spinal metastatic tumors is well established, and radiotherapy is often the initial treatment modality (17,18). Rapid pain relief and neurologic improvement can be expected in most radiosensitive tumors. The main limitation of external-beam radiation therapy is the radiosensitive nature of the spinal cord. Radiation exposure to the spinal cord limits the treatment dose to surrounding spinal column tumors to a level that is often below the optimal therapeutic dose (19,20).

Advanced imaging and stereotactic localization techniques of spinal column lesions have also evolved during the past decade. As a result, the advances in stereotactic radiosurgery as used for brain metastases may also be applied to the spine (21,22).

Stereotactic radiosurgery systems use an orthogonal pair of x-ray cameras coupled with a dynamically manipulated, robot-mounted linear accelerator (Fig. 16.1). This accelerator has six degrees of freedom that guide the therapy beam to the intended target without the use of frame-based fixation. Real-time imaging allows the tracking of patient movement. Cervical spine lesions are localized and tracked relative to cranial bony landmarks, whereas lower spinal lesions are tracked relative to fiducial bone markers. These markers must be implanted in a separate procedure and are seen as one of the disadvantages of this technique. The accuracy of such systems has been shown to be from 0.6 mm to 1.3 mm $\pm$ 0.11 of the targeted isocenter of the lesion (23,24). It is this level of accuracy that can be relied on to spare the spinal cord and neural elements and still allow precise delivery of high-dose radiation to the pathologic vertebrae. Before treatment, the spinal lesions are mapped, and the treatment plan and radiotherapy dose are calculated (Fig. 16.2). Although radiosurgery does not prevent further collapse, it can control the local tumor, contribute to an improved quality of life, and can be performed on an outpatient basis, all while minimizing the morbidity to the patient.

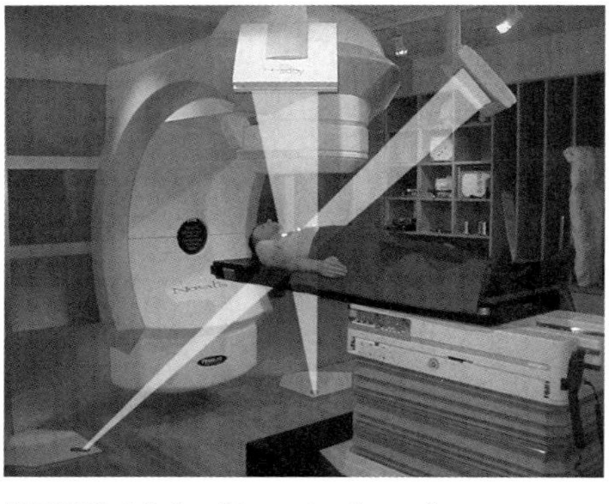

FIGURE 16.1 Stereotactic radiosurgery systems use an orthogonal pair of x-ray cameras coupled with a dynamically manipulated, robot-mounted linear accelerator.

CURRENT APPROACH

Historically, in the treatment of patients with spinal metastasis, the physician's armamentarium was limited. Surgery was usually offered to patients with a reasonable life expectancy and evidence of neurologic involvement or instability or both. These surgical procedures, often associated with a significant morbidity, were poorly tolerated in this subgroup of critically ill patients. The vast majority of patients, including those who were too ill or unwilling to undergo surgery, were offered radiation therapy, often in combination with steroids.

Patchell et al. (25) randomly assigned patients with spinal cord compression caused by metastatic cancer to either surgery followed by radiotherapy (n = 50) or radiotherapy alone (n = 51) (25). The primary end point was the ability to walk. Significantly more patients in the surgery group (42 of 50, 84%) than in the radiotherapy group (29 of 51, 57%) were able to walk after treatment (p = 0.001). Patients treated with surgery also retained the ability to walk significantly longer than did those with radiotherapy alone (median, 122 days *vs.* 13 days; p = 0.003). The need for corticosteroids and opioid analgesics was significantly reduced in the surgical group. The authors concluded that direct decompressive surgery plus postoperative radiotherapy is superior to treatment with radiotherapy alone for patients with spinal cord compression caused by metastatic cancer.

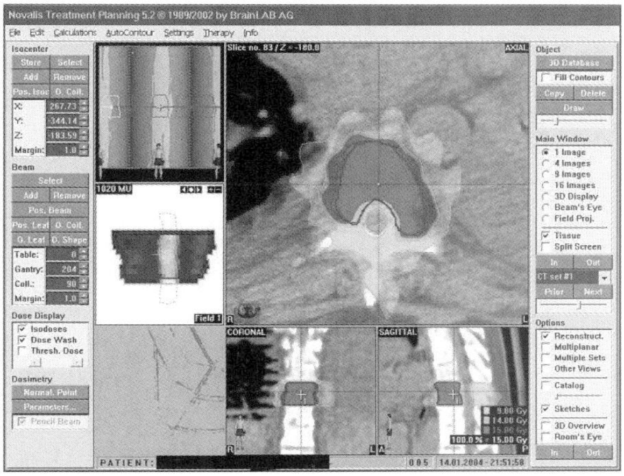

FIGURE 16.2 Example of lesion mapping and dose determination.

Until recently, few minimally invasive alternatives existed that would offer the patient reasonable pain control while addressing spinal biomechanics. The current approach to patients with spinal lesions at our institution involves coordinated efforts between the Department of Radiation Oncology and the Spine Institute, where we use these least-invasive methods of treatment. An algorithm dictates treatment based on neurologic status, vertebral collapse, and the general health of the patient (Fig. 16.3). Neurologically intact patients are often spared debilitating operative procedures, provided that no gross spinal instability is demonstrated. In these patients, treatment begins with three-dimensional mapping of the lesion (Fig. 16.2). This is followed by precise administration of radiation via the Novalis (BrainLab, Germany) stereotactic system. This system has been shown to be accurate up to 0.7 mm ± 0.2 mm (24). These patients are then followed up clinically and radiographically for evidence of endplate collapse. If the endplate shows signs of collapse, the patient is then treated with a vertebral augmentation procedure.

Patients with metastatic lesions and vertebral body collapse undergo a two-stage procedure. First, they undergo a vertebral augmentation as clinically indicated. This is followed by lesion mapping and radiosurgery. These patients benefit from advances in minimally invasive techniques. The tumor is locally controlled via radiosurgery with few systemic effects. The vertebral body is augmented with PMMA, which maintains spinal biomechanics and prevents deformity progression. As radiosurgery is tissue sparing when compared with conventional external-beam radiation (XRT), surrounding tissues retain their normal consistency, and potential future procedures, surgical or otherwise, will not be as challenging as those after XRT. Furthermore, because the radiation dose is localized to the involved vertebral body, wound-healing complications are not as severe as those after XRT. The vertebral augmentation procedures also do not significantly complicate future surgical procedures.

This treatment algorithm does not provide a "cure," nor does it prevent recurrences. However, in our experience, this approach affords excellent pain control while maintaining spinal biomechanics and offers these patients a meaningful quality of life. It spares the patient from an open procedure and the associated recovery. Most of our vertebral augmentations are performed on an outpatient basis, and our patients have few postoperative restrictions on their activities.

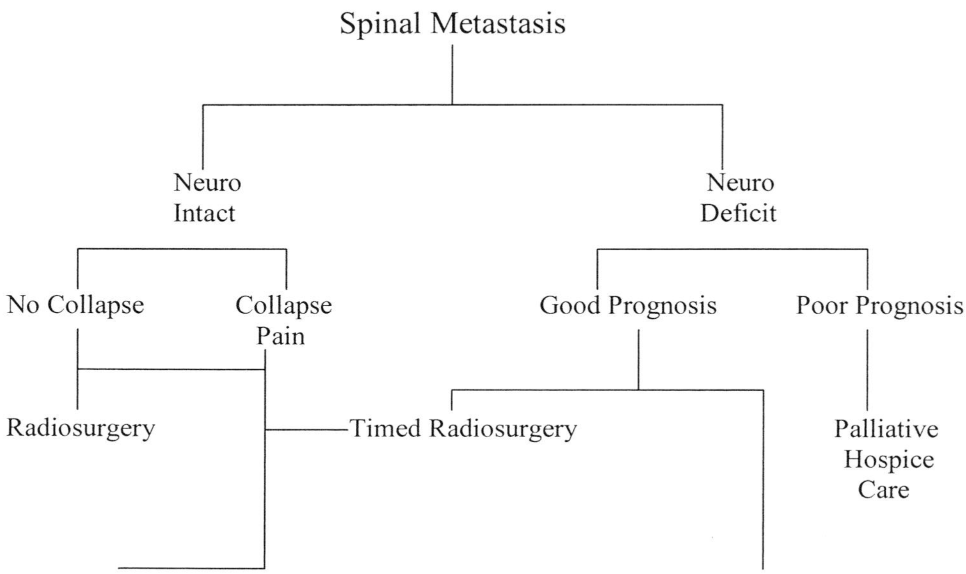

FIGURE 16.3 A spinal metastasis treatment algorithm based on neurologic status, vertebral collapse, and the general health of the patient.

The challenging patients are those with neurologic involvement and instability. These patients usually require surgical intervention to decompress the neural elements and stabilize the spine. This usually commits them to a large open procedure and exposes them to potentially significant complications, including death. Patients who are too ill or unwilling to undergo surgery will undergo a trial of radiation therapy followed by hospice care.

OUTCOMES OF RADIOSURGERY AND COMBINED VERTEBRAL AUGMENTATION AND RADIOSURGERY

Ryu et al. (23) tested the clinical feasibility of intensity-modulated radiosurgery in a series of 10 patients who had spinal metastasis with or without spinal cord compression. The majority of patients had prompt pain relief within 2 to 4 weeks of treatment. Complete and partial recovery of motor function also was achieved in patients with spinal cord compression. The average maximum dose of radiation to the anterior edge of the spinal cord was 50% of the prescribed dose, and no acute radiation toxicity was detected clinically during the 6-month follow-up. One of the major limitations of radiosurgery is its inability to address spinal stability. Although effective tumor control leads to pain relief and neurologic improvement, the weakened vertebra remains without any structural support. This frequently leads to vertebral collapse and initiates a cascade of pain and deformity progression.

Gerszten et al. (26) prospectively treated 125 spinal lesions with a single-fraction radiosurgery technique. Axial and radicular pain improved in 74 of 79 patients, and no acute radiation toxicity or new neurologic deficits occurred during the follow-up period. These results verify those reported by Ryu.

Gerszten et al. (27) further reported on a prospective series of 26 patients with pathologic compression fractures (16 thoracic and 10 lumbar). Seven lesions had received prior external-beam radiation therapy. All patients underwent kyphoplasty with the percutaneous transpedicular technique. At time of the kyphoplasty, fiducial markers were placed in pedicles at adjacent levels. Patients then underwent outpatient, single-fraction Cyberknife radiosurgery, at a mean time of 12 days after kyphoplasty. No acute radiation-induced toxicity or new neurologic deficit occurred during the follow-up period (range, 11 to 24 months; median, 16 months), and axial pain improved in 24 (92%) of 26 patients. The authors concluded that combined kyphoplasty and spinal radiosurgery treatment was clinically effective in patients with pathologic fractures.

Jang et al. (28) reported on the use of vertebroplasty and conventional radiotherapy to treat 28 patients with metastatic spinal tumors. Radiotherapy was performed immediately after the vertebroplasty in 22 patients. Pain levels were assessed before and after the procedure by using a visual analogue scale (VAS), and follow-up assessment was conducted at 1, 3, 6, and 9 months. On postoperative day 3, marked to complete VAS score–based pain relief was achieved in 13 (48%) patients, and moderate relief was demonstrated in 11 (41%). The mean VAS pain score was reduced from 8.2 to 3, and major complications were absent in all cases. Follow-up plain radiography was performed to assess vertebral column stability. Neither additional vertebral collapse in the treated vertebrae nor neurologic deterioration was observed.

SUMMARY

Vertebral augmentation and radiosurgery are minimally invasive options for the treatment of metastatic lesions of the spine. Radiosurgery offers the patient excellent pain relief and local tumor control. In addition to pain relief, vertebral augmentation restores spinal biomechanics and prevents deformity progression. Both of these procedures can be performed on an outpatient basis, sparing the patient the need for an extensive open procedure and extended hospital stays. We perform the two procedures in a staged fashion in selected patients. The goal in this challenging population is improved quality of life and patient satisfaction.

CASE EXAMPLES

Case 1

A 60-year-old, previously healthy man, had a 1-year history of chronic, progressive, mid-back pain, which occasionally radiated to his left hip. Workup revealed an L-3 pathologic compression fracture with some nerve root compression, as well as a 3.5-cm mass on the left kidney (Figure 16.4A–D). A biopsy of the kidney was performed, and pathologic evaluation revealed atypical cells favoring a low-grade renal neoplasm. The renal lesion was treated with chemotherapy. The patient then underwent Novalis (BrainLab) shaped-beam stereotactic radiosurgery with computer-assisted dose planning and body-frame application for treatment of his painful L-3 spinal metastasis. He noted immediate improvement in his pain. After the eighth radiosurgery session, the patient reported an acute, dramatic increase in his back pain, which prevented him from ambulating. This prompted an urgent computed tomography (CT) scan and a surgical

A B C D

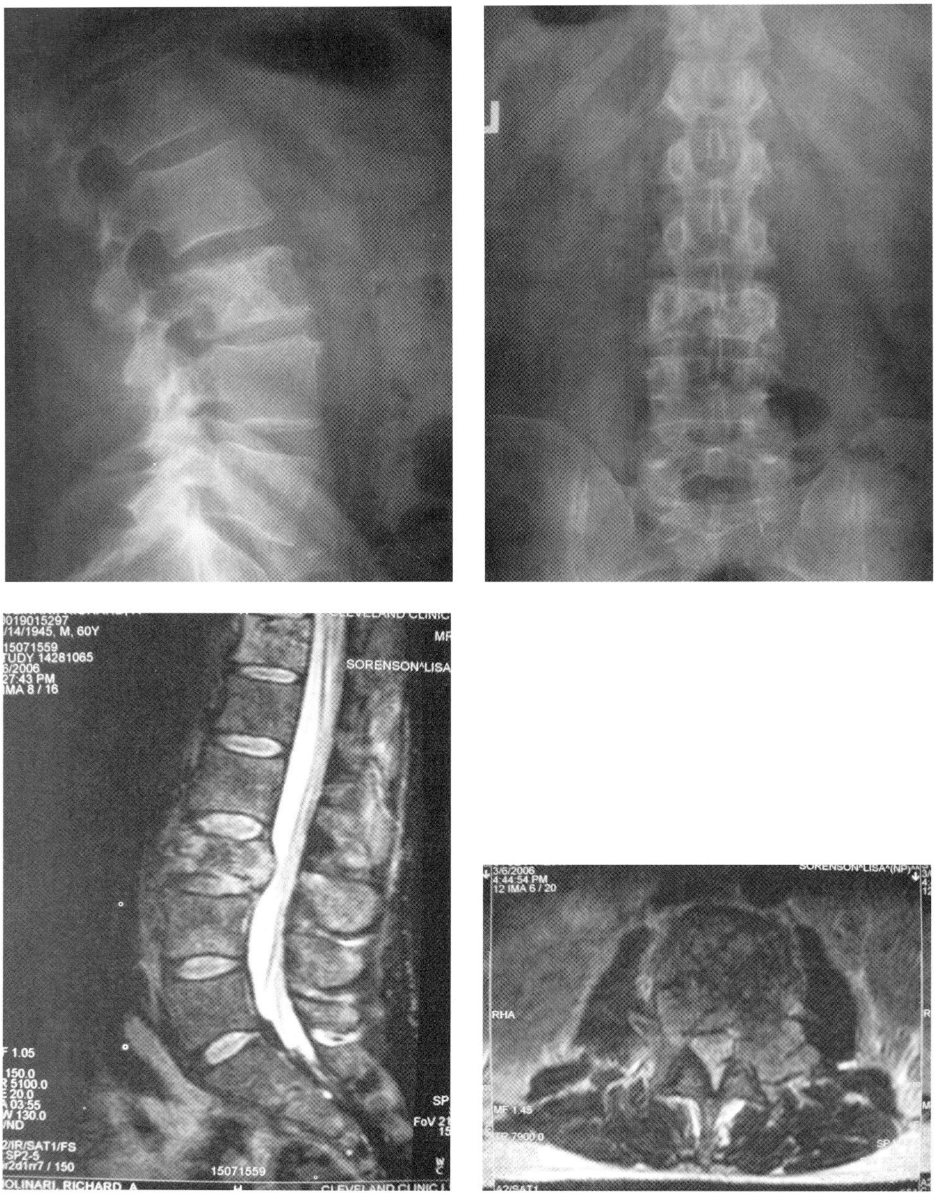

FIGURE 16.4 **A:** A 60-year-old man with 1-year history of progressive low back pain. Lateral radiograph demonstrating a lytic lesion of the L-3 vertebral body. **B:** Anteroposterior radiograph demonstrating mild L-3 vertebral body collapse. **C:** T_2-weighted sagittal image of the lumbar spine demonstrates a moderate compression fracture involving the L-3 body with bony retropulsion effacing the ventral thecal sac. **D:** T_2-weighted axial image demonstrates an extension of metastatic disease into the left pedicle and the left superior articular facet. A small amount of soft tissue extending into the superior aspect of the left neural foramen at L-3 to L-4 also was noted.

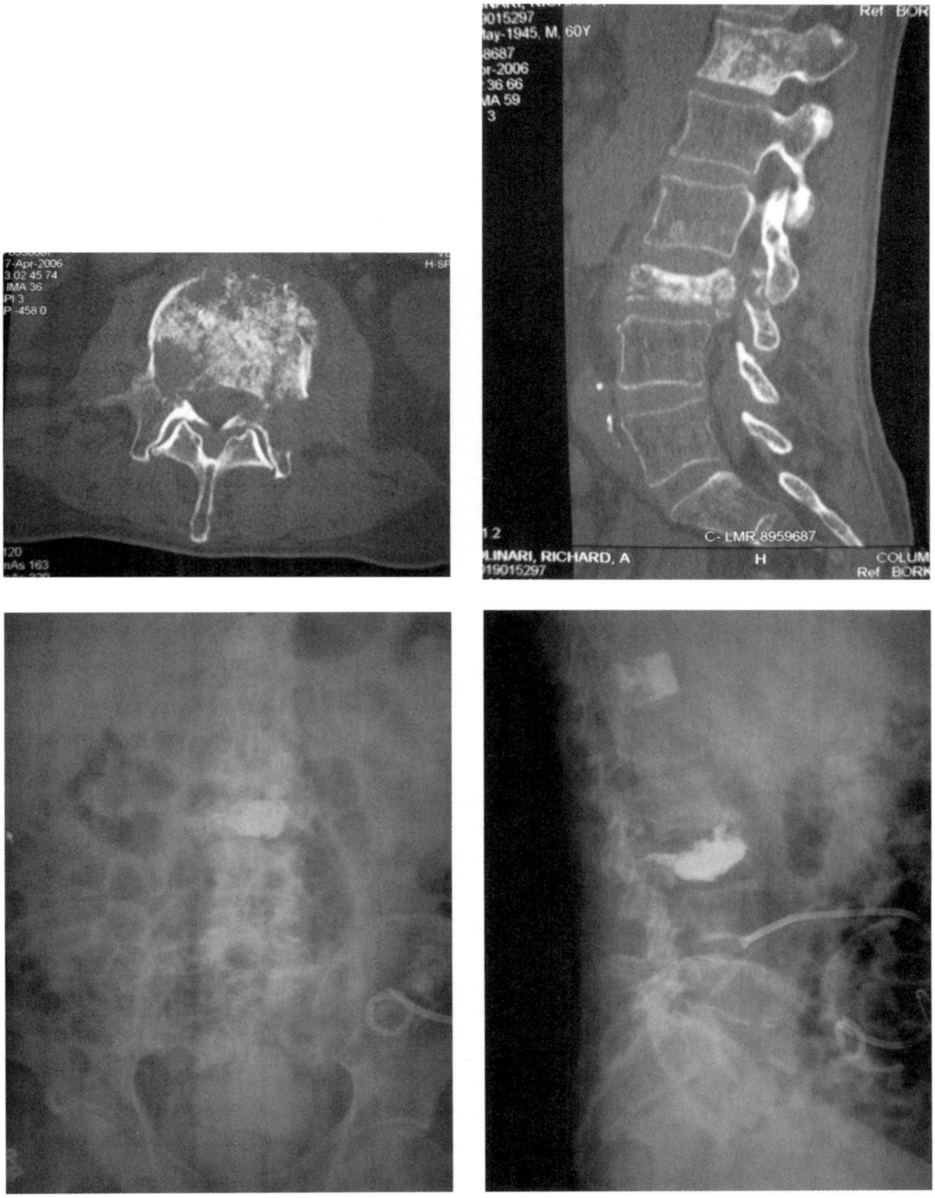

E F G H

FIGURE 16.4 *(Continued)* **E:** Axial CT scan through the L-3 vertebral body demonstrating lytic destruction of the left pedicle, left facet joint, and vertebral body. **F:** Sagittal CT scan obtained after acute exacerbation of back pain after a radiosurgery session. Marked progression of the L-3 vertebral body collapse is noted. Changes suggestive of metastatic disease are seen at T-12. **G, H:** Anteroposterior and lateral radiographs of the lumbar spine after T-12 and L-3 vertebral augmentation. The spinal column height and alignment are well maintained. A pigtail catheter was inserted percutaneously to drain the left psoas abscess. *(Continued)*

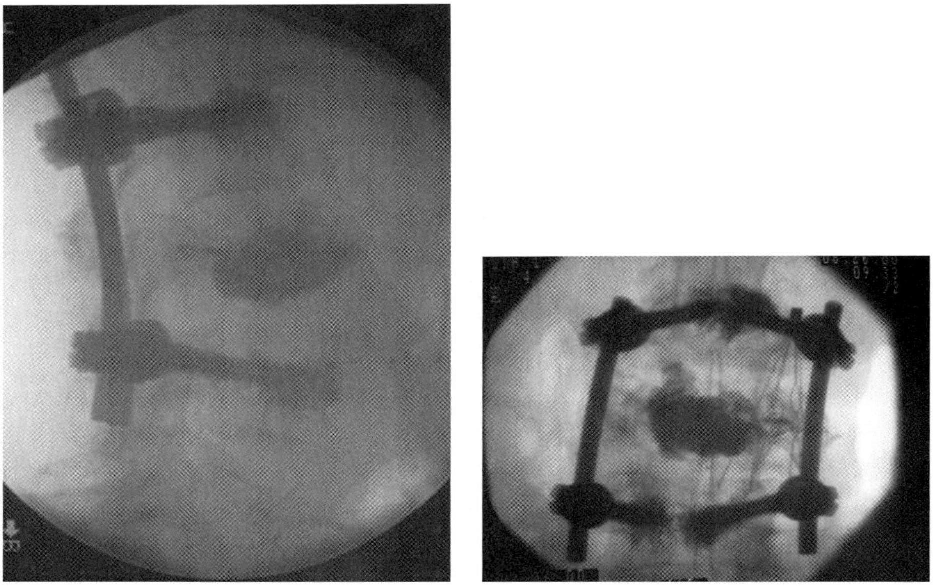

I J

FIGURE 16.4 *(Continued)* **I, J:** Posterior percutaneous pedicle screw stabilization performed for symptoms of mechanical instability. This procedure was performed 1 week after vertebral augmentation and allowed the patient to ambulate and participate in therapy on postoperative day 3.

consultation (Fig. 16.4E and F). The patient was diagnosed with osteonecrotic collapse of L-3 and a new T-12 metastasis. He underwent vertebral augmentation at both levels (Fig. 16.4G and H). The acute component of his pain resolved postoperatively. However, about 1 week after the vertebral augmentation, the patient began complaining of pain with even mild activity, consistent with instability, which ultimately prevented him from ambulating. During the same hospitalization, the patient was diagnosed with a psoas abscess of undetermined etiology, which was treated with percutaneous drainage and intravenous antibiotics. It was thought at the time that he also needed have his L-3 vertebral body stabilized. This was performed in a percutaneous fashion 2 weeks after treatment initiation for the psoas abscess. The spine stabilization was performed percutaneously, with L-2 to L-4 pedicle screw instrumentation (Pathfinder; Abbott Laboratories, Illinois) (Fig. 16.4I and J). This provided him with adequate pain relief and allowed him to participate in physical therapy on the third postoperative day. The patient's symptoms improved, and he was discharged home.

Case 2

A 49-year-old man had a 3-week history of back pain after a mild fall while at work. The patient was referred for a surgical consultation after lumbar radiographs revealed an inferior endplate fracture of the L-3 vertebral body (Fig. 16.5A and B). The patient had a history of bladder cancer as well as a presumptive diagnosis of multiple myeloma, although his protein counts were within normal limits. His workup revealed a L-3 osteolytic lesion (Fig. 16.5C and D). He underwent an L-3 biopsy followed by a vertebral-augmentation procedure. The patient noted immediate postoperative pain relief. The

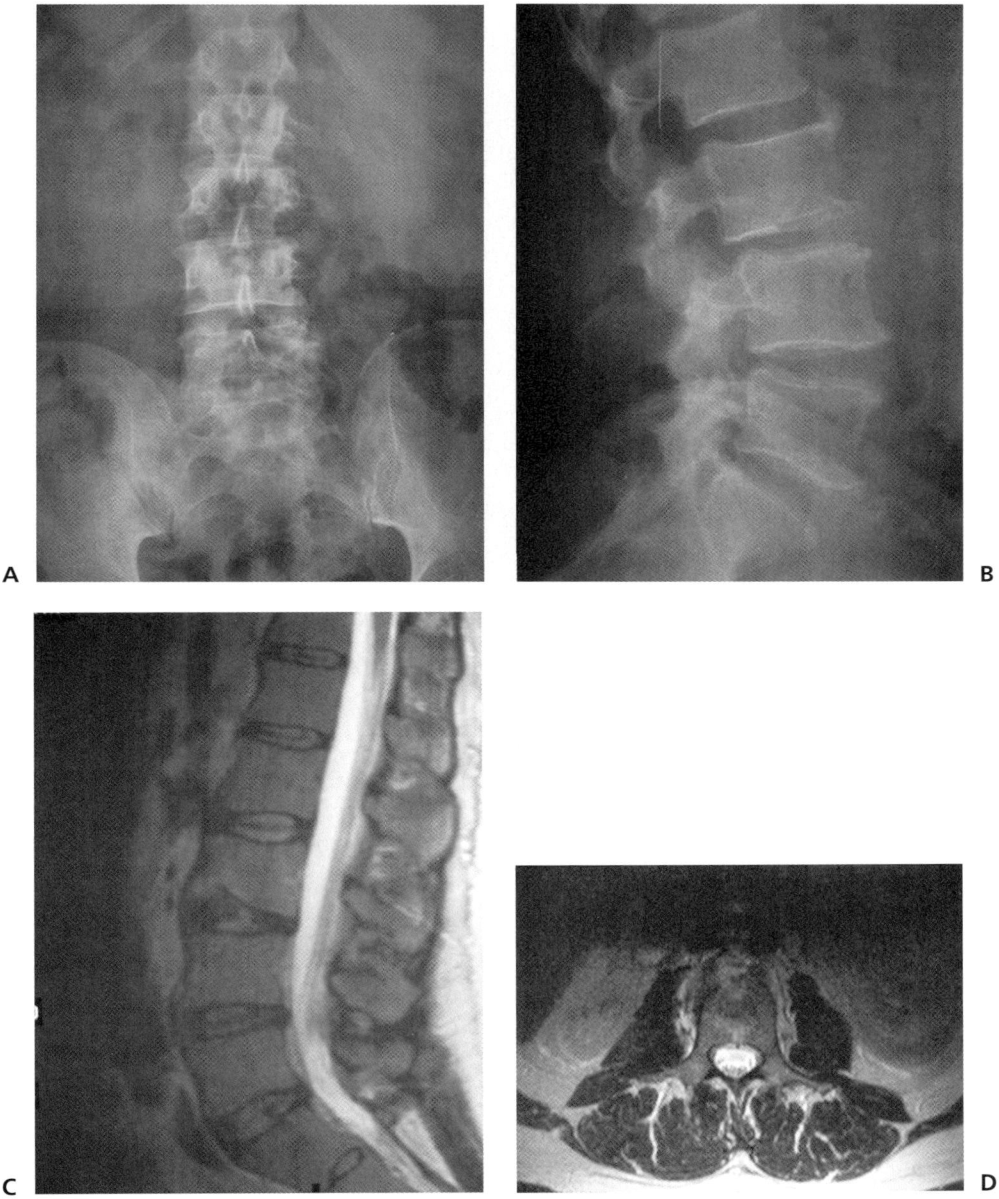

FIGURE 16.5 **A, B:** A 49-year-old man with 3-week history of back pain after a mild accident at work. Lateral radiograph demonstrating a fracture of the inferior endplate of the L-3 vertebral body. **C:** T_2-weighted sagittal image demonstrating inferior endplate fracture of L-3 vertebral body. **D:** T_2-weighted axial image demonstrating anterior cortical breakthrough and an associated right paravertebral soft tissue mass. *(Continued)*

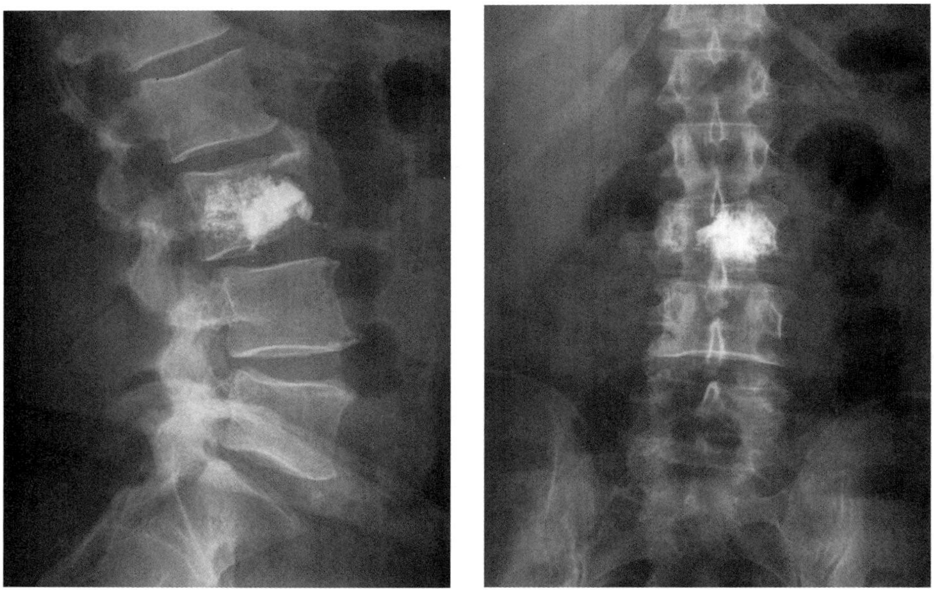

E F

FIGURE 16.5 *(Continued)* **E, F:** 8-week follow-up radiographs of L-3 vertebral augmentation showing preserved vertebral body height and lumbar lordosis.

biopsy revealed the presence of plasma cells consistent with multiple myeloma. The patient subsequently underwent stereotactic radiosurgery. At his 8-week follow-up visit, the patient's pain was well controlled, and he returned to his regular activities (Fig. 16.5E and F).

REFERENCES

1. Sundaresan NKG, Digiacinto G, Hughes J. Metastatic tumors of the spine. In: Sundaresan N, Schmidek H, Schiller A, Rosenthal D, eds. Tumors of the spine: diagnosis and clinical management. Philadelphia: WB Saunders, 1990:279–304.
2. McLain R, WJ. Tumors of the spine. In: Herkowitz H, Garfin S, Balderston R, eds. The spine. Philadelphia: WB Saunders, 1999:1171–1206.
3. Black P. Spinal metastasis: current status and recommended guidelines for management. Neurosurgery 1979;5:726–746.
4. Schaberg J, Gainor BJ. A profile of metastatic carcinoma of the spine. Spine 1985;10:19–20.
5. Carter DR, Hayes WC. Bone compressive strength: the influence of density and strain rate. Science 1976;194:1174–1176.
6. Kayanja MM, et al. The biomechanics of 1, 2, and 3 levels of vertebral augmentation with polymethylmethacrylate in multilevel spinal segments. Spine 2006;31:769–774.
7. Galibert P, DH, Rosat P, Le Gars D. (Preliminary note on the treatment of vertebral angioma by percutaneous acrylic vertebroplasty). Neurochirurgie [French] 1987;33:166–168.
8. Lieberman IH, et al. Initial outcome and efficacy of "kyphoplasty" in the treatment of painful osteoporotic vertebral compression fractures. Spine 2001;26:1631–1638.
9. Bai B, et al. The use of an injectable, biodegradable calcium phosphate bone substitute for the prophylactic augmentation of osteoporotic vertebrae and the management of vertebral compression fractures. Spine 1999;24:1521–1526.

10. Cotten A, et al. Percutaneous vertebroplasty: state of the art. Radiographics 1998;18:311–320; discussion 320–323.
11. Khanna AJ, et al. Functional outcomes of kyphoplasty for the treatment of spinal metastases. Abstract of papers, 72nd annual meeting of American Academy Orthopaedic Surgeons, Washington, DC: 2005.
12. Dudeney S, et al. Kyphoplasty in the treatment of osteolytic vertebral compression fractures as a result of multiple myeloma. J Clin Oncol 2002; 20:2382–2387.
13. Khanna AJ, et al. Clinical and functional outcomes of kyphoplasty for vertebral compression fractures. Presented at the North American Spine Society (NASS), October 29, 2004.
14. Fourney DR, et al. Percutaneous vertebroplasty and kyphoplasty for painful vertebral body fractures in cancer patients. J Neurosurg 2003; 98(1 suppl):21–30.
15. Weill A, et al. Spinal metastases: indications for and results of percutaneous injection of acrylic surgical cement. Radiology 1996;199:241–247.
16. Cotten A, et al. Percutaneous vertebroplasty for osteolytic metastases and myeloma: effects of the percentage of lesion filling and the leakage of methyl methacrylate at clinical follow-up. Radiology 1996;200:525–530.
17. Gerszten PC, WW. Current surgical management of metastatic spinal disease. Oncology 2000; 14:1013–1030.
18. Faul CM, FJ. The use of radiation in the management of spinal metastases. J Neurooncol 1995; 23:149–161.
19. Kondziolka D, et al. Stereotactic radiosurgery plus whole brain radiotherapy versus radiotherapy alone for patients with multiple brain metastases. Int J Radiat Oncol Biol Phys 1999;45:427–434.
20. Loblaw DA, LN. Emergency treatment of malignant extradural spinal cord compression: an evidence-based guideline. J Clin Oncol 1998;6: 1613–1624.
21. Kondziolka D, et al. KonStereotactic radiosurgery plus whole brain radiotherapy versus radiotherapy alone for patients with multiple brain metastases. Int J Radiat Oncol Biol Phys 1999;45:427–434.
22. Chang SD. The clinical use of radiosurgery. Oncology 1998;12:1181–1191.
23. Ryu S, et al. Image-guided and intensity-modulated radiosurgery for patients with spinal metastasis. Cancer 2003;8:2013–2018.
24. Yan H. A phantom study on the positioning accuracy of the Novalis Body system. Med Phys 2003;12:3052–3060.
25. Patchell RA, et al. Direct decompressive surgical resection in the treatment of spinal cord compression caused by metastatic cancer: a randomised trial. Lancet 2005;366:643–648.
26. Gerszten PC, et al. CyberKnife frameless stereotactic radiosurgery for spinal lesions: clinical experience in 125 cases. Neurosurgery 2004;1:89–98; discussion 98–99.
27. Gerszten PC, et al. Combination kyphoplasty and spinal radiosurgery: a new treatment paradigm for pathological fractures. Neurosurg Focus 2005;18:e8.
28. Jang JS, Kim DY, Lee SH. Efficacy of percutaneous vertebroplasty in the treatment of intravertebral pseudarthrosis associated with noninfected avascular necrosis of the vertebral body. Spine 2003;28:1588–1592.

Intraoperative Radionuclide Localization for Osteoid Osteoma and Osteoblastoma of the Spine

17

Brian J.C. Freeman and Samuel W. Judd

ABSTRACT

Osteoid osteomas and osteoblastomas are relatively rare bone-forming tumors that infrequently affect the spine. Complete surgical excision of the nidus is a prerequisite for curative treatment. However, intraoperative localization of the small nidus is often difficult. Incomplete resection leads to local recurrence with persistent pain, requiring revision surgery. As a result, surgeons often resort to wide local excision to ensure complete excision. This may result in long surgery times, significant blood loss, spinal instability, and subsequent need for posterior instrumentation and fusion. We describe a series of nine cases in which an intraoperative gamma probe was used in conjunction with intraoperative fluoroscopy to assist with localization of the primary tumor and to confirm complete excision of seven osteoid osteomas and two osteoblastomas affecting the spine. The technique allows accurate localization, a less-invasive approach, less bone resection, less resultant instability, less blood loss, and perhaps most important, confirmation of complete excision of the tumor.

Osteoid osteoma is a benign tumor of bone first described by Jaffe in 1935 (1). It consists of a small nidus (up to 15 mm in diameter) of highly vascularized osteoblasts producing osteoid surrounded by dense sclerotic bone (2,3). Osteoid osteoma can occur in cancellous or cortical bone and has been described in all four limbs and the axial skeleton (4–6). Patients typically are first seen between the ages of 10 and 25 years (7), complaining of night pain that is relieved by nonsteroidal antiinflammatory drugs (NSAIDs) or salicylates (8). It has been proposed that this typical pain is related to production of prostaglandin by the nidus (9,10). Osteoid osteoma of the spine is less common than that of the long bones, accounting for just 10% of cases (11). It usually affects the posterior elements of the spine, including the lamina, pars interarticularis, pedicles, and transverse and spinous processes (4,8). A handful of cases originating from the vertebral body have been described (12,13). Spinal osteoid osteomas cause axial back or neck pain, depending on location, but may also cause radicular pain, paraspinal muscle spasms, and reactive deformity, notably scoliosis (14,15).

Osteoblastomas are histologically very similar to osteoid osteomas, but are larger, with a nidus bigger than 15 mm in diameter, and behave in a more aggressive way. They may not necessarily have a well-defined sclerotic border and do not always occur with pain that is responsive to salicylates and NSAIDs (16–18). Apart from this, they can be regarded in a similar light as osteoid osteoma, and the management principles and difficulties are the same (2,7,18,19).

Curative treatment of osteoid osteoma and osteoblastoma involves the complete surgical excision of the nidus. Incomplete excision results in local recurrence, requiring further surgery (19,20). As a result, to ensure complete excision, many surgeons previously used *en bloc* resection, potentially leading to spinal instability and the need for posterior instrumentation and fusion (21).

In recent years, various minimally invasive treatments have gained popularity, including computed tomography (CT)-guided percutaneous procedures with intralesional drill excision (22,23), or radiofrequency thermal ablation (24–26). However, both techniques have been associated with relatively high rates of recurrence (24,27–29).

Both the vascular nature of the nidus and the rapid bone turnover surrounding it mean that osteoid osteomas and osteoblastomas *concentrate* radionuclide. This in turn makes them readily identifiable with nuclear scintigraphy (21). Rinsky (30) observed this and wrote an influential article on the use of intraoperative radiopharmaceuticals to assist with localization of such tumors.

The use of radionuclides for intraoperative localization of tumors has steadily increased over the past 15 years at our institution (31–33). By using the appropriate radiopharmaceutical together with a suitably designed detector system that can be sterilized for use during surgery, it has been possible *both* to localize the tumour and to confirm complete clearance of the nidus, thereby eliminating the risk of recurrence.

CURRENT TECHNIQUE

All patients have a conventional workup with plain-film radiography, computed tomography, magnetic resonance imaging, and a preoperative ^{99m}technitium bone scan to identify and localize the lesions (Figs. 17.1 and 17.2). A prerequisite for use of the intraoperative probe is a *positive* preoperative isotope bone scan.

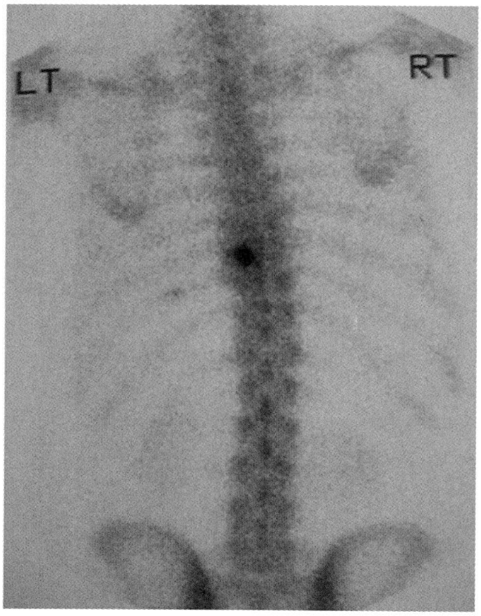

FIGURE 17.1 Radionuclide bone scan showing increased uptake posterior elements on the left in T-9 vertebra (Case 5, Table 17.1). Histology confirmed osteoid osteoma.

On the day of surgery, 600 MBq of ^{99m}Tc HMDP (hydroxy-methylene-diphosphate) is administered intravenously 3 hours before surgery with appropriate reductions in dose for children (34). The surgical team gown with lead aprons. The patient is anesthetized and placed on a radiolucent operating table in the appropriate position. Fluoroscopy is used to confirm the appropriate anatomic level, and a permanent mark is made on the skin. The patient is then prepared and draped. An incision is made, and the posterior elements of the spine are exposed.

We use a 5-mm-diameter cadmium telluride (Cd Te) solid-state detector (Radiation Monitoring Devices, Watertown, MA, U.S.A.) that has been sterilized in ethylene oxide (Fig. 17.3A). The nuclear probe converts gamma radiation directly into an electrical signal, read by a battery-operated digital counter and rate meter (Fig. 17.3B). The sterile probe is passed to the surgeon. The correct operation of the probe system is checked by directing the detector over an area of known high uptake, for example, the urinary bladder. The probe is then used to scan the area containing the lesion, and the counts per

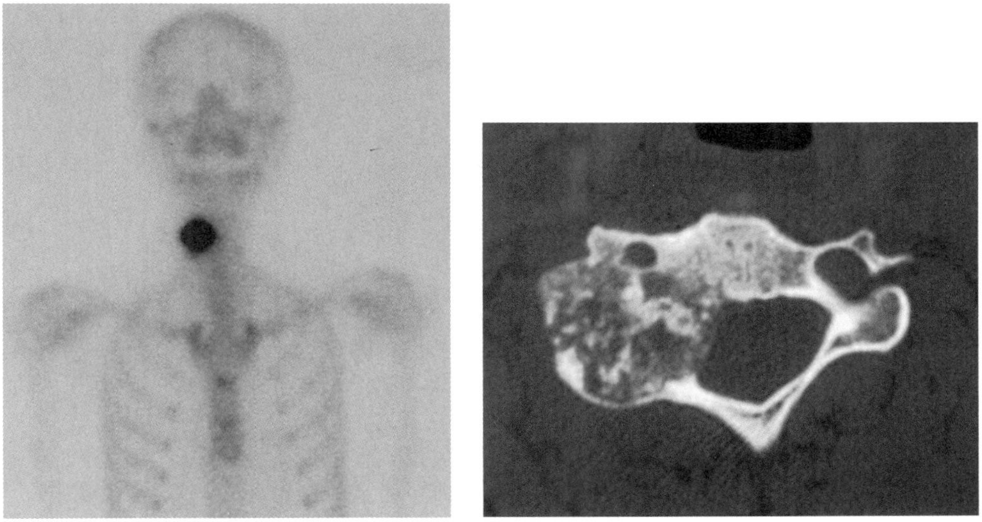

A B

FIGURE 17.2 **A:** Radionuclide bone scan showing increased uptake in the region of the right C-5 vertebra (case 8, Table 17.1). Histology confirmed an osteoblastoma. **B:** Axial computed tomography showing expansive lesion on right C-5 vertebra (case 8, Table 17.1). Histology confirmed an osteoblastoma.

second (cps) are recorded. After this, the posterior elements of the normal bone *adjacent* to the site of the lesion are scanned and the cps recorded to provide a "background count" for direct comparison. The tumor is then excised (Fig. 17.4), and the cps are recorded from the tumor bed. Ideally the cps should now have fallen to the same level as the surrounding normal tissues. A second check can be made by recording the cps from the excised specimen, which should register "high" if the specimen contains the nidus (Fig. 17.5). All surgical specimens are then sent for histologic evaluation. If a large amount of bone has been excised, reconstruction with bone graft and posterior instrumentation may be required. After surgery, the operating theater is checked for radioactive contamination.

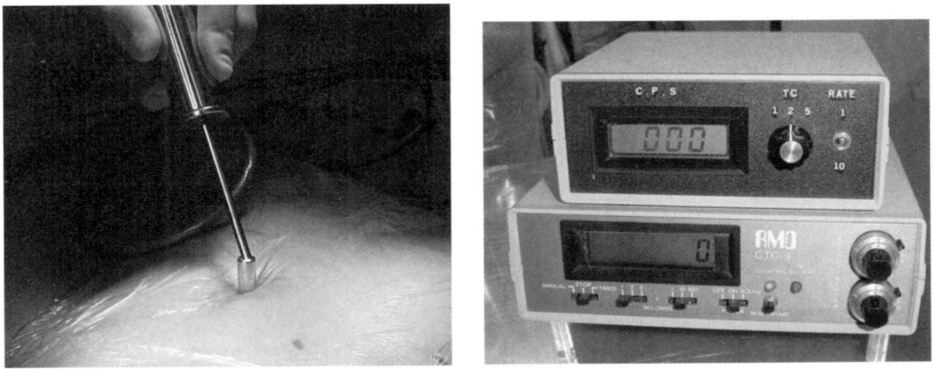

A B

FIGURE 17.3 **A:** Sterile cadmium telluride solid-state detector in position over thorax, confirming position of T-9 osteoid osteoma. The nuclear probe converts gamma radiation directly into an electrical signal. **B:** Digital counter and ratemeter converts electrical signal into counts per second (cps).

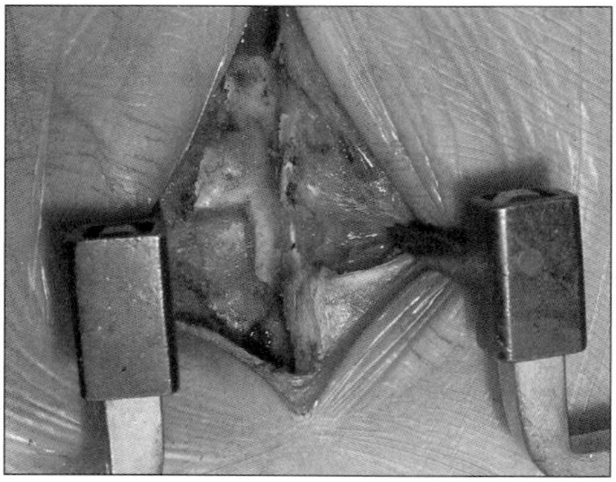

FIGURE 17.4 Operative picture (case 5, Table 17.1). Posterior elements of T-9 (left side), including the osteoid osteoma, have been removed. Counts per second dropped from 330 to 25 cps in the tumor bed after excision.

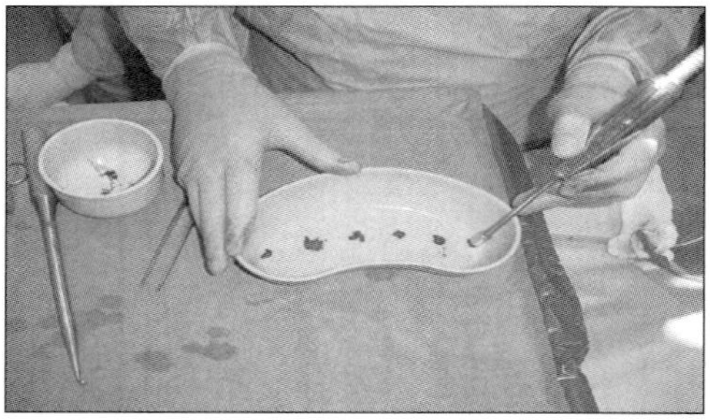

FIGURE 17.5 Specimens of bone are separated as shown in the kidney dish. Counts per second for *each* specimen are measured. Often one specimen shows very high cps. This is labeled the "probable nidus." All specimens are labeled and sent for histologic examination.

RESULTS

Between October 1995 and September 2006, nine patients were seen at our institution, with a diagnosis of spinal osteoid osteoma in seven and spinal osteoblastoma in two (Table 17.1). All had a history of back or neck pain of varying duration (range, 6 to 48 months; mean, 19.7 months), two of whom also had a thoracolumbar scoliosis. The seven male and two female patients had an age range of 9 to 31 years (mean age, 19.1 years). All tumors involved posterior elements of the spine, with two arising in the cervical spine, four in the thoracic spine, two from the lumbar spine, and one from the sacrum.

Treatment had failed for three of the nine patients, including CT-guided radiofrequency ablation in one and surgical excision under fluoroscopic control in two. No case had previously used an intraoperative gamma probe for localization.

In all cases, the cps were measured just before excision and after excision. A considerable decrease in the cps was noted in all cases after excision (Table 17.1). For the osteoid osteoma cases, the mean cps before excision was 203.8 (range, 60 to 515) decreasing to a mean of 72.5 cps (range, 10 to 220) after excision. For the osteoblastoma cases, the mean cps before excision was 373.5 (range, 67 to 680), decreasing to a mean of 40.5 cps (range, 16 to 65) after excision. Two cases required reconstruction with bone graft and posterior spinal instrumentation (one C5 osteoblastoma, one L-2 osteoid osteoma, and failed previous excision).

Histologic examination confirmed the diagnosis of osteoid osteoma in seven cases and osteoblastoma in two cases. Complete excision was recorded in *all* cases. The mean follow-up was 4.5 years (range, 0.5 to 11 years; eight of nine patients had a follow-up exceeding 2 years). All patients reported disappearance of the characteristic preoperative pain. All patients had discontinued analgesic medication by 3 months and returned to normal activities.

DISCUSSION

The accurate localization of the osteoid osteoma, in particular, remains a challenge. Plain radiographs are of little value in the spine and may not show the lesion at all (35).

TABLE 17.1 Details of the Nine Cases Undergoing Surgery with the Assistance of the Sterile Gamma Probe

Case	Sex	Age (yr)	Presenting Symptoms	Duration of Symptoms	Site	Procedure	CPS Pre-Op	CPS Post-Op	Previous Surgery	Histology
1	F	30	Midthoracic pain	18 mo	Right T-6 transverse process	Excision	123	80	Failed CT-guided excision biopsy	Osteoid osteoma
2	M	9	Cervical pain	6 mo	Left C-6 pars	Excision	80	10	No	Osteoid osteoma
3	M	19	L thoracolumbar pain + scoliosis	3 yr	Left T-10 lamina	Excision	515	220	No	Osteoid osteoma
4	M	31	Thoracolumbar pain	1 yr	Left T-11 pedicle	Excision	115	55	Failed surgical excision	Osteoid osteoma
5	F	18	Dorsal spine and chest pain	3 yr	Left T-9 lamina	Excision	330	25	No	Osteoid osteoma
6	M	15	L thoracolumbar pain + scoliosis	18 mo	Left L-2 lamina	Excision + instrumented fusion	134	50	Failed excision biopsy	Osteoid osteoma
7	M	12	Lumbar pain	12 mo	L-4 pedicle	Excision	60	45	No	Osteoid osteoma
8	M	21	Right neck and shoulder pain	4 yr	Right C-5 lamina + pedicle	Excision + instrumented fusion	680	65	No	Osteoblastoma
9	M	17	Left lower back pain.	3 yr	Left side of sacrum	Excision	60	15	Harlow Wood biopsy	Osteoblastoma

cps, counts per second.

Radiopharmaceutical compounds have been used with great success to aid detection of occult bony tumors. Introduced in 1971 by Subramanian and McAfee (36), phosphate compounds labeled with technetium-99m have become well established for the imaging of bone tumors and infections. The isotope's high uptake and rapid blood clearance make it ideally suited to this task. Osteoid osteomas and osteoblastomas concentrate radiopharmaceuticals, allowing localization by scintigraphy (21,31–33). Osteoid osteomas induce much more reactive bone formation in *cortical* bone compared with *cancellous* bone, the latter being more difficult to localize. However, even taking this into account, *no* confirmed false-negative nuclear scans have been noted (30).

Once the area of interest has been identified, computed tomography (CT) is extremely useful in allowing visualization of the nidus and any perilesional sclerosis (37). CT is extremely sensitive and enables the surgeon to localize the tumor before surgery (38,39).

Recently, magnetic resonance imaging (MRI) has been used to assist in the diagnosis. It can demonstrate soft-tissue and bone-marrow abnormalities such as unilateral neural arch edema and may even reveal the nidus (40). Others suggest that it is useful to identify a region of interest and subsequently to guide a detailed CT scan (41).

When conservative treatment with an antiinflammatory agent fails for these tumors, surgery is recommended (42). The surgical treatment of osteoid osteoma and osteoblastoma requires *complete* excision of the central nidus to prevent local recurrence (6,11,18). However, as the lesion is usually *not* visible to the naked eye, wide local excision is still recommended by some to ensure complete removal. Osebold et al. (43) and Faraj et al. (44) both advised additional fusion of the spine after *en bloc* resection of these tumors to prevent instability.

Recent attention has focussed on less-invasive treatments. The use of CT guidance in *percutaneous* resection of osteoid osteoma of the lumbar spine has been successfully reported with minimal soft tissue disruption (23,45–47). However, Sans et al. (27) reported incomplete excision and local recurrence after this technique. Van Royen et al. (8) used CT-based electrooptical navigation systems with high-speed intralesional drill excision. However, the use of a toothed drill under CT guidance to excise a lesion that, by definition, consists of sclerotic bone in the spine could be considered dangerous. The risk of breaching the spinal canal is increased because of the hard, brittle nature of the bone surrounding an osteoid osteoma or osteoblastoma.

CT-guided radiofrequency ablation has been used for the treatment of osteoid osteoma throughout the appendicular skeleton (24–26,48–50). Success rates reported range from 77% and 100% (28). Typically the lesion is heated up to 90°C for a period of 4 minutes, producing a zone of necrosis of osteoid tissue measuring 5 mm in radius adjacent to the noninsulated tip of the electrode. Recurrence rates after this technique of between 5% (48) and 16% (24) have been reported in the literature. Osteoid osteomas in a nondiaphyseal location are statistically more likely to recur than are those in a diaphyseal location when treated with this method, and, not surprisingly, the success rates decreases to approximately 60% for recurrent lesions treated this way (28). The technique has been used much less frequently for lesions in the spine, presumably because of the risk of thermal damage to adjacent neural structures. The other disadvantage of this technique is that histologic confirmation of the diagnosis is not always achieved.

The fact that osteoid osteomas and osteoblastomas concentrate radiopharmaceuticals allows accurate localization with nuclear scintigraphy when they are not readily apparent on standard radiographs. This property has been taken a step further with the advent of the mobile gamma camera to assist in intraoperative localization of such tumors. Osebold et al. (43) report on *three* cases in which such a device was used to assist in the localization of osteoid osteomas occurring in the lumbar spine. However, the authors still performed *en bloc* resection followed by local fusion with internal fixation in all three cases.

We have extended the use of a sterile nuclear gamma probe in combination with fluoroscopy to assist with cases occurring *throughout* the spine. Three of our nine cases had had previous interventions, including surgery, in which the nidus was quite clearly *not* removed and one case in which radiofrequency ablation had failed. Use of the gamma probe allows accurate localization before making an incision, meaning smaller incisions and less soft tissue disruption. Operations are undoubtedly shorter with less blood loss. Using a guided open approach such as this allows the structures of the spine to be visualized directly, permitting safe excision of the lesion and minimizing the risk of neural injury.

In our technique, the gamma probe is also used to *confirm* complete excision of the tumor. We believe that this is particularly important in the cases of osteoblastoma, in which localization is not necessarily an issue, but complete excision through an intralesional excision may well leave cells behind. We have had no recurrence of tumor in our series, with a mean follow-up of 4.5 years (eight of nine cases have exceeded the 2-year follow-up). The more accurate localization means that the surgeon can be more conservative in the excision and preserve more of the surrounding normal bone. The need for fusion and spinal instrumentation is decreased, as stability is less likely to be sacrificed. We had two cases of nine in which reconstruction was required; the first was a recurrent case in which the original nidus had been missed; the second was an osteoblastoma arising from the lamina of the fifth cervical vertebra, and the excision of this large tumor clearly destabilized the cervical spine.

CONCLUSION

The administration of radiopharmaceuticals and an intraoperative mobile gamma probe does much to help in the localization and confirmation of complete excision of osteoid osteoma and osteoblastoma affecting the spine. The more-accurate localization results in the safe excision of the tumor with maximal conservation of surrounding normal bone, while minimizing operative time, blood loss, and hospital stay. This is a guided open procedure that allows safe excision of spinal tumors that may be lying adjacent to important neural structures and minimizes the risk of local recurrence. It has much to commend it.

REFERENCES

1. Jaffe HL. Osteoid osteoma: a benign osteoblastic tumour comprised of osteoid and atypical bone. Arch Surg 1935;31:709–728.
2. Frassica FJ, Waltrip RL, Sponsellar PD, et al. Clinico-pathological features and treatment of osteoid osteoma and osteoblastoma in children and adolescents. Orthop Clin North Am 1996;27:559–574.
3. Jackson RP, Reckling FW, Mants FA. Osteoid osteoma and osteoblastoma: similar histological lesions with different natural histories. Clin Orthop 1977;128:303–313.
4. William R, Osebold MD, Edward L, et al. Intraoperative use of the mobile gamma camera in localizing and excising osteoid osteoma of the spine. Spine 1993;18:1816–1828.
5. Golding JSR. The natural history of osteoid osteoma: a report of twenty cases. J Bone Joint Surg 1954;36B:218–229.

6. Moberg E. The natural course of osteoid osteoma. J Bone Joint Surg 1951;33A:166–170.
7. Ozaki T, Liljenqvist U, Hillmann A, et al. Osteoid osteoma and osteoblastoma of the spine: experiences with 22 patients. Clin Orthop 2002: 397:394–402.
8. Van Royen BJ, Baayen JC, Pijpers R, et al. Osteoid osteoma of the spine: a novel technique using combined computer-assisted and gamma probe-guided high-speed intralesional drill excision. Spine 2005;30:369–373.
9. Greco F, Tamburrelli F, Ciabattoni G. Prostaglandins in osteoid osteoma. Int Orthop 1991;15:35–37.
10. Wold LE, Pritchard DJ, Bergert J, et al. Prostaglandin synthesis by osteoid osteoma and osteoblastoma. Mol Pathol 1988;1:129–131.
11. MacLellan DI, Wilson FC. Osteoid osteoma of the spine: a review of literature and report of six new cases. J Bone Joint Surg 1967;49A:111–121.
12. Heiman ML, Cooley CWJ, Bradford DS. Osteoid osteoma of a vertebral body. Clin Orthop 1976;118:159–163.
13. Fielding JW, Kein MA, Hawkins RJ, et al. Osteoid osteoma of the cervical spine. Clin Orthop 1977;128:163–164.
14. Haibach H, Farrell C, Gaines RW. Osteoid osteoma of the spine: a surgically correctable cause of painful scoliosis. Can Med Assoc J 1986; 135:895–899.
15. Keim HA, Reina EG. Osteoid osteoma as a cause of scoliosis. J Bone Joint Surg 1975;57A:159–163.
16. Boriani S, Capanna R, Donati D, et al. Osteoblastoma of the spine. Clin Orthop 1992;278:37–45.
17. Mcleod RA, Dahlin DC, Beabout JW. The spectrum of osteoblastoma. AJR Am J Roentgenol 1976;126:321–325.
18. Unni KK. Benign osteoblastoma. In: Unni KK, Dahlin DC (eds). Dahlin's bone tumors: General Aspects and Data on 11087 Cases, 5th ed. Philadelphia: Lippincott–Raven, 1996:131–142.
19. Pettine KA, Klassen RA. Osteoid osteoma and osteoblastoma of the spine. J Bone Joint Surg Am 1986;68:354–361.
20. Marcove RC, Heelan RT, Huvos AG, et al. Osteoid osteoma: diagnosis, localisation and treatment. Clin Orthop 1991; 267:197–201.
21. Bradford DS, Ulrich Bueff H. Benign and malignant tumors of the spine. In Lonstein JE, Bradford DS, Winter RB, Ogilvie JW (eds). Moe's Textbook of Scoliosis and Other Spinal Deformities, 3rd ed. Philadelphia: WB Saunders, 1995:485–487.
22. Assoun J, Railhac JJ, Bonnevaille P, et al. Osteoid osteoma: percutaneous resection with CT guidance. Radiology 1993;188:541–547.
23. Labbe JL, Clement JL, Duparc B, et al. Percutaneous extraction of vertebral osteoid osteoma under computed tomography guidance. Eur Spine J 1995;4:368–371.
24. Cribb GL, Goude WH, Cool P, et al. Percutaneous radiofrequency thermocoagulation of osteoid osteomas: factors affecting therapeutic outcome. Skeletal Radiol 2005;34:702–706.
25. Yip PS, Lam YL, Chan MK, et al. Computed tomography-guided percutaneous radiofrequency ablation of osteoid osteoma: local experience. Hong Kong Med J 2006;12:305–309.
26. Rosenthal DI, Hornicek FJ, Torriani M, et al. Osteoid osteoma: percutaneous treatment with radiofrequency energy. Radiology 2003;229:171–175.
27. Sans N, Galy-Foucade D, Assoun J, et al. Osteoid osteoma: CT-guided percutaneous resection and follow up in 38 patients. Radiology 1999;212: 687–692.
28. Hadjipavlou AG, Lander PH, Marchesi D, et al. Minimally invasive surgery for ablation of osteoid osteoma of the spine. Spine 2003;28: E472–477.
29. Vanderschueren GM, Taminiau AH, Obermann WR, et al. Osteoid osteoma: clinical results with thermocoagulation. Radiology 2002;224:82–86.
30. Rinsky LA, Goris M, Bleck EE, et al. Intraoperative skeletal scintigraphy for localisation of osteoid osteoma in the spine. J Bone Joint Surg Am 1980;62:143–144.
31. Colton CL, Hardy JG. Evaluation of a sterilizable radiation probe as an aid to the surgical treatment of osteoid osteoma. J Bone Joint Surg 1983;65A: 1019–1021.
32. Szypryt EP, Hardy JG, Colton CL. An improved technique of intra-operative bone scanning. J Bone Joint Surg 1986:68B:643–66.
33. Perkins AC, Hardy JG. Intra-operative nuclear medicine in surgical practice. Nucl Med Commun 1996;17:1006–1015.
34. Paediatric Task Group of the European Association of Nuclear Medicine. A radiopharmaceutical schedule for imaging in paediatrics. Eur J Nucl Med 1990;17:127–129.

35. Osti OL, Sebben R. High frequency radio-wave ablation of osteoid osteoma in the lumbar spine. Eur Spine J 1998;7:422–425.
36. Subramanian G, McAfee JG. A new complex of 99m technitium for skeletal imaging. Radiology 1971;99:192–196.
37. Bassi P, Piazza P, Cusmano F, et al. The role of computerised tomography in the diagnosis of osteoid osteoma. Radiol Med (Torino) 1988;75: 470–475.
38. Sim FH, Dahlin DC, Beabout JW. Osteoid osteoma: diagnostic problems. J Bone Joint Surg 1975;57A:154–159.
39. Steinberg GG. Pre-operative localization of osteoid osteoma: a new technique that uses CT. AJR Am J Roentgenol 1990;155:883–885.
40. Harish S, Saifuddin A. Imaging features of spinal osteoid osteoma with emphasis on MRI findings. Eur Radiol 2005;15:2396–2403.
41. Hachem K, Haddad S, Aoun N, et al. MRI in the diagnosis of osteoid osteoma. J Radiol 1997;78: 635–641.
42. Kneisl JS, Simmons MA. Medical management compared with operative management for osteoid osteoma. J Bone Joint Surg Am 1992;74:179–185.
43. Osebold WR, Lester EL, Hurley JH, et al. Intraoperative use of the mobile gamma camera in localizing and excising osteoid osteomas of the spine. Spine 1993;18:1816–1828.
44. Faraj A, Byrne P, Mehdian H. Osteoid osteoma of the lateral mass of C5: should excision be combined with fusion? Eur Spine J 1998;7:242–245.
45. Mazoyer JF, Kohler R, Bossard D. Osteoid osteoma: CT-guided percutaneous treatment. Radiology 1991;181:269–271.
46. Roger B, Bellin MF, Wioland M, et al. Osteoid osteoma: CT guided percutaneous excision confirmed with immediate follow-up scintigraphy in 16 outpatients. Radiology 1996;201:239–242.
47. Voto SJ, Cook AJ, Weiner DS, et al. Treatment of osteoid osteoma by computed tomography guided excision in the paediatric patient. J Pediatr Orthop 1990;10:510–513.
48. Lindner NJ, Ozaki T, Roedl R, et al. Percutaneous radiofrequency ablation in osteoid osteoma. J Bone Joint Surg 2001;83B:391–396.
49. Cove JA, Taminiau AH, Obermann WR, et al. Osteoid osteoma of the spine treated with percutaneous computed tomographically-guided thermocoagulation. Spine 2000;25:1283–1286.
50. Gangi A, Dietermann JL, Guth S, et al. Percutaneous laser photocoagulation of spinal osteoid osteomas under CT guidance. AJNR Am J Neuroradiol 1998;19;1995–1998.

En Bloc Resection of Tumors of the Thoracolumbar Spine: Surgical Techniques

P.I.J.M. Wuisman

18

ABSTRACT

Although the best chance for cure (local recurrence, disease-free survival) of aggressive benign and malignant tumors of the spine is realized through a wide *en bloc* resection, the surgical technique is demanding and not yet standardized. Usually the surgical procedure includes a staged removal of the tumor with a healthy soft-tissue cover as a barrier and an adequate reconstruction. Three different types of *en bloc* resection of the spine can be identified: *en bloc* resection of the dorsal elements, a sagittal *en bloc* resection, and a total spondylectomy. To perform these resections, careful planning is mandatory and consists of an adequate oncologic and surgical staging of the tumor, choosing of appropriate surgical approaches and techniques, and the use of optimal reconstruction materials and spinal-fixation systems. Principles of wide *en bloc* surgical resection should be applied to primary aggressive benign and malignant spinal tumors, and some selected secondary malignant tumors of the spine with anticipated acceptable morbidity and satisfactory survival.

INTRODUCTION

To date, adequate surgical intervention in combination with multimodal therapy are the cornerstones for the treatment of primary aggressive benign and malignant tumors, some secondary malignant tumors arising in the extremities and the pelvis, and also in the spine. However, the topographic vicinity of vital organs, vessels, and neural structures to the vertebral column profoundly complicates the management of these tumors with respect to planning, surgical procedure, and reconstruction. To reduce the tumor spillage and spread during surgery, the chance of local recurrence, and to improve the survival time, an algorithm has been developed to map the tumor adequately, to choose the optimal surgical approach and surgical techniques, and to perform a sound reconstruction. Equally important is the careful pre- and postoperative care and choice of adjuvant treatment.

Usually the investigation starts with a thorough anamnesis: pain (skeletal and/or caused by nerve root irritation) constitutes the most frequent complaint with which vertebral neoplasm is presented (1). At the onset, it is usually mild and then becomes subcontinuous and continuous, finally not depending on posture or rest. Much less frequently (less than 5%), the clinical onset is characterized by the occurrence of disorders due to myeloradicular compression (paresthesia, hypesthesia, sphincter disorders) that are frequent in advanced stages of disease.

After conventional radiographs (at the onset often negative) and persistence of pain and/or possible occurrence of myeloradicular symptoms, additional imaging investigations [CT, magnetic resonance imaging (MRI), and/or positron emission tomography (PET) or bone scans] are initiated, which usually identifies a lesion and establishes its topographic features. Once the radiologic features of the lesion have been defined, biopsy is performed, either image-guided (CT or C-arm guided) or open.

Anamnesis, imaging, and biopsy allow appropriate terminology, classification, and choice of surgical techniques and materials to perform an *en bloc* resection of spinal tumors. For example, sophisticated imaging methods allow both an appropriate oncologic staging, introduced by Enneking, and the now widely used surgical staging system for the spine, the WBB system (2,5). According to the oncologic classification system of Enneking, an *en bloc* resection is an attempt to remove the whole tumor in one piece, together with a layer of healthy tissue (5). The specimen can be subjected to histologic analysis, and the margins can be categorized as "intralesional," "marginal," or "wide." In 1997, Weinstein-Boriani-Biagini described a surgical staging system for the spine, the WBB system. It is a standardized simple aid: a vertebra is divided into 12 radiating zones, which can be used for the optimal selection of any spinal column tumor (4). In addition, sophisticated anesthesiologic, surgical techniques, and modern spinal-fixation techniques allow challenging procedures, restoring stability and avoiding severe neurologic injury.

Indications for *en bloc* resection of spinal tumors include aggressive benign tumors, primary malignant tumors, and isolated spinal metastases in the setting of controlled systemic disease, although the latter is controversial (2,3,17,18). Recurrent tumors previously treated unsuccessfully with surgery are also suitable for an attempt at an *en bloc* resection. One or more consecutive vertebrae can be removed as a single *en bloc* specimen. Contraindications include distant metastases, uncontrolled systemic disease, and encasement of adjacent or vascular structures that cannot be excised.

Various surgical procedures and spinal materials have been developed to perform not only multilevel posterior and/or anterior fixation but also to replace vertebral bodies (4,6–8,10,11,17). Based on these reports, several other surgical techniques have been described, encompassing variable indications, approaches, stabilization techniques, and yielding promising results in view of local control and overall prognosis (2,10,16,17,19). Before surgery, an outline of the surgery should be made and discussed with the participating disciplines. Quite often an interdisciplinary team consisting of general or vascular surgeons, neurosurgeons, and plastic surgeons is needed to perform the surgery. Appropriate reconstruction materials should be ordered. When a vascularized graft is used to reconstruct the osseous defect, the type of graft and the acceptor and donor vessels for anastomosis should be discussed. The same applies to free or pedunculated muscle flaps to reconstruct soft-tissue defects.

SURGICAL RESECTION TECHNIQUES

The three types of *en bloc* resection are a one-stage posterior resection and reconstruction when only the dorsal elements are involved; a staged surgical procedure for both a sagittal resection when the tumor occupies one side of the vertebra; and a spondylectomy or vertebrectomy when the tumor involves the vertebral body.

Posterior *en bloc* Resection

This type of surgery is performed when the tumor is confined to the radices 10 to 3 and layers A and B, according to the WBB system (4). The patient is placed on a Jackson table with chest, hip, and thigh supports, and a dorsal midline incision is made over the spinous process, usually two to three levels below and above the involved segment(s). The subcutaneous soft tissues are dissected subperiosteally laterally to the transverse process above and below the involved segments, to allow pedicle screw placement. Over the involved segments, the soft tissue is kept intact to assure wide surgical margins. After pedicle screw placement, the superior and inferior uninvolved facet articulations are dissected at the junction areas, followed by both a hemilaminectomy and a piecemeal removal of the rostral and caudal uninvolved laminae and facets, respectively.

Next, a thread-wire saw or an osteotome can be used to perform the *en bloc* resection. When using a thread-wire saw, pass the saw from rostral to caudal in a sublaminar fashion so that the tool is becoming wrapped around the pedicle(s). Repeating the procedure for the contralateral side completes the release of the entire dorsal complex. Alternatively, osteotomes are used to perform the pedicle osteotomies. By using blunt dissectors, the undersurface of the lamina can be dissected, with special attention given to the course of dura mater and the nerve roots. If the tumor is attached to the dura mater, the dura can be cut at the appropriate sides to assure healthy margins.

Subsequently, histologic probes of the soft tissues and bony margins are taken. Bone wax can be used to seal the cut bony surfaces.

Subsequently, the spinal framework is mounted, the surgical field thoroughly irrigated, posterolateral material applied to induce fusion, and thereupon, the wound is closed.

Sagittal *en bloc* Resection

A sagittal split osteotomy is performed if the tumor occupies one side of the vertebral body with or without involvement of the ipsilateral pedicle/articular process. Ideal distribution for performing a sagittal *en bloc* resection is a tumor confined to the radices (12) 11 through 6 (7) or (1) 2 through 5 (6).

Depending on the size of the extraosseous tumor extension, a staged anteroposterior or a posteroanterior and posterior approach is chosen. For tumors affecting L-5, the approach will be a staged ipsilateral pararectal, retroperitoneal, and a posterior midline incision. In case of a small or no extraosseous tumor extension, we usually choose a combined lateral and posterior approach. The patient is positioned laterally, and a lateral transthoracic, thoracoabdominal, or a retroperitoneal approach is performed. In the chest, the parietal pleura is incised above and below the tumor, assuring that the tumor will be covered by the parietal pleura. Subsequently, the intercostal veins and arteries are ligated. The uninvolved intervertebral disc(s) or the vertebral body(ies) is (are) incised or osteotomized above and below the tumor. The anterior part of the dissection is finished by performing an osteotomy through the healthy part(s) of the corpus(ora) vertebra perpendicular to the axis of the spine toward the dorsal elements.

Then a midline dorsal vertical incision is made over the spinous processus and is extended one to three levels above and below the involved segment(s) of the thoracolumbar spine. The paraspinal muscles are elevated in a subperiosteal fashion. Exposure must be completed to the tips of the transverse processes of the affected vertebra and all adjacent vertebrae.

Subsequently, pedicle screws are placed two levels above and below the affected levels, followed by a laminectomy at the healthy side of the affected vertebra. If needed, at the site of the affected vertebra the pedicle(s) can leave intact as part(s) of the specimen. At this site involved nerve roots should be dissected and ligated near the dura. The next step is the ipsilateral incision of the discs at the appropriate levels. Under amplifier control, the posterior osteotomy is performed perpendicular to the axis of the spine, followed by removal of the specimen.

Depending on the resected part of the vertebra, a biologic reconstruction of the defect (e.g., fibula parts, rib parts) or even a cage reconstruction can be performed.

Vertebrectomy

Ideal distribution for performing a vertebrectomy is a tumor confined to the radices (5) 6 through 9 (10) and layers A, B, or C. However, most tumors are already growing into the canal (layer D). Various surgical techniques have been developed for the different anatomic areas of the thoracolumbar spine. At the cervicothoracic level, a staged posteroanterior approach with partial or total sternotomy can be performed. Usually, we first perform a dorsal decompression and stabilization, followed by a combined anterior low cervical approach, including a (partial) sternotomy, enabling an exposure of the C-5/-6 to T-4. (8)

At the lower thoracic levels (T-3 to T-11), we can perform either a combined posterolateral approach, an endoscopic anterior release followed by a dorsal approach, or a dorsal approach alone (Fig. 18.1) Thoracoscopic release can replace the open thoracotomy only in small and medium-sized tumors. For the thoracolumbar level, we usually perform a combined anterolateral and posterior approach, either in a staged surgical intervention (first anterolateral followed by an posterior approach) or as a one-stage procedure.

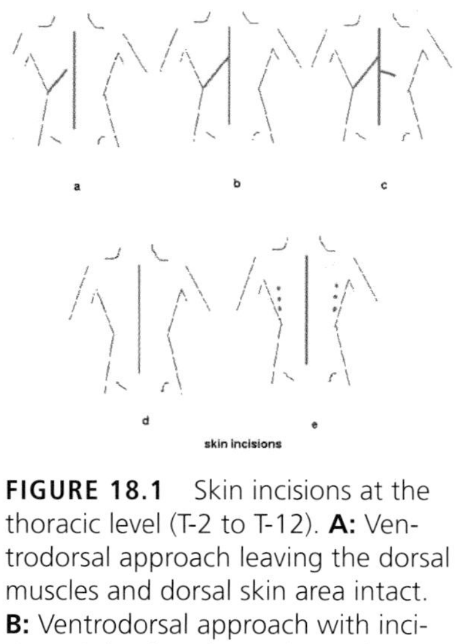

FIGURE 18.1 Skin incisions at the thoracic level (T-2 to T-12). **A:** Ventrodorsal approach leaving the dorsal muscles and dorsal skin area intact. **B:** Ventrodorsal approach with incision of the dorsal muscles and skin. **C:** Bilateral thoracotomies and dorsal midline approach. **D:** Dorsal midline approach. **E:** Ventral thoracoscopic approach and dorsal midline approach.

At the lumbar level (L-1 to L-4), depending on the site and extension of the tumor, we opt for a dorsal approach alone or a combined anterolateral and dorsal approach. Because of the anatomy (mainly the location of the common iliac vessels and the pelvis), an L-5 resection is performed by a combined anterior approach (pararectal incisions) followed by a dorsal procedure, including the removal of the tumor and the reconstruction.

A wide anterior and/or posterior exposure at the affected level is essential because it facilitates release of the vertebra and dorsal elements, respectively. For example, in a case with a primary tumor located in the thoracic spine and having an ipsilateral, subperiosteal extension of the tumor involving several ribs (Fig. 18.2), a staged anterolateral and posterior approach can be performed to resect the tumor and reconstruct the defect. First, a thoracotomy is performed at the side of the extraosseous extension of the tumor, with partial rib resection, leaving the pleura over the tumor intact. Subsequently, the segmental vessels are dissected and ligated over the tumor area, and the discs incised above and below the tumor. The wound is closed. After repositioning the patient (prone position), the dorsal elements of the affected vertebra are completely skeletonized. The proximal portions of the ribs at the affected levels are bilaterally freed from

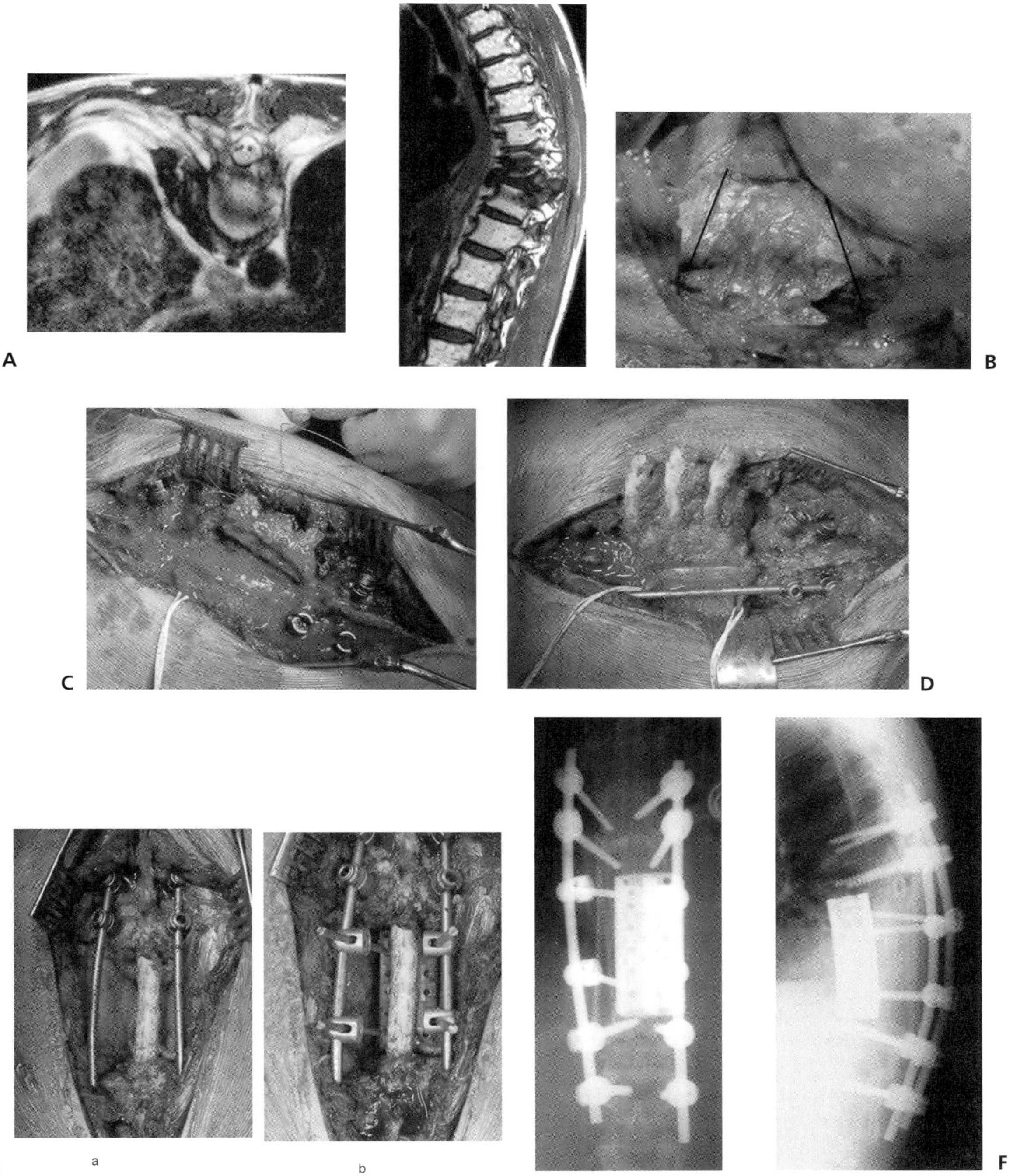

FIGURE 18.2 Male, 24 years old, Ewing sarcoma T-8, -9, -10. WBB radices 4–10 (T-9), layers A–D. **A:** T_1-weighted MRI imaging in the axial (a) and sagittal (b) view at the T-9 level showing enhanced signal intensity at the corpus vertebra T-8, T-9, T-10, collapse of T-9, and an extraosseous tumor extension. **B:** Intraoperative anterior view showing cut ends of three ribs; the tumor is covered by the pleura parietalis and drawing lines for incision through the intervertebral discs at the levels T-7, -8 and T-10, -11, respectively. **C:** Posterior view after *en bloc* removal of three dorsal lamina by using a T-saw. **D:** Removal of the tumor around the cord. **E:** Situs after tumor removal (a) and after reconstruction (b) of the ventral defect with a modular tumor system connected with pedicles to the dorsal rod–screw system. **F:** Postoperative radiographs in AP and lateral views showing the reconstruction after *en bloc* resection of T-8, -9, and -10. *(Continued)*

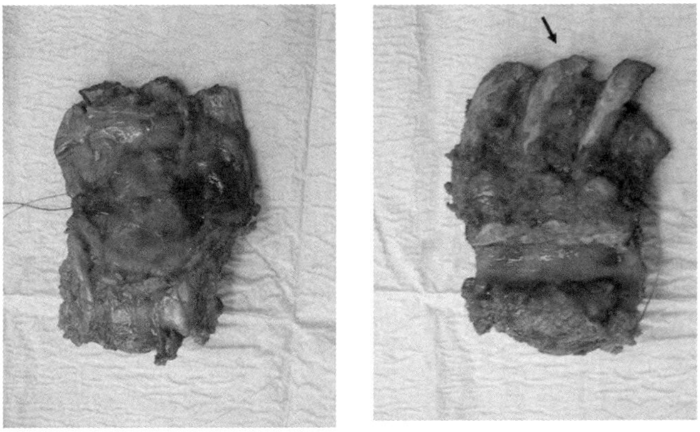

a b

FIGURE 18.2 *(Continued)* **G:** Specimen in anterior (a) and posterior (b) views.

the underlying pleura, transected at the healthy side approximately 3 cm lateral to the vertebral articulation, and removed.

Subsequently, pedical screws are inserted two levels above and below the affected levels, followed by disruption of the superior and inferior facet articulations of the affected vertebra by stripping the capsular ligaments completely. Next, partial piecemeal removal of the posterior elements and ligamentum flavum of the adjacent unaffected rostral and caudal vertebrae is performed to create an extradural working space above and below the affected vertebra. This allows the dura to be dissected free from the involved vertebra, permitting a clear view of the pedicle and adjacent disc spaces. Either a thread-wire saw or an osteotome can be used to perform the desired osteotomy and release of the dorsal elements. After removal of the dorsal elements, the paraspinal soft tissues can be safely elevated in a plane between the vertebra and the parietal pleura at both sides.

Subsequently, at the healthy side, the dorsolateral and ventral two thirds of the vertebral bodies are dissected free from the paraspinous anatomy and pleura by blunt dissection, followed by dorsal dissection of the discs at the appropriate levels. In the thoracic spine, unaffected and affected exiting nerve roots can be sacrificed at the dura level to make the exposure easier.

Now the specimens are freed and loose from the surrounding tissues and rolled out around the dura. In the lumbar spine up to the L-5 level, similar approaches can be used; however, muscular attachments of the psoas muscle and diaphragm must be released from the vertebra carefully. In the lumbar spine, care must be taken not to injure unaffected exiting lumbar roots. Nevertheless, if a lumbar nerve root is encased by tumor, it should be ligated and included with the specimen, because attempts to preserve the nerve root by intralesional tumor dissection will inevitably lead to disease recurrence and, as a result, to eventual loss of the nerve root.

Special attention should be drawn to the surgical approach of both the cervicothoracic and the lumbosacral junctions. Access to these regions is complicated by the presence of major vascular elements as well as important visceral and soft-tissue structures. The cervicothoracic junction can be defined as an area extending from vertebral segments C-7 to T-4 and includes the lower brachial plexus, thoracic outlet, and superior mediastinum. The lumbosacral junction includes the elements L-5 and S-1, the lumbosacral plexus, the common iliac veins and arteries, the vena cava and aorta, and the peritoneum and other structures occupying the retroperitoneal fossa (e.g., psoas muscle, ureter, lymph nodes and channels, autonomous nerve plexus). Both areas are unique in that it is a transition area from a mobile, lordotic spine to a rigid, kyphotic thoracic spine and sacrum, respectively. Furthermore, both junctions represent an area under stress, as the transfer of weight occurs between levels of the spinal column.

Several surgical approaches to both junctions have been described in the literature; these include posterior, anterior, posterolateral, and anterolateral approaches. Posterior approaches, such as laminectomy and pediculectomy, are common approaches that provide poor exposure of the anterior spinal elements and have limited use in the management of complex spinal diseases states such as tumors. The limitations imposed by a purely posterior exposure have resulted in the development of various combined anterior and posterior approaches. We use these combined posteroanterior approaches for all vertebrectomies. (8,20) The anterior approach at both levels allows not only excellent and adequate exposure for a safe resection, but also a stable reconstruction by using fibular autograft or allograft, iliac crest autograft, or expandable cages. All are suitable options for anterior column reconstruction and can be supplemented with anterior plating.

Reconstruction Techniques

Various reconstruction techniques can be used after dorsal, sagittal, or total *en bloc* resection of a spinal segment(s). These are generally divided into three groups: biologic reconstructions (autologous and/or allogenous grafts), prosthetic reconstructions (cement, prosthesis), and composite reconstructions (prosthesis and grafts). The reconstruction can be completed by a self-blocking system (prosthesis with anchorage systems) and/or can be associated with anterior anchorage systems or with circumferential systems (anterior systems with anchorage by artificial pedicles to posterior instrumentation). Another important feature for anterior instrumentation is its modularity (that is, the possibility of adapting, directly during surgery, the specific needs of the reconstruction with a broad spectrum of possibilities with respect to the anterior replacement of the vertebral body(ies) and of the fixation techniques).

After removal of the *en bloc* specimen, the vertebral endplates of recipient vertebra are prepared to accept appropriate-sized expandable cages, strut grafts, or even vascularized grafts. The prone position not only allows adaptation of the posterior column stabilization system (usually by mild compression) to fixate firmly the anterior column reconstruct, but also connection of a ventral cage by artificial pedicles with the dorsal-fixation system. Wounds are closed in a standard fashion.

Postoperative Care

Mobilization starts after hemodynamic stabilization of the patient (usually, the patient stays 1 or more days on an intensive care unit). Adequate enteral or parenteral nutrition, external support (external orthoses are prescribed on an as-needed basis), and early mobilization help to avoid complications associated with prolonged bed rest, including poor wound healing, pneumonia, decubitus ulcers, and deep-vein thrombosis. If patients have difficulties due to neurologic deficits or a prolonged recovery is expected, usually they are sent to specialized rehabilitation centers for physical and mental recovery and guidance, respectively. Follow-up imaging to assess for hardware stability is performed during the first postoperative week and at further routine intervals, not only to document fusion but also to rule out local and or systemic spread of the disease in time. Adjunctive radiotherapy and/or chemotherapy are administered if necessary, depending on the final surgical margin and histopathologic findings, as soon as the wounds are healed, usually approximately 2 to 3 weeks after surgery.

DISCUSSION

Primary malignant spinal tumors are quite rare in the spine, as solid metastases of solid neoplasms prevail: in order of frequency, they come from breast, prostate, lung, kidney, intestinal cancer, and from unknown sites. Frequently, primary localizations or manifestations of systemic disease of malignant hematologic disorders such as myelomas and lymphomas occur. With regard to primary disease of the vertebral column, a clear prevalence of intradural pathologies exists, both extra- and intramedullary, making up 90%. Extradural pathologies of exclusive and/or prevalent orthopaedic interest cover the remaining 10% and are represented by giant cell tumor, chordoma, osteosarcoma, Ewing sarcoma, and some others with minor frequencies, such as schwannoma and malignant fibrous histiocytoma.

The neurologic deficits and histiotypes of the tumors often guide therapy, which may be exclusively chemotherapy with or without radiotherapy or embolization, exclusive surgery, and more often, integration of the methods. However, the main problems encountered in the treatment of primary aggressive benign or malignant tumors of the spine include (a) incorrect diagnosis and misjudgment of the overall medical condition of the patient; (b) incorrect choice of the appropriate adjuvant treatment and surgical procedure, which is not matched to the patient's prognosis and disease; (c) misjudgment of the type and extent of surgical stabilization; (d) failing to obtain appropriate surgical margins; and (e) technical pitfalls, including infection, hardware failure, and pseudarthrosis.

The prognosis associated with and the treatment of primary aggressive benign and malignant tumors of the spine is influenced by many factors, such as age, location, type and extension of the tumor, general condition of the patient, drug resistance of the tumor, the severity of neurologic deficit at time of presentation, existence of spinal deformity and/or impending increase of deformity, and the time and onset of symptoms. Paralysis, for example, occurring in children generally has a better prognosis compared with that in adults, and deficits arising in the cervicothoracic spinal column are associated with a dismal prognosis. Severe neurologic deficit (Frankel A and B) has a bad prognosis and probably constitutes an indication for urgent decompression.

Several studies described the surgical *en bloc* resection of primary malignant or aggressive benign vertebral tumors (2,3,10–15,17). The unique anatomic structure of the vertebra makes it difficult to obtain complete excision of the tumor, and most surgeries before the 1990s were amendable only to curettage or piecemeal resection. However, conclusive evidence has showed the superiority of *en bloc* resection over piecemeal resection with respect to local recurrence and overall survival for primary malignant spinal tumors (3). Whereas wide resections for tumor not penetrating the cortex of the vertebra are definitively feasible, attainment of wide *en bloc* resections for extracompartmental tumors (most frequently encountered) is profoundly complicated and may require additional resection of adjacent tissue layers functioning as a biologic border for invading tumor cells. For example, extracompartmental tumor growth in the spinal canal with invasion of or attachment to the dura can necessitate *en bloc* resection, including a part of the dura (9). In some cases, however, for example, in extracompartmental tumor growth with circumferential dura invasion, it may be impossible to avoid at least some intralesional dissection for tumors affecting the spine. In these cases, however, recent reports have shown that outcomes of *en bloc* resections that left partial contaminated margins are better than those for entirely intralesional resections (2,3,17).

The histology of surgical margins of spinal malignancies indicates that a wide surgical margin can be achieved around an affected vertebra if the lesion is intracompartmental (layers B or C, according to the WBB system). For a tumor extending into the spinal canal (layer D) or one invading the paravertebral areas (layer A), most often a marginal resection is possible when the lesion is well encapsulated with a fibrous membrane.

Potential risks during and after surgery include major vessel surgery, excessive bleeding, spinal cord injury, tumor spillage, and spinal material–related failures. Wound-healing problems and deep infections are serious postoperative problems, often needing repeated multiple surgeries. These complications are probably due to soft-tissue manipulation during surgery, long surgery times, marked blood loss, and the health state of the patient before surgery. However, recent surgical and technical refinements contribute to a significant decrease in complications and technical failures.

In conclusion, therapeutic conduct in the treatment of aggressive benign and primary malignant tumors of the spine must take into account the general conditions and the life expectancy of the patient. Although the aim of such procedures is obtaining a wide resection, only in a minority can these margins be achieved. However, the long-term outlook of primary malignant tumors of the spine has been improved significantly by an aggressive surgical approach with or without effective adjuvant treatment modalities. Surgery should always be considered as a part of the overall judgment of the physical and mental health state of the patient.

REFERENCES

1. Algra PR. MR and CT of spinal metastases. 1992. Thesis, Vrije Universiteit, Amsterdam.
2. Boriani S, Biagini R, De Iure F, et al. En bloc resections of bone tumors of the thoracolumbar spine: a preliminary report on 29 patients. Spine 1996;21:1927–1931.
3. Boriani S, De Iure F, Bandiera S, et al. Chondrosarcoma of the mobile spine: report on 22 cases. Spine 2000;25:804–812.
4. Boriani S, Weinstein JN, Biagini R. Primary bone tumors of the spine: terminology and surgical staging. Spine 1997;22:1036–1044.
5. Enneking WF, Spanier SS, Goodman MA. A system for the surgical staging of musculoskeletal sarcoma. Clin Orthop Relat Res 1980;153:106–120.
6. Fourney DR, Abi-Said D, Rhines LD, et al. Simultaneous anterior-posterior approach to the thoracic and lumbar spine for the radical resection of tumors followed by reconstruction and stabilization. J Neurosurg 2001;94:232–244.
7. Gokaslan ZL, York JE, Walsh GL, et al. Transthoracic vertebrectomy for metastatic spinal tumors. J Neurosurg 1998;89:599–609.
8. Hu H, Winters HA, Paul RM, Wuisman PI. Internal thoracic vessels used as pedicle graft for anastomosis with vascularized bone graft to reconstruct C7-T3 spinal defects: a new technique. Spine 2007;32:601–605.
9. Krepler P, Windhager R, Toma CD, et al. Dura resection in combination with en bloc spondylectomy for primary malignant tumors of the spine. Spine 2003;28:E334–E338.
10. Magerl F, Coscia MF. Total posterior vertebrectomy of the thoracic or lumbar spine. Clin Orthop Relat Res 1988;232:62–69.
11. Roy-Camille R, Saillant G, Bisserie M, et al. Resection vertebrale totale dans la chirurgie

tumorale au niveau du rachis dorsal par voie posterieure pure: technique, indications. [Total excision of thoracic vertebrae (author's transl)]. Rev Chir Orthop Reparatrice Appar Mot 1981;67: 421–430.

12. Savini R, Gherlinzoni F, Morandi M, et al. Surgical treatment of giant-cell tumor of the spine: the experience at the Istituto Ortopedico Rizzoli. J Bone Joint Surg Am 1983;65:1283–1289.
13. Shives TC, Dahlin DC, Sim FH, et al. Osteosarcoma of the spine. J Bone Joint Surg Am 1986;68: 660–668.
14. Shives TC, McLeod RA, Unni KK, et al. Chondrosarcoma of the spine. J Bone Joint Surg Am 1989;71:1158–1165.
15. Sturm PF, Abramovitz J, Wagner C, et al. Malignant fibrous histiocytoma of the spine: a case report and review of the literature. Spine 1992;17: 975–977.
16. Sundaresan N, Rosen G, Huvos AG, et al. Combined treatment of osteosarcoma of the spine. Neurosurgery 1988;23:714–719.
17. Tomita K, Kawahara N, Baba H, et al. Total en bloc spondylectomy: a new surgical technique for primary malignant vertebral tumors. Spine 1997; 22:324–333.
18. Tomita K, Kawahara N, Kobayashi T, et al. Surgical strategy for spinal metastases. Spine 2001;26: 298–306.
19. Weinstein JN, McLain RF. Primary tumors of the spine. Spine 1987;12:843–851.
20. Wuisman P, Harle A, Matthiass HH, et al. Twostage therapy in the treatment of sacral tumors. Arch Orthop Trauma Surg 1989;108:255–260.

Surgical Outcomes and Guidelines for Management of Metastatic Spinal Cancer (A Point-of-View Review)

A.G Hadjipavlou, M. Szpalski, R. Gunzburg, M. Aebi, K.N. Kakavelakis, and P. Katonis

19

ABSTRACT

The effectiveness and safety of surgery for metastatic cancer of the spine can be evaluated only through patient-outcome studies. Review of the literature reveals that certain outcome instruments have been validated for metastatic spinal disease, such as EORTC, QLQ-L30, EQ-SD, HUI-MARK 3, ESAS, McGill pain questionnaire, VAS, MPAC, and so on. The results of the following reported parameters should be considered important when assessing surgical outcomes: neurologic improvement 55% to 87%; restoration of ambulation, 40% to 100%; restoration of sphincter control, 36% to 89%; pain relief, 47% to 100%; local recurrences, 8% to 31%; complication rates, 16% to 32%; reoperation rates for complications, 7% to 24%; patient satisfaction, 55% to 80%; mortality rates (4 to 6 weeks after surgery), 3% to 10.2%; and mean survival (months), 8% to 15.9%. This information should form the basis for what should be considered acceptable outcomes. Furthermore, certain facts that can influence the final outcomes may be considered prognostic factors (origin of tumor, visceral metastasis, number of affected vertebrae, and state of neurologic dysfunction). The combination of surgical outcomes and prognostic factors is important when considering the construction of clinical guidelines for management of metastatic spinal disease. The combination of the Tokuhashi prognostic scoring system, the Harrington structural and neurologic classification, the Tomita classification of spinal metastasis spread, and the Kostuik instability system form a reasonable and clinically easily applicable guideline system.

INTRODUCTION

It has been reported that in 5% to 10% of all cancer patients, during the course of their disease, spinal metastasis will develop (4,108). The spine is the most common site for skeletal metastasis (50). The original report by Jaffee (50) in 1958, claiming that the incidence of spinal metastasis is 70%, has not been substantiated. Other publications assert that spinal involvement ranges from 56% (82) to 30.6% (77) and 33.4% (21). The frequency of spinal metastasis from different types of cancer that were treated surgically is shown in Table 19.1. The data are gathered from a total of 22 articles (7,16,23,26,36,43,45,47,51,60,64,76,83,89,92–94,101,107,110,112) that include 1,517 patients. Obviously this information is skewed by the surgical selection and does not

TABLE 19.1 Origin of Metastatic Spinal Cancer (Data from 22 Reports, 1,517 pts)

Tumor	*N*	%	
Breast	295	19.4	I: Hosono N et al. (1995) Spine (47)
Lung	258	17.0	II: Sundaresan N et al. (1985) J Neurosurg (92)
Miscellaneous	108	7.1	III: Hatrick N et al. (2000) Radiother Oncol (43)
Renal	214	14.1	VI: Wise JJ et al. (1999) Spine (112)
Thyroid	69	4.5	V: Onimus M et al. (1996) Eur Spine J (76)
Unknown	90	5.9	VI: Weigel B et al. (1999) Spine (110)
Multiple myeloma	70	4.6	VII: Enkaoua E A et al. (1997) Spine (23)
Lymphoreticular system	28	1.8	VIII: Chataigner H et al. (2000) Eur Spine J (16)
Prostate	109	7.2	IX: Bilsky MH et al. (2000) Spine (7)
GI	85	5.6	X: Hertlein H et al. (1992) Eur Spine J (45)
Sarcomas	83	5.5	XI: Wai E K et al. (2003) Spine (107)
Chondrosarcoma	8	0.5	XII: Kocialkowski A et al. (1992) Eur Spine J (60)
+ Ewing + chordoma			XIII: Tomita T et al. (1994) Int Orthop (101)
Uterus + cervix	25	1.6	XIV: Gokaslan Z L et al. (1998) J Neurosurg (36)
Melanoma	13	0.9	XV: Sundaresan N et al. (1991) J Neurosurg (93)
Ovary	2	0.1	XVI: Sundaresan N et al. (1991) J Neurosurg (93)
Hepatobiliary	34	2.2	XVII: Sundaresan N et al. (2002) Spine (94)
Nasopharynlaryngeal	15	1.0	XVIII: Falicov A et al. (2006) Spine (26)
Genitourinary	9	0.6	XIX: Schoeggl A et al. (2002) Spinal Cord (83)
Pancreas	2	0.1	XX: Sioutos PJ et al. (1995) Cancer (89)
TOTAL	1,517	100	XXI: Lewandrowski K et al. (2004) Spine (64)
			XXII: Jansson K A et al (2006) Eur Spine (51)

depict the entire spectrum of spinal metastases. However, it illustrates the gravity of the condition that necessitated surgery. Less-biased statistics may derive from a pool of patients unselected for any particular treatment. Unfortunately, even in this situation, most patients' data are collected from symptomatic patients who underwent various treatments. Only research from extensive numbers of autopsies can indicate the true incidence of spinal metastasis, and even these are very few (Table 19.2) (21,77,78,99). Various reports suggest that in 10% to 25% of treated patients with preexisting spinal metastasis, spinal cord compression will develop (4,6,12,34,44,81,82,114). Some assert that metastatic disease of the spine, if left untreated, may eventually lead to paraplegia (35,37,67,79). Pain and neurologic deficit are the most dreadful complications of metastatic cancer of the spine. Intractable pain may become a horrific experience, and spinal cord compromise may lead to the devastating consequences of paraplegia. In this situation, surgery plays an important role. Several surgical options exist; however, their indications and outcomes must be scrutinized for better medical care.

INSTRUMENTS FOR OUTCOMES ASSESSMENT

In recent years, patient-outcome studies have been introduced to assess the results of treatment to provide patients, physicians, insurance providers, and government agencies with a tool with which to evaluate the different treatment methods. When assessing impaired body function caused by metastatic spinal tumors, health care providers should accumu-

TABLE 19.2 Origin of Metastatic Spinal Cancer

	Unselected Treatment[a]		Autopsy[b]	
Tumor	***N***	**%**	***N***	**%**
Lung	74	21.3	169	40.5
Breast	39	11.2	64	15.3
Kidney	24	6.9	2	0.5
Genitourinary	11	3.2	0	0.0
Liver	15	4.3	9	2.2
Prostate	34	9.8	31	7.4
Stomach	15	4.3	21	5.0
Rectum	10	2.9	5	1.2
GI	6	1.7	14	3.4
Thyroid	7	2.0	0	0.0
Uterus	6	1.7	8	1.9
Lymphoreticular	0	0.0	40	9.6
Colon	5	1.4	0	0.0
Melanoma	6	1.7	0	0.0
Head & neck	3	0.9	0	0.0
Osteosarcoma + Ewing	4	1.2	0	0.0
Unknown	42	12.1	6	1.4
Other	46	13.3	48	11.5
TOTAL	347	100	417	100

[a]Tokuhashi Y et al. (2005) Spine (99)
[a]Patchel RA et al. (2005) Lancet (78)
[b]Ortiz Gomez et al. (1995) Int Orthop (77)
[b]Drury RAB et al. (1964) J Clin Pathol (21)

late "reproducible objective data" that will form the basis for outcome studies. The objective is to measure how well the results approach the goals of treatment (i.e., restore function and control pain). Clinical examination alone cannot make this determination.

Psychometric instruments are practical tools for evaluating disability from metastatic cancer of the spine. The goals for grading the functional status of the patient should be based on pain assessment, profile of mood states, and overall performance status. The latter depends on the neurologic status, pain, and disability. Therefore a complete neurologic assessment is considered an integral part of the evaluation of patients with metastatic tumor to the spine. Although the neurologic assessment provides reliable and straightforward clinical documentation, the assessment of pain disability and bodily functional performance of the patient can be appreciated only through psychometric questionnaires. The latter should be simple and reproducible (39). Pain is an alarming consequence of metastatic cancer of the spine. Specific efforts should be made to avoid crude assessment and try to quantify and locate the pain. The McGill pain questionnaire is a sensitive tool. A visual analogue scale (VAS) for pain measurement combined with a pain diagram indicating the original site of pain and its spread is a very simple and reliable method for quantifying and depicting pain. The VAS, although a subjective assessment of pain, has been shown to be more reliable than other types of pain assessment (52).

Cancer patients are fraught with emotional and psychological problems. Because anxiety and depression have a direct correlation with pain intensity, these two factors may need to be addressed. The Zung anxiety scale (117) and the Hamilton Depression scale (40) are suitable instruments in this situation. The Memorial Pain Assessment Card (MPAC) (30) is a modified visual analogue with multidimensional characteristics, practically equivalent to a full assessment combining the McGill pain questionnaire, the Hamilton depression scale, and the Zung anxiety scale (17).

A distinction should be made between radicular pain and axial pain. Even the surgical approach may be responsible for severe pain. A report (36) detailing outcomes of pain demonstrated that in 72 patients who underwent an anterior approach through thoracotomy, 90% had postoperative pain (only 23% achieved complete resolution, 60% had significant improvement, and 8%, no change or worsening of thoracotomy pain). Quantification of pain is useful in monitoring the effectiveness of pain management, as well as in helping establish pain-control goals for the individual patient (17).

Pain and neurologic deficit contribute to disability of everyday activities. Therefore instruments to evaluate the quality of life should also be included when assessing patients with metastatic disease to the spine. As surgical procedures to treat metastatic disease to the spine have increased, a greater interest has been expressed in the overall quality-of-life assessment and outcomes studies. However, few published reports exist on the assessment of these patients' health-performance status after surgery. The treating physician should keep in mind that patients with spinal metastasis differ from noncancer patients or cancer patients undergoing potentially curative treatment (14), therefore limiting the sensitivity of these instruments to monitor changes (11,15). Instruments for assessing the patient's function and guidelines for treatment should be flexible and applicable to all sorts of cancer-treatment modalities available in the armamentarium of medicine, not only to evaluate the surgical aspects of tumor management but also to better compare the different treatments. A number of instruments are available to measure global quality of life in patients with cancer.

The Edmonton Symptom Assessment Scale (ESAS) is a validated patient-centered questionnaire designed specifically to address the overall quality of life in patients with terminal cancer (11,15,53). The questionnaire is multidimensional and measures nine domains (pain, tiredness, nausea, depression, anxiety, drowsiness, appetite, well-being, and shortness of breath). After surgery, the largest improvement is seen in the domain of pain (107).

The Townsend questionnaire is a physician-determined categories assessment of the patient's physical disability. Patients are classified into one of the four categories: (a) normal, pain-free function, (b) normal function with pain, (c) significantly limited function requiring some type of assistance (e.g., a walker, cane), and (d) nonfunctional (e.g., wheelchair bound, or bedridden) (104).

Other validated outcome measures in cancer patient are EORTC QLQ-C30 (27), HUI-MARK 3 (28), and EQ-5D (20). These have been successfully applied in cancer patients with metastases to the spine (26). The HUI-MARK 3 contains one question relating to pain and measures pain on a scale 1 to 5 (Table 19.3). Two studies (26,84) compared the VAS pain scale with HUI pain, demonstrating that on the VAS pain scale, 1 to 4 corresponds to mild pain, 5 to 6 to moderate pain, and 7 to 10 to severe pain.

The overall distribution of HUI-MARK 3 utility calculated quality-adjusted life years (QALY) during

TABLE 19.3 HUI-MARK 3

Description	Scale
• Free of pain and discomfort	1
• Mild to moderate pain	2
• Pain does not prevent activity	
• Moderate pain	3
• Pain prevents few activities	
• Moderate to severe	4
• Pain prevents some activities	
• Severe pain	5
• Pain prevents most activities	

the 1-year postoperative period (26). The QLQ-C30 measures quality of life and has one global health status (QL2), five functional scales, physical functions (PF2), role functions (RF2), emotional function (EF), cognitive functions (CF), and social functioning (SF), as well as nine symptom scales.

Performance status can be assessed by the Eastern Cooperative Oncology Group (ECOG) grading system or the Karnofsky performance status. The ECOG (Table 19.4) performance status (109) measures functional performance on a scale from 0 to 4 and is a good index of assessing the preoperative functional status (26).

The condition of the patient's health status can be detailed by using the Karnofsky performance status (PS) (54). The rating for the criteria of the PS is shown in Table 19.5. The score ranges from 0 to 100%. Scoring between 0 and 10% indicates poor health and total dependency on others, from 50% to 70%, inability to work and requires assistance, and 80% to 100%, ability to carry on with normal activities. This was successfully applied by Tokuhashi et al. (98) in clinical guidance for predicting cancer patient outcomes.

Functional outcomes for neurologic assessment can be graded by the Frankel (33) or the American Spinal Injury Association (ASIA) impairment scores (2). However, these systems are not specific enough to describe nuances of the physical state of locomotion.

TABLE 19.4 Eastern Cooperative Oncology Group (ECOG) Performance Status Measurement

Description of function
• Fully active. • Able to perform pre-disease activities. • No restrictions • Ambulatory and able to perform light work. • Restricted in physically strenuous activity. • Ambulatory and capable of all self-care. • Unable to perform work activities. • Bedridden less than 50% of the time. • Capable of only limited self-care. • Bedridden more than 50% of the time. • Completely disabled, not capable of any self-care. • Bedridden 100% of the time. • Dead

Oken MM et al. (1982) Am J Clin Oncol [75]

TABLE 19.5 Criteria of Karnofsky Performance Status (PS)

• Dead	0
• Moribund Fatal processes progressing rapidly	10%
• Very sick; hospitalization necessary Active support treatment necessary	20%
• Severely disabled; hospitalization is indicated, although death not imminent	30%
• Disabled Requires special medical care and assistance	40%
• Requires considerable assistance and frequent medical care	50%
• Requires occasional assistance, but is able to care for most needs	60%
• Cares for self Unable to carry on normal activity or to do active work	70%
• Normal activity with effort Some signs or symptoms of disease	80%
• Able to carry on normal activity Minor signs or symptoms of disease	90%
• Normal No complaints No evidence of disease	100%

Karnofsy DA. (1967) Gann Monograph (54).

Four other scales also address the state of ambulation (9,18,33,100). Therefore these Scales can be used as a complementary to ASIA or Frankel scales, such as combining the Cooper and the Frankel grading systems.

Oswestry disability questionnaire and SF-36 are simple tools designed to quantify disability originating from back pain and can have a practical application in this situation as well.

SURGICAL OUTCOMES

The following ten items are considered important for measuring outcomes after surgery, and therefore should be specifically evaluated: the overall neurologic status, ambulation, sphincter control, pain and suffering, survival rates, local recurrences, surgical complications including immediate postsurgery mortality rate, reoperation rates for complications, and overall patient satisfaction.

Furthermore, when managing spinal metastases, guidelines for the decision of the appropriate treatment should take into consideration the patient's anticipated survival period (Table 19.6), the advantages of surgery over other types of treatment, and particularly the benefits that may be expected from surgery.

TABLE 19.6 Overall Survival Rates after Surgery

3 month	50.0%	Kocialkowski A et al. (1992) Eur Spine J (60)
	76.0%	Wai EK et al. (2003) Spine (107)
6 month	58.8%	Klekamp J et al. (1998) Acta Neurochir (Wien) (58)
	72.0%	Rompe JD et al. (1999) Ach Orthop Trauma Surg (80)
	78.0%	Hosono N et al. (1995) Spine (47)
9 month	50.0%	Falicov A et al. (2006) Spine (26)
12 month	25.0%	Kocialkowski A et al. (1992) Eur Spine J (60)
	48.8%	Klekamp J et al. (1998) Acta Neurochir(Wien) (58)
	50.0%	Rompe J D et al. (1999) Ach Orthop Trauma Surg (80)
	65.0%	Villavicencio AT et al. (2005) Neurosurg Focus (106)
	62.0%	Gokalsan ZL et al. (1998) J Neurosurg (36)
19 month	4.7%	Rompe JD et al. (1999) Ach Orthop Trauma Surg (80)
60 month	19.5%	Klekamp J et al. (1998) Acta Neurochir (Wien) (58)
Median month	6.5	Schoeggl A et al. (2002) Spinal Cord (83)
	10	Sioutos PJ et al. (1995) Cancer (89)
	10.6	Hirabayashi H et al. (2003) Cancer (46)
	14	Lewandrowski KU et al. (2004) Spine (64)
	30	Sundaresan N et al. (2002) Spine (94)
Mean month	8	Chataigner H et al. (2000) Eur Spine J (16)
	8.5	Hertlein H et al. (1992) Eur Spine J (45)
	9	O'Neil J et al. (1988) Clin Orthop Relat Res (73)
	9	Livingston KE et al. (1978) J Neurosurg (65)
	11	Atanasiu JP et al. (1993) Spine (3)
	15.6	Ernstbergen et al. (2005) Acta Orthop Belg (25)
	13.1	Weigel B et al. (1999) Spine (110)
	15.9	Wise JJ et al. (1999) Spine (110)
	15.9	Cahill DW et al. (1999) J Neurosurg (13)
	12.0	Kocialkowski A et al. (1992) Eur Spine J (60)

TABLE 19.7 Overall Neurologic Improvement

55%	Kostuik J et al. (1993) Spine (63)
57%	Ernstbergens et al. (2005) Acta Orthop Belg (25)
58%	Weigel B et al. (1999) Spine (110)
60%	King GJ et al. (1991) Spine (56)
60%	Villavicencio AT et al. (2005) Neurosurg Focus (106)
63%	Rompe JD et al. (1999) Ach Orthop Trauma Surg (80)
64%	Atanasiu JP et al. (1993) Spine (3)
68%	O'Neil J et al. (1988) Clin Orthop Relat Res (73)
68%	Harrington KD (1986) J Bone Joint Surg (Am) (42)
69%	Hatrick N et al. (2000) Radiother Oncol (43)
73%	Tomita T et al. (1994) Int Orthop (101)
74%	Hammerberg KW (1992) Spine (41)
76%	Bauer HCF (1997) J Bone Joint Surg (Am) (5)
76%	Gokalsan ZL et al. (1998) J Neurosurg (36)
79%	Onimus M et al. (1996) Eur Spine J (76)
81%	Hosono N et al. (1995) Spine (47)
88%	King GJ et al. (1991) Spine (56)
88%	Hertlein H et al. (1992) Eur Spine J (45)
87%	Shimizu K et al. (1992) Spine (85)

More specifically, the anticipated improvements after surgery are for overall neurologic deficit, 55% to 87% (Table 19.7); for restoration of sphincter control, 36% to 89% (Table 19.8); for pain relief; 47% to 100% (Table 19.9); and for restoration of ambulation, 40% to 100% (Table 19.10; data combining results from anterior and posterior decompression). Apparently restoration of ambulation after posterior decompression alone fares worse. Other outcomes such as complication rates, including 4- to 6-week mortality rates after surgery and reoperation rates for complications and local recurrences after surgery, are listed in Tables 19.11, 19.12, 19.13, and 19.14. Local tumor recurrence is more likely in patients with certain tumors and particularly in those resistant to chemotherapy and radiation therapy, such as renal cell carcinoma. In this instance, the recurrence was reported as high as 40% to 50% (16,47,56,110). The overall patient satisfaction was rated in the range of 55% to 80% (72,110).

In our series of 70 patients, the complication rate was 25%, including two deaths. In one case, surgery was aborted, while in progress, because of massive intraoperative bleeding, despite preoperative transarterial embolization of the region (69). Other complications were profuse bleeding in nine patients, infections in three patients, wound dehiscence in three patients, and incomplete surgery in three patients.

TABLE 19.8 Restoration of Sphincter Control

36%	King G J et al. (1991) Spine (56)
43%	Kocialkowski A et al. (1992) Eur Spine J (60)
47%	Kostuik J et al. (1993) Spine (63)
51%	Sinardet D et al. (2000) Neurochirurgie (88)
77%	Tomita T et al. (1994) Int Orthop (101)
89%	Klekamp J et al. (1998) Acta Neurochir (Wien) (58)

TABLE 19.9 Pain Relief

47%	Sinardet D et al. (2000) Neurochirurgie (88)
71%	Touboul E et al. (1986) Sem Hôp Paris (103)
77%	Hirabayashi H et al. (2003) Cancer (46)
79%	Kocialkowski A et al. (1992) Eur Spine J (60)
81%	Kostuik J et al. (1993) Spine (63)
85%	Sundaresan N et al. (1985) J Neurosurg (92)
85%	Ernstberger T et al. (2005) Acta Orthop Belg (25)
85%	Villavicencio AT et al. (2005) Neurosurg Focus (106)
88%	King GJ et al. (1991) Spine (56)
89%	Weigel B et al (1999) Spine (110)
90%	Hatrick N et al. (2000) Radiother Oncol (43)
91%	Hammerberg KW (1992) Spine (41)
92%	Gokalsan ZL et al. (1998) J Neurosurg (36)
92%	Hertlein H et al. (1992) Eur Spine J (45)
94%	Harrington KD (1986) J Bone Joint Surg (Am) (42)
94%	O'Neil J et al. (1988) Clin Orthop Relat Res (73)
94%	Hosono N et al. (1995) Spine (47)
95%	Atanasiu JP et al. (1993) Spine (3)
95%	Tomita T et al. (1994) Int Orthop (101)
100%	Shimizu K et al. (1992) Spine (85)
100%	Bilsky HM et al. (2000) Spine (7)

TABLE 19.10 Restoration of Ambulation from Anterior and Posterior Approaches

40%	Livingstone KE et al. (1978) J Neurosurg (65)
44%	Kostuik J et al. (1993) Spine (63)
51%	Gokalsan ZL et al. (1998) J Neurosurg (36)
52%	Sinardet D et al. (2000) Neurochirurgie (88)
60%	Tomita T et al. (1994) Int Orthop (101)
62%	Patchel RA et al. (2005) Lancet (78)
64%	Hosono N et al. (1995) Spine (47)
64%	King GJ et al. (1991) Spine (56)
70%	Weigel B et al. (1999) Spine (110)
70%	Onimus M et al. (1996) Eur Spine J (76)
76%	Hammerberg KW (1992) Spine (41)
78%	Hatrick NC et al. (2000) Radiother Oncol (43)
80%	Siegel T et al. (1985) Neurosurgery (86)
82%	O'Neil J et al. (1988) Clin Orthop Relat Res (73)
100%	Villavicencio AT et al. (2005) Neurosurg Focus (106)
100%	Sundaresan N et al. (1985) J Neurosurg (92) (1991) Neurosurgery (93)
	Restoration of Ambulation after Laminectomy alone
23%	Klekamp J et al. (1998) Acta Neurochir (Wien) (58)
23%	Kennady JC et al. (1962) Am J Surg (55)
33%	Schoeggl A et al (2002) Spinal Cord (84)
35%	Wright RL (1963) Ann Surg (116)
36%	White WA (1971) Cancer (113)
47%	Siegel T et al. (1985) Neurosurgery (86)

TABLE 19.11 Complication Rates

12%	Bilsky MH et al. (2000) Spine (7)
12%	Wai EK et al. (2003) Spine (107)
16%	Hosono N et al. (1995) Spine (47)
19%	Weigel B et al. (1999) Spine (110)
20%	Jansson KA et al. (2006) Eur Spine J (51)
25%	Wise JJ et al. (1999) Spine (112)
23%	Review of 24 surgical reports: Klimo P Jr et al. (2005) Neuro-oncol (59)
29%	Falicov A et al. (2006) Spine (26)
32%	Gokalsan ZL et al. (1998) J Neurosurg (36)

TABLE 19.12 Postsurgery Mortality Rates (4 to 6 wk)

3.0%	Gokalsan ZL et al (1998) J Neurosurg (36)
6.3%	Klimo P Jr et al. (2005) Neuro-oncol (59)
6.0%	Wise JJ et al (1999) Spine (112)
6.0%	Siegal TJ et al. (1985) J Bone Joint Surg (Am) (87)
7.0%	Weigel B et al. (1999) Spine (110)
8.0%	Sundaresan N et al. (1991) Neurosurgery (93)
8.0%	Harrington KD (1986) J Bone Joint Surg (Am) (42)
9.0%	Sinardet D et al. (2000) Neurochirurgie (88)
11.0%	Sioutos PJ et al. (1995) Cancer (89)
10.0%	Turner PL et al. (1988) J Bone Joint Surg (Br) (105)
10.0%	Hertlein H et al. (1992) Eur Spine J (45)
10.2%	Chataigner H et al. (2000) Eur Spine J (16)
12.0%	Bilsky HM et al. (2000) Spine (7)
13.0%	Jansson KA et al. (2006) Eur Spine J (51)
16.0%	Kocialkowski A et al. (1992) Eur Spine J (60)
18.0%	Fidler MW (1986) J Bone Joint Surg (Br) (29)

TABLE 19.13 Reoperation Rates for Complications or Local recurrences

7.0%	Weigel B et al. (1999) Spine (110)
10.2%	Jansson KA et al. (2006) Eur Spine J (51)
12.1%	Hertlein H et al. (1992) Eur Spine J (45)
24.0%	Bauer HCF. (1997) J Bone Joint Surg (Am) (5)
15.8%	Chataigner H et al. (2000) Eur Spine J (16)
56.2%	King GJ et al. (1991) Spine (56)

TABLE 19.14 Local Recurrences after Surgery

3.5%	Falicov A et al. (2006) Spine (26)
8.0%	Review of 9 surgical reports: Klimo P Jr et al. (2005) Neuro-oncol (59) 1. Bilsky MH et al. (2000) Spine (7) 2. Fourney DR et al. (2001) J Neurosurg (31) 3. Hammerberg KW (1992) Spine (41) 4. Hosono N et al. (1995) Spine (47) 5. King G J et al. (1991) Spine (56) 6. Muhlbauer M et al. (2000) Acta Neurochir (Wien) (68) 7. Siegal T et al. J Bone Joint Surg (Am) (87) 8. Weigel B et al. (1999) Spine (110)
8.4%	Chataigner H et al. (2000) Eur Spine J (16)
11.0%	Nazarian S (1997) Rev Chir Orthop Reparatrice Appar Mot (71)
12.1%	King G J et al. (1991) Spine (56)
21.0%	Hirabayashi H et al. (2003) Cancer (46)
22.0%	Weigel B et al. (1999) Spine (110)
31.6%	Bridwell KH et al. (1988) Spine (10) (after laminectomy)
32.0%	Sundaresan N et al. (2002) Spine (94)
49.0%	Hertlein H et al. (1992) Eur Spine J (45)

PROGNOSTIC FACTORS

Conventional wisdom dictates that to construct reasonable guidelines for managing metastatic tumors of the spine, it is important to understand what constitutes prognostic factors and what the reported results are after surgery. These data would form the basis for what should be considered acceptable outcomes.

It has been observed that certain factors, irrespective of treatment selection, may influence the prognosis when malignant tumors develop spinal metastases.

The original claim that the histopathology of the tumor had no bearing on the ultimate prognosis (57) has not been duplicated by others (see Table 19.1). Several authors concluded that the origin of the primary tumors can influence the ultimate prognosis (Table 19.15). In general, metastatic spinal tumors from unknown adenocarcinoma, stomach, esophagus, pancreas, and lungs, portend the worse possible prognosis, and carcinoid, thyroid, breast, prostate, and myeloma carry the best prognosis. Distinction should also be made between the different types of lung cancer (74). In general, non–small cell lung cancer (NSCLC) patients with spinal metastases had survival rates of 37.1%, 14.6%, and 2.1% at follow-up of 6 months, 1 year, and 2 years, respectively. The median survival time was 4.5 months, and the mean, 6.2 months. However, for small cell lung cancer (SCLC), the corresponding survival rates were 36.8%, 5.3% and 0% at 6 months, 1 year, and 2 years' follow-up respectively. In both NSCLC and SCLC with spinal metastases, the presence of hypercalcemia or hypoalbuminemia was indicative of a gloomy prognosis, with a survival period of less than 3 months (74).

The aggressiveness of cancer can also be classified as slow growth (breast, thyroid, prostate), moderate growth (kidney, uterus), and rapid growth (lung, stomach, liver, colon, unknown) (23,46,97,99,102).

The survival with visceral metastasis was also observed by Tokuhashi et al. (99) and Tomita et al. (102). The average survival with no visceral metastases was 36.8 months

TABLE 19.15 Survival Period (mo)

	Mean							Median					
Histopathology	I	II	III	IV	V	VI	VII	VIII	IX	X	XI	XII	XIII
Carcinoid	30.0												
Thyroid	25.6					21.0				25.5		51.1	25.5
Breast	18.6	8.9	4.5					21.2	10.5 (13)	18.6	36	21.3	21.2
Prostate	17.9	10.1	6.6					7.3		20.1			20.1
Rectum	17.7									15.2			15.7
Kidney	9.8	6.8		8.0		13.0		13.1	11	8.8	36	34.2	8.8
Uterus	8.7		11.0					7.4	6				
Miscellaneous	6.7		7.0							7.0			
Liver	6.5									8.7			8.7
Gallbladder	6.1												
Unknown	6.0				2.5						15		
Lung	5.2	2.8	7.1				6.0		6.0	4.5		9.9	2.1
Sarcoma	4.5										27	10.9	
Stomach	2.8												
Bladder	2.5												
Esophagus	2.0												4.5
Pancreas	1.5									5.7			5.7
Myeloma		33	5					35.2	13	44.4		54.2	44.4
Colon												12.9	
GI			2					8.1	4	2.1	12	15	2.1
Melanoma			9					1.5					
Lymphoma			9										
Other								8			30		

I. Tokuhashi Y et al. (2005) Spine (99)
II. Kocialkowski A et al. (1992) Eur Spine J (60)
III. Wai EK et al. (2003) Spine (107)
IV. King GJ et al. (1991) Spine (56)
V. Saengnipanthkul S et al. (1992) Spine (81)
VI. Enkaoua EA et al. (1997) Spine (23)
VII. Ogihara S et al. (2006) Spine (74)
VIII. Weigel B et al. (1999) Spine (110)
IX. Sioutos PJ et al. (1995) Cancer (89)
X. Hirabayashi H et al. (2003) Cancer (46)
XI. Sundaresan N et al. (2002) Spine (94)
XII. Hosono N et al. (2005) Clin Orthop Relat Res (48)
XIII. Weigel B et al (1999) Spine (110)

(range, 5 to 84 months), treatable visceral metastases, 16.5 months (4 to 31 months), and untreatable visceral metastases, 8.9 months (range, 1 to 24 months).

The influence of an extraskeletal metastatic lesion on the survival rate is also in agreement with Weigel et al. (110), who demonstrated that a patient's survival period without extraskeletal metastases at surgery was significantly longer than with extraskeletal metastases (23.5 months vs. 5.8 months; $p < 0.0001$).

The location of the metastatic lesion was also implicated as a survival factor. Atanasiu et al. (3) reported that lesions in the upper cervical spine had an adverse effect on life expectancy, with average survival of 1.8 months; however, this was challenged by Klekamp et al. (58), who found no differences in prognosis between the upper and lower spine.

The number of affected vertebrae demonstrated an influence on survival. Patients with single level involvement (average survival, 12.9 months) had a better survival rate than did patients with multiple-level involvement (average, 7.9 months) (73,89,102). This was also confirmed by others who reported gloomy prognoses for multiple-level involvement, even after effective surgical treatment (85).

Neurologic dysfunction was observed to be associated with the survival time. Some believe that ambulatory patients survive longer than nonambulatory patients with sphincter incontinence (56,89). The state of sphincter incontinence as a bad prognostic sign is also emphasized by some (70). The rate of neurologic deterioration was related to prognosis; slow progression had a good prognosis as opposed to rapid progression, which had dismal results. The latter was compounded when the onset of treatment was delayed (42,70). However, the notion of preoperative intact neurologic status (ambulatory vs. nonambulatory) as a predictor of longer survival was challenged by others (90,110).

Likewise, timing for adjunctive radiation treatment (preoperative radiation vs. postoperative radiation) was also questioned as a significant prognostic predictor for outcomes (92). Weigel (110) and Hirabayashi (46) emphasized that postoperative ambulation definitely has a positive prognostic influence on survival, rather than preoperative ambulation.

Weigel et al. (110) also reported that the patient's age can be considered as a prognostic factor for survival, because patients younger than 60 years survived significantly longer than older patients (20.1 months vs. 6.2 months; $p = 0.028$). The age as a prognostic factor has not been incorporated into the Tokuhashi scoring system and deserves to be duplicated by others. A report indicates that when more than two of the "prognostic factors" are present, they have a compounding adverse effect on survival (89). For example, lung cancer, neurologic deficit, and involvement of multiple vertebrae in the same patient would have a greater adverse effect on survival than the combined effect of the same type of lung cancer involving a single vertebra and without neurologic deficit.

One should take into consideration that when estimating survival, invariably, most of the data from different reports were based on metastatic tumor of the spine that became symptomatic.

Clinical practice in surgical results and prognostic factors of metastatic spinal tumors have not undergone adequate scrutiny. The surgical information provided in this article must be available and known to everyone concerned with spinal tumors (physicians, patients, insurance, etc.) to form the basis of what should be considered acceptable surgical outcomes. Inferior results, therefore, are not acceptable, and well-designed guidelines should strive to achieve the best possible outcomes.

SURGICAL GUIDELINES

The rationale of guidelines is to achieve better treatment outcomes than would have been achieved otherwise. Their scientific strength depends on how well evidence-based knowledge is used (115). It is reasonable to assume that consensus-based guidelines supported by available evidence are more convincing than individual ones. Unfortunately, no such reported guidelines are available for the management of metastatic spinal tumors. Certain published guidelines are based on individual experiences without enough clinical evidence to support their effectiveness. These guidelines do not cover an integrated approach for the management of metastatic spinal tumors but are concerned with different aspects of the problem.

In 1990, Tokuhashi et al. (98) published a guideline-scoring system for the preoperative evaluation of metastatic spine tumor based on the general condition of the patient, as graded by the Karnofsky performance status and five of the aforementioned prognostic factors: (a) the number of extraspinal bone metastases, (b) the number of metastases in the vertebral body, (c) metastases to the major internal organs (lungs, liver, kidneys, and brain), (d) the primary site of the cancer, and (e) the severity of spinal cord palsy. Each parameter has a score ranging from 0 to 2 points. The maximum score that can be obtained is 12. The final score is related to the patient's prognosis: the higher the score, the better the prognosis. The authors advocate that excisional surgery should be performed on the patients who score above 9 points, and palliative surgery, on those who score less than 5 points. The patients who score between 5 and 9 points fall into a gray area.

Table 19.16 demonstrates the Tokuhashi prognostic scoring system for preoperative evaluation of the metastatic spinal lesions. The general condition is based on the Karnofsky performance status (PS) (54). The rating to determine the preoperative health status is as follows: the score is 0 for poor condition (*p* values, 10% to 40%); 1 for moderate (50% to 70%), and 2 for good (80% to 100%). For extraspinal bone metastatic foci more than three, the score is 0; between one and two metastatic foci, the score is 1; and for nonmetastatic lesions, 0. For the number of metastases in the spine, the score is 0 for more than three vertebral metastases; 1, for one or two metastases; and 2, for no more than one vertebra. For metastasis to a major internal organ, which indicates feasibility for concurrent resectability with the spinal tumor, the score is: 0 for unremovable lesions; 1 for removable lesions, and 3 for no metastases. For the primary site of the cancer, the score is: 0 when the expected survival is less than 3 months (lung amd stomach); 1 for expected survival rate of 3 to 12 months (kidney, liver, uterus,

TABLE 19.16 Tokuhashi System for Preoperative Evaluation of Metastatic Spine Tumors

Parameters	Score
General condition (performance status)	0, 1, 2
> Extraspinal bone metastatic foci	0, 1, 2
> No. of metastases in the spine (vertebrae)	0, 1, 2
> Metastasis to major internal	0, 1, 2
> Primary site of the cancer (Histopathology)	0, 1, 2
> Spinal cord Palsy	0, 1, 2

Indications for Type of Surgery

Indications	Score
Excisional Surgery	>9
Palliative Surgery	<5

Tokuhashi Y et al. (1990) Spine (98).

others, unidentified), and 2 for expected survival rate of more than 12 months (thyroid, prostate, breast, rectum). Finally, the severity of spinal cord palsy was rated as 0, 1, and 2 for Frankel grades A and B (complete paraplegia); Frankel C and D (incomplete paraplegia), and Frankel E (none) respectively.

In 1997, Tokuhashi et al. (99) reported that the reliability for predicting the prognosis was 63.3%, tested in 128 patients with metastatic spinal tumors.

The Tokuhashi scoring system was tested by Enkaoua et al. (23) for three types of metastatic tumors: renal cell carcinoma, thyroid cancer, and unknown primary cancer. The median survival period was 5.3 months for a score of 7 or less and 23.6 months for a score of 8 or more. The authors concluded that for a cancer of unknown primary site, the score should be zero, because the prognosis is invariably gloomy.

Subsequently, Tokuhashi et al. (99) revised the original scoring system to improve its accuracy by providing more-detailed prognostic value based on the origin of primary tumor. The score was modified to range between 0 and 5 points. The score was designated as 0 for metastases originating in the lungs, osteosarcoma, stomach, bladder, esophagus, or pancreas; 1 for metastases from the liver, gallbladder, and unidentified sources; 2 for other sites; 3, from kidney or uterus; 4, from rectum; 5, from thyroid, breast, prostate, or carcinoid tumor. Therefore in the revised system, a total of 15 scores can be obtained. In the patients with a total score of less than 8 or multiple vertebral metastases, the authors indicate conservative or palliative procedure (predicted survival period is less than 6 months), whereas they advocate excisional procedure when the score is 12 or more (predicted survival period, 1 year or more) and for score between 9 and 11 (predicted survival period, 6 months or more) and with metastases in a single vertebra. The consistency rate between the criteria for predicted prognosis and the actual survival period was high in patients within each score range (0 to 8, 9 to 11, 12 to 15), 86.4% in 118 patients evaluated prospectively after 1998, and 82.5% in all 246 patients evaluated retrospectively.

No reports exist in the literature indicating that the actual value of each scoring point (0, 1, and 2) in each factor has been analyzed statistically.

Ogihara et al. (74) reported that the Tokuhashi preoperative scoring system for patients with lung cancer did not correlate with the survival period. The authors found that only a performance status ECOG (PS) (Table 19.4) (75) which is similar to the Karnofsky test was correlated with the survival rate. However, this test was predictive only when applied postoperatively. The average survival rate of patients with postoperative PS 0 to 2 was 13.9 months, whereas that of patients with postoperative PS 3 or 4 was 2.0 months.

By using the Karnofsky performance index, Weigel et al. (110) found that postoperatively, the general state of health was 55%, a state of health that lies halfway between total dependency (50%) and partial dependency on others (60%). No one achieved 100%. Best scores were achieved with breast tumors (80% on the index), the second best results were seen in renal cell carcinoma patients, with 30% of the patients scoring 80% to 90%, and the poorest scores were seen in patients with melanoma (mean index, 48%), tumors of other sites (43%), and lungs (38%).

Chantaigner et al. (16) asserted that when deciding for a surgical option, in nonneurologic patients, the Karnofsky performance status alone was more effective than the Tokuhashi score, which also included the Karnofsky performance status.

Some of the authors are more selective than others and apply more vigorous selection of indications in their inclusion criteria for surgery. Therefore the overall survival period after surgery is not accurate. In some series, surgery is not indicated when the

TABLE 19.17 Harrington Classification Based on Structural Defect and Neurologic Deficit

Class	Neurologic Status	Structural Changes
I	Not significant	No vertebral collapse
II	Not significant	Vertebral involvement without collapse or instability (lytic or blastic lesion)
III	Major (sensory or motor)	No significant bone destruction or instability (lytic tumor)
IV	Not significant	Mechanical pain from vertebral collapse ± instability
V	Major	Retropulsion of hard discovertebral elements ± kyphotic deformity

estimated survival rate is 3 months, whereas in others, the criterion for surgery is longer than 6 months. This explains the longer survival rates with different cancer patients and particularly in lung cancer (6 to 12 months) in some reports (41,91).

Harrington (42) put forward a classification system based on bone destruction and neurologic involvement. He distinguished five classes of spinal metastatic lesions (see Table 19.17) and suggested nonsurgical treatment for class I and II, surgical intervention for class IV and V lesions, and for class III, which lies in the gray zone, treatment depends on various circumstances. This is a practical guideline system for managing metastatic tumors to the spine, but it does not make provisions for the choice of surgery from the vast armamentarium of surgical techniques, nor does it discuss the merit of each surgical intervention. In addition, this system does not take into account the biology of the origin of tumor, the radiosensitivity of the lesion, and the performance status of the patient. The applicability of the Harrington classification system for selecting the appropriate treatment in metastatic cancer of the spine was also reported by others (112).

Harrington (42) alluded to instability as one of the deciding factors for surgical stabilization. It is reasonable to assume that vertebral instability caused by bone destruction would provoke pain. However, he has not determined what constitutes instability in destructive metastatic lesions.

Kostuik et al. (61,62) devised a vertebral-body stability model by dividing the vertebral body into six segments. More specifically, the vertebral body is divided into an anterior column consisting of the vertebral body and a posterior column consisting of the pedicles, laminae, and spinous processes. The anterior column is further subdivided into four segments: anterior right, anterior left, middle right, and middle left. The posterior column is also subdivided into right and left segments. If no more that one or two of the six segments are destroyed, the spine is considered stable. If three or four of the segments are destroyed, the spine is considered probably unstable, and if five or six segments are affected, the spine is considered markedly unstable.

Although this has not been biomechanically tested or clinically substantiated, it may have potential applications when describing instability in the Harrington classification.

According to Taneichi et al. (96) impending collapse is indicated when either a greater that 50% to 60% destruction of the vertebral body or 25% to 30% destruction of the vertebral structure is present when an associated destruction of the costovertebral junction in thoracic spine is found, or when the destruction in the thoracolumbar spine anteriorly is 35% to 40% or 20% to 25% involves the posterior elements.

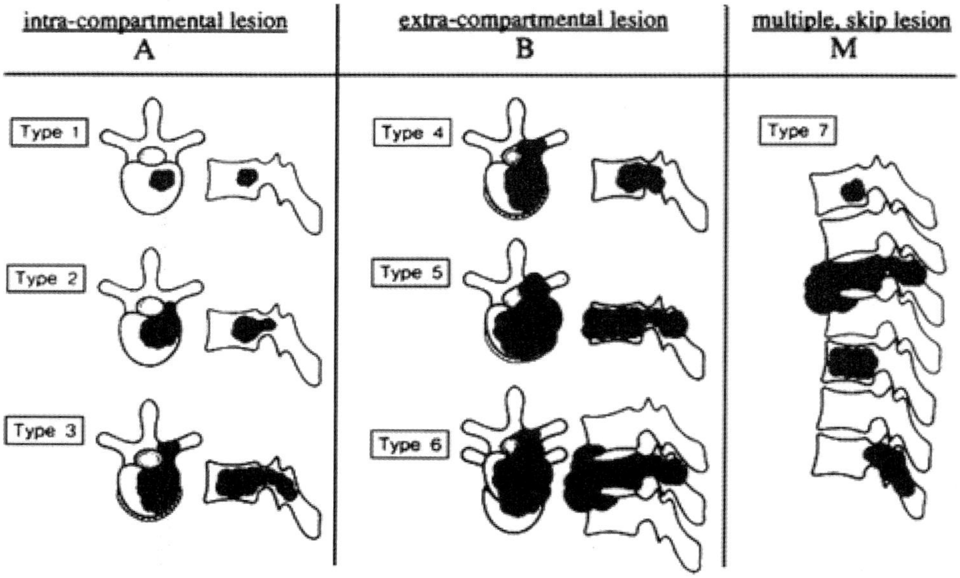

FIGURE 19.1 Tomita classification based on vertebral spread of metastasis. (Tomita K et al. Intern Orthop,1994)

Bridwell et al. (10) are of the opinion that, if less than 50% of vertebral body has been resected, vertebral body reconstruction may not be necessary.

Tomita K et al. (101), based on Enneking's grading of skeletal resection (24), Denis's three-column classification of fracture of the spine (19), and Weinstein's zone classification (111) (intraosseous, extraosseous, and distant spread) proposed a classification consisting of seven types of lesions (Fig. 19.1). This seems a reasonable classification for allowing the surgeon to choose the extent of surgical intervention, such as radical excision versus stabilization alone.

The most recent topographic classification system reported by Boriani, Weinstein, and Biagnini (8) provides an excellent guideline for surgical excision of primary tumors of the spine and therefore is not applicable for metastatic tumors.

A system that would encompass all these criteria would form a more comprehensive approach for the management of metastatic spinal malignancies. For this reason, we constructed a guideline system combining the Harrington's classification (neurologic status and structural changes), Tokuhashi's prognostic scoring system, Tomita's spread of spinal metastasis, and Kostuik's instability model (Table 19.18). The system starts by evaluating the neurologic deficit (Frankel grading, Cooper ambulation), the Karnofsky performance status, and vertebral body structural changes according to a modified Harrington classification. For class I and II without significant neurologic involvement and without vertebral collapse, the management is nonsurgical and consists of chemotherapy, hormonal manipulation, and radiation therapy (Fig. 19.2) (42). However, the treatment is contingent on the origin of the metastatic tumor. For example, in renal cell carcinoma, which is resistant to radiation therapy and chemotherapy, radical excision is indicated (Fig. 19.3) even in class I. For class II tumors, as in the case of multiple myeloma or small lytic metastatic lesion (Fig. 19.4), considerable and immediate relief of pain can be obtained by combining of chemotherapy and cement-augmentation procedure (vertebroplasty or balloon kyphoplasty).

TABLE 19.18 Treatment Guidelines

Class I		CHEMOTHERAPY OR HORMONAL TX OR RADIATION
Class II		CHEMOTHERAPY OR HORMONAL TX OR RADIATION
		± CEMENT AUGMENTATION (for lytic lesions)
Class III		RADIATION ± CEMENT AUGMENTATION
Class IV	SURGERY / TOKUHASHI	<5 → CONSERVATIVE TX OR PALLIATIVE STABILIZATION SURGERY (Stabilization ± Augmentation) >9 → RADICAL EXCISION + RECONSTRUCTION
Class V	SURGERY / TOKUHASHI	<5 → DECOMPRESSION + STABILIZATION >9 → RADICAL EXCISION + RECONSTRUCTION
Class VI or V	SURGERY / TOKUHASHI	>9 + TOMITA M → RADICAL EXCISION + RECONSTRUCTION ± AUGMENTATION

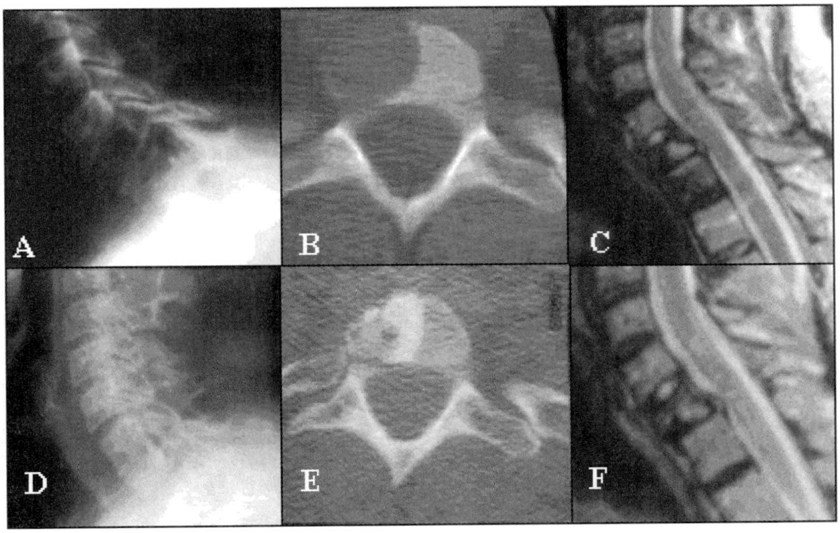

FIGURE 19.2 Metastatic lytic breast cancer in the cervical spine, with restricted daily living activities. Radiograph **(A)**, axial CT **(B)**, and sagittal MRI **(C)** before treatment. Radiograph **(D)**, axial CT **(E)**, and sagittal MRI **(F)** after radiation combined with chemotherapy and hormonal therapy. Complete restoration of daily activities was achieved.

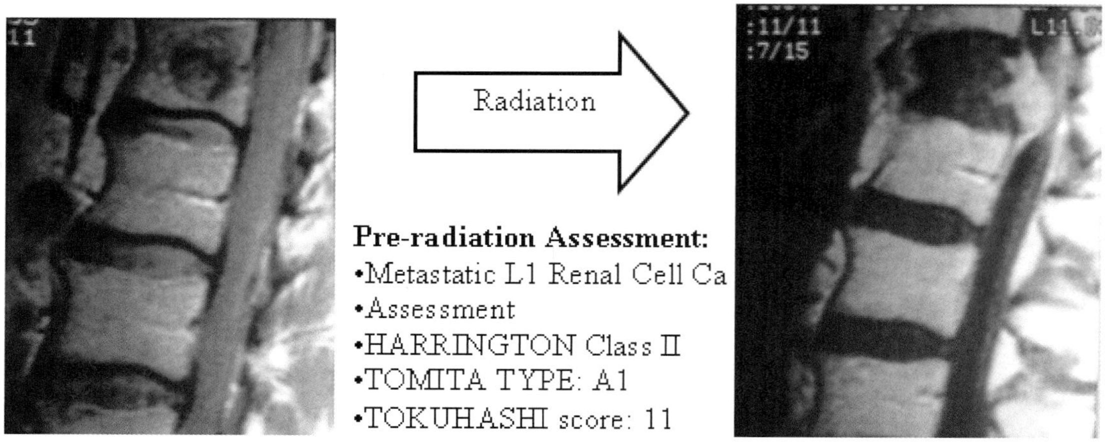

FIGURE 19.3 Ineffectiveness of radiation for renal cell carcinoma, which is notoriously radioresistant. A serious neurologic deficit developed.

For category III lesions, with neurologic deficit in the absence of major destruction of bone or spinal instability, surgery should not be entertained unless the tumor is radioresistant or unresponsive to chemotherapy (Fig. 19.5) (42).

For class IV and V, surgery is the treatment of choice. The Tokuhashi scoring system is valuable for estimating the prognosis and making decisions for the type of surgery. We incorporate into the decision making also the local spread of tumor, as suggested by Tomita. For Harrington class IV, consisting of mechanical pain caused by vertebral collapse and/or instability, with a Tokuhashi score of less than 5 with the old system, or 8 with the revised system, the indications for treatment would be either conservative treatment or palliative surgery, consisting of stabilization and/or cement augmentation (Figs. 19.6 and 19.7). For a Harrington class IV or V, a Tokuhashi score greater than 9 (old system) or 12 (revised system) and a Tomita B IV score (widespread metastases), local radical excision, if feasible combined with stabilization, is indicated (Fig. 19.8). When the score lies in the gray zone of 5 and 9 (estimated survival, 6

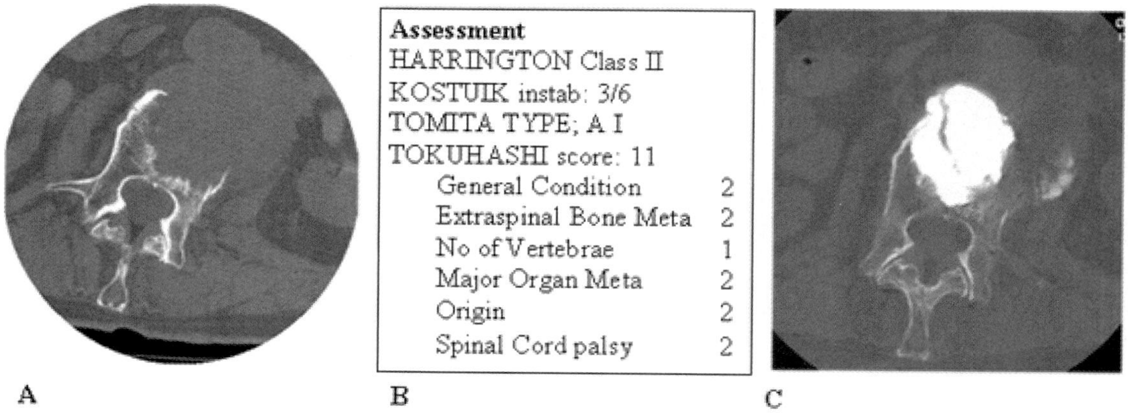

FIGURE 19.4 A lytic metastasis lesion from cancer of the breast causing severe back pain **(A)**. Preoperation clinical assessment before treatment **(B)**. Successful treatment with vertebroplasty **(C)**.

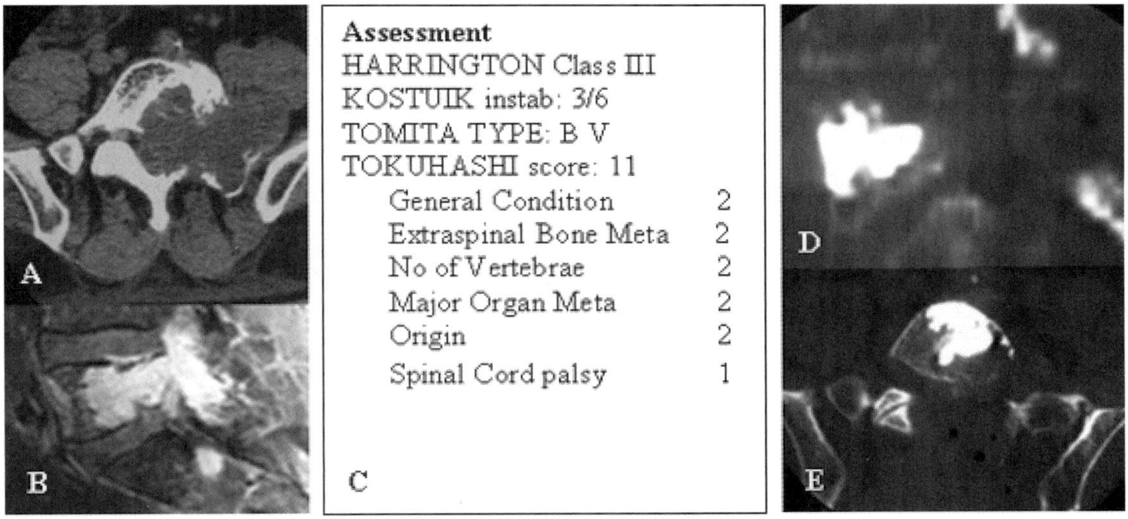

FIGURE 19.5 A 63-year-old man with intractable back pain and radiculopathy resistant to radioiodine and external beam radiation **(A)**. Axial MRI imaging and **(B)** sagittal enhanced gadolinium images revealing vascular metastatic thyroid cancer. Clinical assessment before treatment **(C)**. The patient underwent successful decompression, laminectomy, and kyphoplasty with immediate relief of back and leg pain. Postoperative sagittal **(D)** and axial **(E)** CT images. Outcome: survival longer than 5 years.

months), conservative or surgical treatments may be used, depending on several factors, to which we alluded earlier, that may influence the decision. For class V, characterized by intrusion of hard discovertebral elements into the spinal canal, compromising the spinal cord, the choice is only surgical. Spinal kyphotic deformity with cord compromise should be categorized as class V. In this situation, radiation has no logical place, and surgery would be the treatment of choice.

We also used the Kostuik instability rating as depicted on an axial CT scan as a descriptive documentation of the vertebral destruction by the tumor.

In a series of 75 patients, treated at the University Hospital in Crete, Greece, the effectiveness of the Tokuhashi prognostic scoring system combined with modified

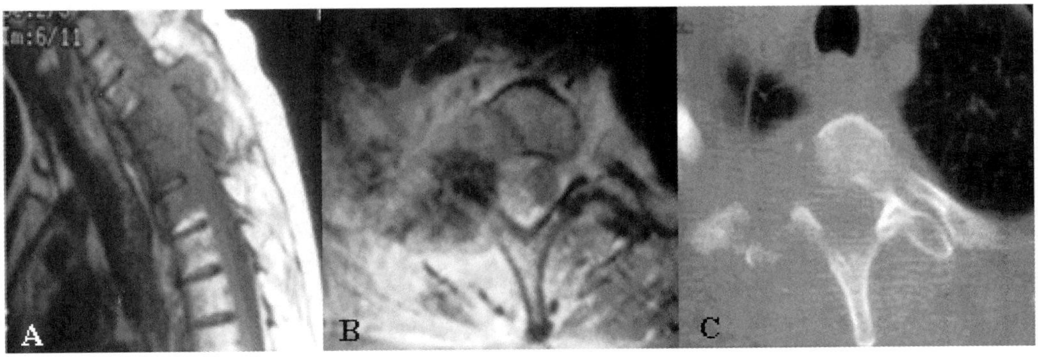

FIGURE 19.6 Metastatic cancer of the breast with spinal cord compression, as seen on sagittal MRI **(A)**, axial MRI **(B)**, and axial CT scan **(C)**.

Assessment
HARRINGTON Class V
KOSTUIK instab: 1/6
TOMITA TYPE: M V II
TOKUHASHI score: 7

General Condition	1
Extraspinal Bone Meta	2
No of Vertebrae	0
Major Organ Meta	2
Origin	2
Spinal Cord palsy	0

A

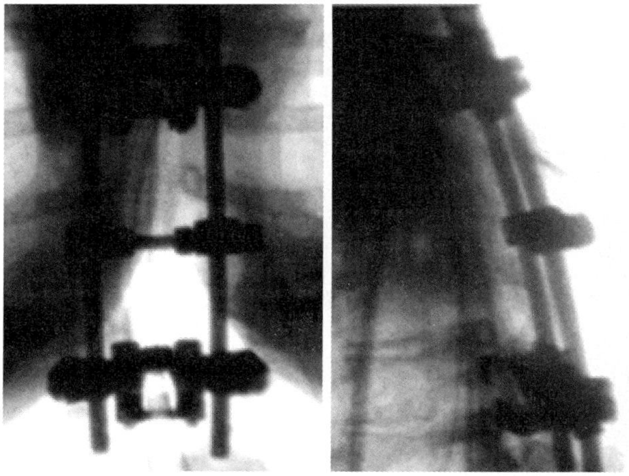

B C

FIGURE 19.7 Preoperative clinical assessment **(A)**. Postoperative AP **(B)** and lateral **(C)** radiographs. Outcome: Ambulation was restored with a survival rate of 12 months after posterior decompression and stabilization.

Harrington and Tomita classifications for selecting the appropriate surgery, had a predictive outcome (when patients in the gray zone were excluded) of 79.3% (50 of 63) and failure rate of 20.6% (13 of 63). In the gray zone, the favorable results (longevity greater than 9 months) were 60% (six of ten), and unfavorable, 40% (four of ten).

The scope of this article is not to compare the effectiveness of treatments between radiation therapy and surgery. However, we briefly touch this subject. In a meta-analysis

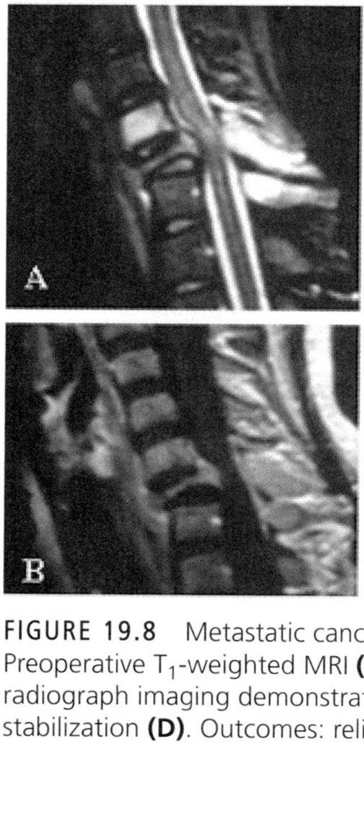

Assessment
HARRINGTON Class: IV
KUSTUIK stability : 6/6
TOMITA TYPE : B VI
TOKUHASHI score : 12

General Condition	2
Extraspinal Bone Meta	2
No of Vertebrae	2
Major Organ Meta	2
Origin	2
Spinal Cord palsy	2

C

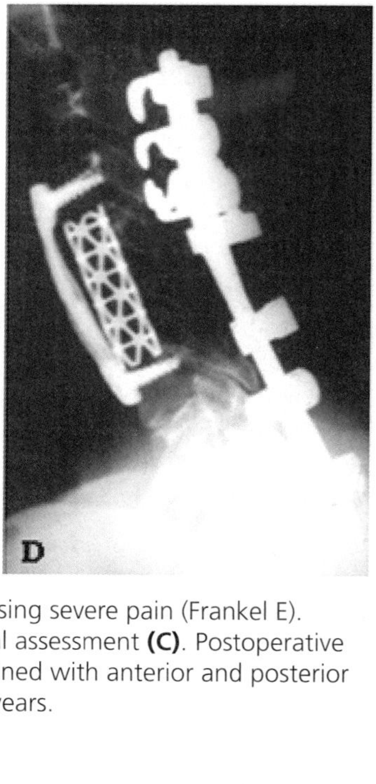

FIGURE 19.8 Metastatic cancer of the breast in a 60-year-old woman, causing severe pain (Frankel E). Preoperative T_1-weighted MRI **(A)**, T_2-weighted MRI **(B)**. Preoperation clinical assessment **(C)**. Postoperative radiograph imaging demonstrating successful anterior decompression combined with anterior and posterior stabilization **(D)**. Outcomes: relief of pain and survival period longer than 4 years.

study of surgery versus conventional radiotherapy for the treatment of metastatic spine epidural tumor (59), 24 surgical articles (n = 999) and four radiation articles (n = 543) were reviewed. The overall success rates for ambulation after surgery and radiation treatment were 85% and 64%, respectively.

It is obvious that radiation therapy cannot provide stability and cord compression to a metastatic lesion causing bone destruction and osseous neurocompression (41).

Regarding pain, review of the literature (Klimo et al.) (59) revealed that the overall improvement of pain after surgery was 90% (71% to 100%) compared with 70% (54% to 83%), as indicated by the radiation literature.

Patchel R et al. (78), in a randomized trial study comparing surgery alone versus radiation therapy alone, concluded that the percentage of patients able to walk after treatment was significantly higher in the surgical group (84%) than in radiotherapy patients (57%). Other outcomes were also significantly better in the surgical group: The ability to walk (median, 122 days with surgery, versus 13 days with radiation), restoration of ambulation (62% with surgery versus 19% in the radiation group), greater improvement in pain, muscle strength, functional status, and survival rates (median survival, 126 days in the surgery group versus 100 days in the radiation-alone group).

Because irradiation therapy adversely affects the response to chemotherapy (1,38, 49,95), painful destructive vertebral lesions with instability without neurologic compromise can effectively be managed with chemotherapy combined with cement-enhancement techniques (vertebroplasty or kyphoplasty). This experience may prevent the accumulated toxicity of combining radiation with chemotherapy. The analgesic effect for vertebral cement enhancement in metastatic tumors is about 84% (32).

The ultimate intent of surgical management for metastatic spinal disease is to improve the overall quality of life of the patient; and this is definitely apparent from the cited reports. The greatest effect substantially occurs in the reduction of the level of the pain. In general, a minimum life expectancy of 3 to 6 months has been accepted as a prerequisite for surgical indication (112). However, even in a life expectancy shorter than 3 months, performing surgical intervention may be justified (66). In this situation, palliative surgery is indicated, and the anticipated surgical intervention should be performed with the expectation of improving the remaining global quality of life, notwithstanding the morbidity of the procedure (105). Some of the procedures, such as cement augmentation (vertebroplasty, balloon kyphoplasty) and neuroaugmentation (morphine pump) for alleviating pain are associated with minimal morbidity. Surgery is also indicated for patients who have reached spinal cord tolerance after external radiation beam treatment.

Furthermore, it is not the purpose of this chapter to describe the available surgical techniques. In brief, the decision to use a particular approach (anterior or posterior) depends on the location of the tumor (vertebral body, extension into the epidural space, paraspinal, posterior vertebral elements, etc.), the type of reconstruction and stabilization, and ultimately the extent and aggressiveness of the tumor. Anterior transcavitary exposure through a posterolateral transpedicular approach provides sufficient access for aggressive tumor resection and anterior and posterior reconstruction similar to total "*en bloc* spondylectomy" technique (7,101,102). If negative histologic margins are feasible, indicating possibly curative outcomes, then *en bloc* resection rather than piecemeal excision should be selected. Tomita K et al. (102) demonstrated that *en bloc* resection can increase the postoperative survival period of metastatic spinal tumors. An appropriate choice of surgical treatment may extend the survival time by 3 to 6 months (98).

In conclusion, survival outcomes for managing metastatic spinal tumors are still gloomy. However, life expectancy can be improved when performed in a timely fashion;

appropriate surgical intervention is based on reasonable guidelines. Surgery is very effective for managing metastatic spinal tumors that produce pain, neurologic deficit, paralysis, and sphincteric incontinence. Pain shows the greatest response. It is important to quantify the patient's pain, psychological distress, and performance status before establishing treatment goals. The modified Harrington classification system combined with the Kostuik instability model, the Tomita grading system for vertebral tumor spread, and the Tokuhashi preoperative scoring system questionnaire are excelled guides for predicting outcomes of metastatic tumors and establish guidelines for selecting the most appropriate treatment. The degree of the clinical validity of these guidelines has not been vigorously tested and therefore scientifically supported. Although they are not consensus or evidence-based guidelines, they are, however, useful tools for selecting the most appropriate surgical intervention. Furthermore, they can form the basis for establishing the standards for more widely acceptable guidelines.

REFERENCES

1. Alderson MR, Hamlin I, Staunton MD. The relative significance of prognostic factors in breast carcinoma. Br J Cancer 1971;25:646–656.
2. American Spinal Injury Association. International standards for neurological classifications of spinal cord injury (revised). Chicago: American Spinal Injury Association, 2000, 1–23.
3. Atanasiu JP, Badatcheff F, Pidhorz L. Metastatic lesions of the cervical spine: a retrospective analysis of 20 cases. Spine 1993;18:1279–1284.
4. Barron KD, Hirano A, Araki S, et al. Experiences with metastatic neoplasms involving the spinal cord. Neurology 1959;9:91–106.
5. Bauer HCF. Posterior decompression and stabilization for spinal metastases: analysis of sixty-seven consecutive patients. J Bone Joint Surg (Am) 1997;79:514–522.
6. Bilsky MH, Lis E, Raizer J, et al. The diagnosis and treatment of metastatic spinal tumor. Oncologist 1999;4:459–469.
7. Bilsky MH, Boland P, Lis E, et al. Single-stage posterolateral transpedicle approach for spondylectomy, epidural decompression, and circumferential fusion of spinal metastases. Spine 2000;25:2240–2249.
8. Boriani S, Weinstein JN, Biagini R. Primary bone tumors of the spine: terminology and surgical staging. Spine 1997;22:1036–1044.
9. Brice J, Mckissock W. Surgical treatment of malignant extradural spinal tumours. Br Med J 1965;22:1341–1344.
10. Bridwell KH, Jenny AB, Saul T, et al. Posterior segmental spinal instrumentation (PSSI) with posterolateral decompression and debulking for metastatic thoracic and lumbar spine disease: limitations of the technique. Spine 1988;13:1383–1394.
11. Bruera E, Kuehn N, Miller MJ, et al. The Edmonton Symptom Assessment System (ESAS): a simple method for the assessment of palliative care patients. J Palliat Care 1991;7: 6–9.
12. Byrne TN. Spinal cord compression from epidural metastases. N Engl J Med 1992;27:614–619.
13. Cahill DW, Kumar R. Palliative subtotal vertebrectomy with anterior and posterior reconstruction via a single posterior approach. J Neurosurg 1999;90(1 suppl):42–47.
14. Cella DF. Quality of life outcomes: measurement and validation. Oncology 1996;10(11 suppl): 233–246.
15. Chang VT, Hwang SS, Feuerman M. Validation of the Edmonton Symptom Assessment Scale. Cancer 2000;88:2164–2171.
16. Chataigner H, Onimus M. Surgery in spinal metastasis without spinal cord compression: indications and strategy related to the risk of recurrence. Eur Spine J 2000;9:523–527.
17. Cleeland CS.The impact of pain on the patient with cancer. Cancer 1984;54(suppl):2635–2641.
18. Cooper PR, Errico TJ, Martin R, et al. A systematic approach to spinal reconstruction after anterior decompression for neoplastic disease of the thoracic and lumbar spine. Neurosurgery 1993;32:1–8.
19. Denis F. Spinal instability as defined by the three-column spine concept in acute spinal trauma. Clin Orthop Relat Res 1984;189:65–76.

20. Dolan P. Modeling valuations for EuroQol health states. Med Care 1997;35:1095–1108.
21. Drury RAB, Palmer PH, Highman WJ. Carcinomatous metastasis to the vertebral bodies. J Clin Pathol 1964;17:448–457.
22. Eastern Cooperative Oncology Group. Eastern Cooperative Oncology Group Performance Status Scale. Revised March 25, 1998. http://ecog.dfci.harvard.edu
23. Enkaoua EA, Doursounian L, Chatellier G, et al. Vertebral metastases: a critical appreciation of the preoperative prognostic Tokuhashi score in a series of 71 cases. Spine 1997;22:2293–2298.
24. Enneking WF. Staging musculoskeletal tumors. In: Enneking WF, ed. Musculoskeletal tumor surgery. New York: Churchill-Livingstone, 87–88.
25. Ernstberger T, Bruning T, Konig F. Vertebrectomy and anterior reconstruction for the treatment of spinal metastases. Acta Orthop Belg 2005;71:459–466.
26. Falicov A, Fisher CG, Sparkes J, et al. Impact of surgical intervention on quality of life in patients with spinal metastases. Spine 2006;31: 2849–2856.
27. Fayers PM. Interpreting quality of life data: population-based reference data for the EORTC QLQ-C30. Eur J Cancer 2001;37:1331–1334.
28. Feeny D, Furlong W, Torrance GW, et al. Multiattribute and single-attribute utility functions for the Health Utilities Index Mark 3 system. Med Care 2002;40:113–128.
29. Fidler MW. Anterior decompression and stabilisation of metastatic spinal fractures. J Bone Joint Surg (Br) 1986;68:83–90.
30. Fishman B, Pasternak S, Wallenstein SL, et al. The Memorial Pain Assessment Card: a valid instrument for the evaluation of cancer pain. Cancer 1987;60:1151–1158.
31. Fourney DR, Abi-Said D, Lang FF, et al. Use of pedicle screw fixation in the management of malignant spinal disease: experience in 100 consecutive procedures. J Neurosurg 2001;94(1 suppl):25–37.
32. Fourney DR, Schomer DF, Nader R, et al. Percutaneous vertebroplasty and kyphoplasty for painful vertebral body fractures in cancer patients. J Neurosurg 2002;98(1 suppl):21–30.
33. Frankel HL, Hancock DO, Hyslop G, et al. The value of postural reduction in the initial management of closed injuries of the spine with paraplegia and tetraplegia. Paraplegia 1969;7:179–192.
34. Gerszten PC, Welch WC. Current surgical management of metastatic spinal disease. Oncology (Williston Park) 2000;14:1013–1024.
35. Gilbert RW, Kim JH, Posner JB. Epidural spinal cord compression from metastatic tumor: diagnosis and treatment. Ann Neurol 1978;3:40–51.
36. Gokaslan ZL, York JE, Walsh GL, et al. Transthoracic vertebrectomy for metastatic spinal tumors. J Neurosurg 1998;89:599–609.
37. Greenberg HS, Kim JH, Posner JB. Epidural spinal cord compression from metastatic tumor: results with a new treatment protocol. Ann Neurol 1980;8:361–366.
38. Greenspan EM. Combination cytotoxic chemotherapy in advanced disseminated breast carcinoma. J Mt Sinai Hosp NY 1966;33:1–27.
39. Hadjipavlou A, Necessary J. Principles of psychometric studies for clinical outcomes and disability evaluation in chronic low back. J Disabil 1988;7: 1–24.
40. Hamilton M. A rating scale for depression. J Neurol Neurosurg Psychiatry 1960;23:56–62.
41. Hammerberg KW. Surgical treatment of metastatic spine disease. Spine 1992;17: 1148–1153.
42. Harrington KD. Metastatic disease of the spine. J Bone Join Surg (Am) 1986;68:1110–1115.
43. Hatrick NC, Lucas JD, Timothy AR, et al. The surgical treatment of metastatic disease of the spine. Radiother Oncol 2000;56:335–339.
44. Healey JH, Brown HK. Complications of bone metastases: surgical management. Cancer 2000; 88(12 suppl):2940–2951.
45. Hertlein H, Mittlmeier T, Piltz S, et al. Spinal stabilization for patients with metastatic lesions of the spine using a titanium spacer. Eur Spine J 1992;1:131–136.
46. Hirabayashi H, Ebara S, Kinoshita T, et al. Clinical outcome and survival after palliative surgery for spinal metastases: palliative surgery in spinal metastases. Cancer 2003;97:476–484.
47. Hosono N, Yonenobu K, Fuji T, et al. Vertebral body replacement with a ceramic prosthesis for metastatic spinal tumors. Spine 1995;15:2454–2462.
48. Hosono N, Ueda T, Tamura D, et al. Prognostic relevance of clinical symptoms in patients with spinal metastases. Clin Orthop Relat Res 2005; 436:196–201.
49. Hurley JD, Trump DS, Flatley TJ, et al. A method of selecting patients for cancer chemotherapy. Arch Surg 1961;83:611–619.

50. Jaffe HL. Tumors and tumorous conditions of the bones and joints. Philadelphia: Lea & Febinger, 1958.
51. Jansson KA, Bauer HC. Survival, complications and outcome in 282 patients operated for neurological deficit due to thoracic or lumbar spinal metastases. Eur Spine J 2006;15:196–202.
52. Jensen MP, Chen C, Brugger AM. Postsurgical pain outcome assessment. Pain 2002;99:101–109.
53. Kaasa T, Loomis J, Gillis K, et al. The Edmonton Functional Assessment Tool: preliminary development and evaluation for use in palliative care. J Pain Symptom Manage 1997;13: 10–9.
54. Karnofsky DA. Clinical evaluation of anticancer drugs: cancer chemotherapy. GANN Monogr 1967;2:223–231.
55. Kennady JC, Stern WE. Metastatic neoplasms of the vertebral column producing compression of the spinal cord. Am J Surg 1962;104: 155–168.
56. King GJ, Kostuik JP, McBroom RJ, et al. Surgical management of metastatic renal carcinoma of the spine. Spine 1991;16:265–271.
57. Kleinman WB, Kiernan HA, Michelsen WJ. Metastatic cancer of the spinal column. Clin Orthop Relat Res 1978;136:166–172.
58. Klekamp J, Samii H. Surgical results for spinal metastases. Acta Neurochir (Wien) 1998;140: 957–967.
59. Klimo P Jr, Thompson CJ, Kestle JR, et al. A meta-analysis of surgery versus conventional radiotherapy for the treatment of metastatic spinal epidural disease. Neurooncology 2005;7:64–76.
60. Kocialkowski A, Webb JK. Metastatic spinal tumours: survival after surgery. Eur Spine J 1992; 1:43–48.
61. Kostuik JP, Errico TJ, Gleason TF, et al. Spinal stabilization of vertebral column tumors. Spine 1988;13:250–256.
62. Kostuik JP, Weinstein JN. Differential diagnosis and surgical treatment of metastatic spine tumors. In: Frymoyer JW, ed. The adult spine. New York: Raven Press, 1991: 861–888.
63. Kostuik JP, Connolly PJ, Esses SI, et al. Anterior cervical plate fixation with the titanium hollow screw plate system. Spine 1993;18: 1273–1278.
64. Lewandrowski KU, Hecht AC, DeLaney TF, et al. Anterior spinal arthrodesis with structural cortical allografts and instrumentation for spine tumor surgery. Spine 2004;29:1150–1158.
65. Livingston KE, Perrin RG. The neurosurgical management of spinal metastases causing cord and cauda equina compression. J Neurosurg 1978;49:839–843.
66. Lord CF, Herndon JH. Spinal cord compression secondary to kyphosis associated with radiation therapy for metastatic disease. Clin Orthop Relat Res 1986;210:120–127.
67. Mones RJ, Dozier D, Berrett A. Analysis of medical treatment of malignant extradural spinal cord tumors. Cancer 1966;19:1842– 1853.
68. Muhlbauer M, Pfisterer W, Eyb R, et al. Noncontiguous spinal metastases and plasmocytomas should be operated on through a single posterior midline approach, and circumferential decompression should be performed with individualized reconstruction. Acta Neurochir (Wien) 2000;142: 1219–1230.
69. Nader R, Alford BT, Nauta HJ, et al. Preoperative embolization and intraoperative cryocoagulation as adjuncts in resection of hypervascular lesions of the thoracolumbar spine. J Neurosurg 2002;97(3 suppl):294–300.
70. Nather A, Bose K. The results of decompression of cord or cauda equina compression from metastatic extradural tumors. Clin Orthop Relat Res 1982;169:103–108.
71. Nazarian S. Place de la chirurgie dans le traitement des metastases du rachis: synthese et conclusion. Rev Chir Orthop Reparatrice Appar Mot 1997;83(suppl III):167–172.
72. Neyt J, Samson M, Hoogmartens M. Surgical treatment of spinal metastases: long term follow-up. Acta Orthop Belg 1993;59:83–86.
73. O'Neil J, Gardner V, Armstrong G. Treatment of tumors of the thoracic and lumbar spinal column. Clin Orthop Relat Res 1988;227:103–112.
74. Ogihara S, Seichi A, Hozumi T, et al. Prognostic factors for patients with spinal metastases from lung cancer. Spine 2006;31:1585–1590.
75. Oken MM, Creech RH, Tormey DC, et al. Toxicity and response criteria of the Eastern Cooperative Oncology Group. Am J Clin Oncol 1982;5:649–655.
76. Onimus M, Papin P, Gangloff S. Results of surgical treatment of spinal thoracic and lumbar metastases. Eur Spine J 1996;5:407–411.
77. Ortiz Gomez JA. The incidence of vertebral body metastases. Int Orthop 1995;19:309–311.
78. Patchell RA, Tibbs PA, Regine WF, et al. Direct decompressive surgical resection in the treatment of spinal cord compression caused by metastatic cancer: a randomised trial. Lancet 2005;366:643–648.

79. Rodriguez M, Dinapoli RP. Spinal cord compression: with special reference to metastatic epidural tumors. Mayo Clin Proc 1980;55: 442–448.

80. Rompe JD, Hopf CG, Eysel P. Outcome after palliative posterior surgery for metastatic disease of the spine-evaluation of 106 consecutive patients after decompression and stabilisation with the Cotrel-Dubousset instrumentation. Arch Orthop Trauma Surg 1999;119: 394–400.

81. Saengnipanthkul S, Jirarattanaphochai K, Rojviroj S, et al. Metastatic adenocarcinoma of the spine. Spine 1992;17:427–430.

82. Schaberg J, Gainor BJ. A profile of metastatic carcinoma of the spine. Spine 1985;10:19–20.

83. Schoeggl A, Reddy M, Matula C. Neurological outcome following laminectomy in spinal metastases. Spinal Cord 2002;40:363–366.

84. Serlin RC, Mendoza TR, Nakamura Y, et al. When is cancer pain mild, moderate or severe? Grading pain severity by its interference with function. Pain 1995;61:277–278.

85. Shimizu K, Shikata J, Iida H, et al. Posterior decompression and stabilization for multiple metastatic tumors of the spine. Spine 1992;17: 1400–1404.

86. Siegal T, Siegal T. Surgical decompression of anterior and posterior malignant epidural tumors compressing the spinal cord: a prospective study. Neurosurgery 1995;17:424–432.

87. Siegal T, Tiqva P, Siegal T. Vertebral body resection for epidural compression by malignant tumors: results of forty-seven consecutive operative procedures. J Bone Joint Surg (Am) 1995; 67:375–382.

88. Sinardet D, Chabane A, Khalil T, et al. Évolution neurologique de 152 patients opérés de métastases. Neurochirurgie 2000;46:4–10.

89. Sioutos PJ, Arbit E, Meshulam CF, et al. Spinal metastases from solid tumors: analysis of factors affecting survival. Cancer 1995;76:1453–1459.

90. Spiegel DA, Sampson JH, Richardson WJ, et al. Metastatic melanoma to the spine: demographics, risk factors, and prognosis in 114 patients. Spine 1995;20:2141–2146.

91. Sundaresan N, Bains M, McCormack P. Surgical treatment of spinal cord compression in patients with lung cancer. Neurosurgery 1985;16:350–356.

92. Sundaresan N, Galicich JH, Lane JM, et al. Treatment of neoplastic epidural cord compression by vertebral body resection and stabilization. J Neurosurg 1985;63:676–684.

93. Sundaresan N, Digiacinto GV, Hughes JEO, et al. Treatment of neoplastic cord compression: results of a prospective study. Neurosurgery 1991;29:645–650.

94. Sundaresan N, Rothman A, Manhart K, et al. Surgery for solitary metastases of the spine: rationale and results of treatment. Spine 2002; 27:1802–1806.

95. Swenerton KD, Legha SS, Smith T, et al. Prognostic factors in metastatic breast cancer treated with combination chemotherapy. Cancer Res 1979;39:1552–1562.

96. Taneichi H, Kaneda K, Takeda N, et al. Risk factors and probability of vertebral body collapse in metastases of thoracic and lumbar spine. Spine 1997;22:239–245.

97. Tatsui H, Onomura T, Morishita S, et al. Survival rates of patients with metastatic spinal cancer after scintigraphic detection of abnormal radioactive accumulation. Spine 1996;21:2143–2148.

98. Tokuhashi Y, Matsuzaki H, Toriyama S, et al. Scoring system for the preoperative evaluation of metastatic spine tumor prognosis. Spine 1990;15:1110–1113.

99. Tokuhashi Y, Matsuzaki H, Oda H, et al. A revised scoring system for preoperative evaluation of metastatic spine tumor prognosis. Spine 2005;30:2186–2191.

100. Tomita T, Galicich JH, Sundaresan N. Radiation therapy for spinal epidural metastases with complete block. Acta Radiol Oncol 1983;22: 135–143.

101. Tomita K, Kawahara N, Baba H, et al. Total en bloc spondylectomy for solitary spinal metastases. Int Orthop 1994;18:291–298.

102. Tomita K, Kawahara N, Kobayashi T, et al. Surgical strategy for spinal metastases. Spine 2001;26:298–306.

103. Touboul E, Camille RR, Guerin RA, et al. Tumeurs extra-durales rachidiennes métastatiques: à propos de cent trente cas. Sem Hôp Paris 1986;62:1785–1794.

104. Townsend PW, Rosenthal HG, Smalley SR, et al. Impact of postoperative radiation therapy and other perioperative factors on outcome after orthopedic stabilization of impending or pathologic fractures due to metastatic disease. J Clin Oncol 1994;12:2345–2350.

105. Turner PL, Prince HG, Webb JK, et al. Surgery for malignant extradural tumours of the spine. J Bone Joint Surg (Br) 1988;70:451–455.

106. Villavicencio AT, Oskouian RJ, Roberson C, et al. Thoracolumbar vertebral reconstruction after surgery for metastatic spinal tumors: long-term outcomes. Neurosurg Focus 2005;19:E8.

107. Wai EK, Finkelstein JA, Tangente RP, et al. Quality of life in surgical treatment of metastatic spine disease. Spine 2003;28:508–512.

108. Walsh GL, Gokaslan ZL, McCutcheon IE, et al. Anterior approaches to the thoracic spine in patients with cancer: indications and results. Ann Thorac Surg 1997;64:1611–1618.

109. Wang JC, Boland P, Mitra N, et al. Single-stage posterolateral transpedicular approach for resection of epidural metastatic spine tumors involving the vertebral body with circumferential reconstruction: results in 140 patients: invited submission from the Joint Section Meeting on Disorders of the Spine and Peripheral Nerves, March 2004. J Neurosurg Spine 2004;1:287–298.

110. Weigel B, Maghsudi M, Neumann C, et al. Surgical management of symptomatic spinal metastases: postoperative outcome and quality of life. Spine 1999;24:2240–2246.

111. Weinstein J. The adult spine: principles and practice. New York: Raven Press, 1991.

112. Wise JJ, Fischgrund JS, Herkowitz HN, et al. Complication, survival rates, and risk factors of surgery for metastatic disease of the spine. Spine 1999;24:1943–1951.

113. White WA, Patterson RH Jr, Bergland RM. Role of surgery in the treatment of spinal cord compression by metastatic neoplasm. Cancer 1971;27:558–561.

114. Wong DA, Fornasier VL, MacNab I. Spinal metastases: the obvious, the occult, and the impostors. Spine 1990;15:1–4.

115. Woolf SH, Grol R, Hutchinson A, et al. Clinical guidelines: potential benefits, limitations, and harms of clinical guidelines. Br Med J 1999;318: 527–530.

116. Wright RL. Malignant tumors in the spinal extradural space: results of surgical treatment. Ann Surg 1963;157:227–231.

117. Zung WW. A rating instrument for anxiety disorders. Psychosomatics 1971;12:371–379.

Index

Note: Page numbers in *italics* denote figures; those followed by a *t* denote tables.